pocket reference

Clinical Pharmacokinetics
2ND EDITION

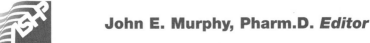

John E. Murphy, Pharm.D. *Editor*

John E. Murphy, Pharm.D., is Professor and Head, Department of Pharmacy Practice and Science, College of Pharmacy, The University of Arizona. Dr. Murphy welcomes comments or suggestions for drugs to be added, deleted, or revised in future editions of this text.

Any correspondence regarding this publication should be sent to the publisher, American Society of Health-System Pharmacists, 7272 Wisconsin Avenue, Bethesda, MD 20814, attn: Special Publishing. Produced in conjunction with the ASHP Publications Production Center.

The information presented herein reflects the opinions of the contributors and reviewers. It should not be interpreted as an official policy of ASHP or as an endorsement of any product.

Drug information and its applications are constantly evolving because of ongoing research and clinical experience and are often subject to professional judgment and interpretation by the practitioner and to the uniqueness of a clinical situation. The authors, editor, and ASHP have made every effort to ensure the accuracy and completeness of the information presented in this book. However, the reader is advised that the publisher, authors, contributors, editors, and reviewers cannot be responsible for the continued currency of the information, for any errors or omissions, and/or for any consequences arising from the use of the information in the clinical setting.

The reader is cautioned that ASHP makes no representation, guarantee, or warranty, express or implied, that the use of the information contained in this book will prevent problems with insurers and will bear no responsibility or liability for the results or consequences of its use.

Managing Editor/Development Editor: Con Ann Ling, Pharm.D.
Production Manager: Bruce Hawkins

Cover design: David Wade

©2001, American Society of Health-System Pharmacists, Inc. All rights reserved.

No part of this publication may be reproduced or transmitted in any form or by any means, electronic or mechanical, including photocopying, microfilming, and recording, or by any information storage and retrieval system, without written permission from the American Society of Health-System Pharmacists.

ASHP® is a service mark of the American Society of Health-System Pharmacists, Inc.; registered in the U.S. Patent and Trademark Office.

ISBN: 1-879907-98-4

Healthfield, Inc.
A Four Season Home Care Co
885 Franklin Road, Suite 330
Marietta, GA 30067
678-290-8101

Contents

Preface xxiii

Contributors xxvii

Reviewers xxxiii

Introduction *by* John E. Murphy xxxv
General Pharmacokinetic Principles...................... xxxv
   Initiating therapy xxxv
   Using population mean values.......................... xxxv
   Considering other factors in pharmacokinetic
      monitoring xxxvi
   Verifying drug concentration measurements xxxviii
   Determining need for dosage adjustments.............. xxxix
   Deciding on monitoring frequency..................... xxxix
A Basic Pharmacokinetic Glossary........................... xl
   Selected pharmacokinetic terminology xl
   Selected pharmacokinetic symbols xlii
General Estimating Equations xliv
   Calculating lean or ideal body weight (IBW) in adults xlv
   Calculating ideal body weight (IBW) in children
      aged 1–18 years xlv
   Calculating surface area (SA) in meters xlv
General Pharmacokinetic Equations xlvi
References xlviii

Chapter 1. Estimating Creatinine Clearance
      by Robert E. Pachorek 1
Estimating Glomerular Filtration Rate by
      Creatinine Clearance............................. 1

Formulas to estimate creatinine clearance in adults 3
Body weight 6
Low serum creatinine/elderly patients 7
Amputations 8
Spinal cord injury 8
Chronic renal insufficiency 8
Dialysis 9
Liver disease 9
Pediatrics 9
Patients with unstable renal function 10
Time to Steady-State Serum Creatinine Concentration 11
Creatinine Clearance Estimation in Unstable
    Renal Function 12
References... 12

Chapter 2. Rational Use of Drug Concentration Measurements *by* James P. McCormack & Glen Brown 15

Evaluating the Need for a Drug Concentration
    Measurement 17
Drug selection 17
Efficacy issues 18
Toxicity issues 19
Adherence issues 19
Approaches to Dosing with Limited Need
    for Drug Concentration Measurements 19
Immediate effect required or expected 19
Immediate effect not required or expected 20
Titrating the dose up 20
Titrating the dose down 21
Conclusion 22

Chapter 3. Aminoglycosides *by* John E. Murphy 23

Usual Dosage Range in Absence of Clearance-Altering
    Factors 23
Loading dose 24
Maintenance dose 25
Dosing interval determination–traditional dosing 27
Dosing and dosing intervals–(LDEI) dosing 27
Dosage Form Availability 29
Bioavailability (*F*) of Dosage Forms 31
General Pharmacokinetic Information 32
Protein binding 32
Clearance (CL) 32

Volume of distribution (V) 33
Half-Life and Time to Steady State 36
Therapeutic Range 38
Suggested Sampling Times and Effect on
    Therapeutic Range 40
Monitoring Aminoglycoside Patients 41
    Aminoglycoside concentration measurements 41
    Assay issues 42
    Initial concentration measurement 42
    Follow-up concentration measurements 43
    LDEI dosing 44
    Approach to monitoring 45
    Renal Function 45
Pharmacodynamic Monitoring—Concentration-Related
    Efficacy.. 46
Pharmacodynamic Monitoring—Concentration-Related
    Toxicity 47
Drug–Drug Interactions.................................... 49
Drug–Disease State or Condition Interactions 50
Summary... 51
References.. 52

Chapter 4. Newer Antiepileptic Drugs
by William R. Garnett 61
Dosage Forms of Newer Antiepileptic Drugs................. 62
Felbamate 62
Gabapentin.. 64
Lamotrigine 67
Tiagabine... 69
Topiramate 71
Use of the New Antiepileptic Drugs 73
References.. 74

Chapter 5. Antirejection Agents *by* Janet Karlix &
    Joe Walker... 79
Cyclosporine: Usual Dosage Range in Absence of
    Clearance-Altering Factors 79
Cyclosporine: Dosage Form Availability 80
Cyclosporine: Bioavailability (*F*) of Dosage Forms.......... 80
Cyclosporine: General Pharmacokinetic Information 81
    Absorption.. 81
    Binding 82
    Metabolism.. 82
    Elimination 82

Cyclosporine: Clearance (CL).............................. 82
Cyclosporine: Volume of Distribution (V) 82
Cyclosporine: Half-Life and Time to Steady State 83
Cyclosporine: Therapeutic Range 83
Cyclosporine: Suggested Sampling Times 84
Cyclosporine: Pharmacodynamic Monitoring 84
   Concentration-related efficacy 84
   Concentration-related toxicity.......................... 85
Cyclosporine: Drug–Drug Interactions..................... 85
Cyclosporine: Drug–Disease State or Condition
   Interactions... 87
Tacrolimus: Usual Dosage Range in Absence of
   Clearance-Altering Factors 87
Tacrolimus: Dosage Form Availability..................... 88
Tacrolimus: Bioavailability (F) of Dosage Forms............ 88
Tacrolimus: General Pharmacokinetic Information 89
   Absorption.. 89
   Distribution... 89
   Metabolism... 89
   Excretion 90
Tacrolimus: Clearance (CL) 90
Tacrolimus: Volume of Distribution (V) 90
Tacrolimus: Half-Life and Time to Steady State 90
Tacrolimus: Suggested Sampling Times 90
Tacrolimus: Therapeutic Range 91
Tacrolimus: Pharmacodynamic Monitoring 91
   Concentration-related efficacy 91
   Concentration-related toxicity 91
Tacrolimus: Drug–Drug Interactions 92
Tacrolimus: Drug–Disease State or Condition
   Interactions 93
References 94

Chapter 6. Carbamazepine *by* William R. Garnett 97
Usual Dosage Range in Absence of Clearance-Altering
   Factors 97
Dosage Form Availability 99
Bioavailability (F) of Dosage Forms 99
General Pharmacokinetic Information 101
   Absorption 101
   Distribution... 102
   Protein binding 102
   Maternal/breast feeding/saliva......................... 103
   Elimination 103

Clearance (CL) 104
Volume of Distribution (*V*) 105
Protein Binding... 105
Half-Life and Time to Steady State 106
Therapeutic Range 106
Suggested Sampling Times and Effect on Therapeutic
    Range 107
Pharmacodynamic Monitoring—Concentration-Related
    Efficacy 108
Pharmacodynamic Monitoring—Concentration-Related
    Toxicity 108
Drug–Drug Interactions 109
Drug–Disease State or Condition Interactions 111
References 112

Chapter 7. Cyclic Antidepressants
    by C. Lindsay Devane 119
Usual Dosage Range in Absence of Clearance-Altering
    Factors 121
Dosage Form Availability 123
General Pharmacokinetic Information 125
Therapeutic Range 128
    Tricyclic antidepressants 128
    Other antidepressants 129
Suggested Sampling Times 132
Further Considerations for Sampling 133
Drug–Drug Interactions 134
Drug–Disease State or Condition Interactions 137
    Adolescence 137
    Advanced age 137
    Alcoholism, alcoholic liver disease 137
    Cardiac disease 138
    Inflammatory disease states 138
    Nutritional status 138
    Renal failure 138
    Smoking status 138
    Thyroid disease 139
References 139

Chapter 8. Digoxin *by* Martin L. Job 143
Usual Dosage Range in Absence of Clearance-Altering
    Factors 143
Dosage Form Availability 144
Bioavailability (*F*) of Dosage Forms 145

General Pharmacokinetic Information 145
Clearance (CL) 146
Volume of Distribution (V) 147
Half-Life and Time to Steady State 147
Therapeutic Range 148
Suggested Sampling Times 149
Pharmacodynamic Monitoring—Concentration-Related
   Efficacy 149
Pharmacodynamic Monitoring—Concentration-Related
   Toxicity 150
Drug–Drug Interactions 150
References 152

Chapter 9. Ethosuximide *by* William R. Garnett 155
Usual Dosage Range in Absence of Clearance-Altering
   Factors 155
Dosage Form Availability 156
Bioavailability (F) of Dosage Forms 156
General Pharmacokinetic Information 156
   Absorption 156
   Distribution 157
   Metabolism 157
Clearance (CL) 158
Volume of Distribution (V) 158
Protein Binding 158
Half-Life and Time to Steady State 159
Therapeutic Range 159
Suggested Sampling Times and Effect on Therapeutic
   Range 159
Pharmacodynamic Monitoring—Concentration-Related
   Efficacy 160
Pharmacodynamic Monitoring—Concentration-Related
   Toxicity 161
Drug–Drug Interactions 161
Drug–Disease State or Condition Interactions 162
References 162

Chapter 10. Heparin and Low Molecular Weight Heparin
   by James B. Groce III 165
Heparin: Usual Dosage Range in Absence of
   Clearance-Altering Factors 165
Treating Thromboembolic Disease 167
Heparin: Dosage Form Availability 168
Heparin: Bioavailability (F) of Routes of Administration ... 169

Heparin: General Pharmacokinetic Information 169
Heparin: Therapeutic Range 172
Heparin: Suggested Sampling Times and Monitoring 175
  Monitoring 176
Heparin: Pharmacodynamic Monitoring—
    Concentration-Related Efficacy 177
Heparin: Pharmacodynamic Monitoring—
    Concentration-Related Toxicity 178
Reversing Heparin's Effect 182
Heparin: Drug–Drug Interactions 182
Heparin: Drug–Disease State or Condition Interactions 183
Heparin: Pharmacokinetic Dosing Approaches............. 184
Summary of Heparin Dosing and Monitoring 188
Low Molecular Weight Heparins (LMWH) 189
LMWH: Usual Dosage Range in Absence of
    Clearance-Altering Factors 191
LMWH: Dosage Form Availability 193
LMWH: Bioavailability (*F*) of Dosage Forms 193
LMWH: General Pharmacokinetic Information 193
LMWH: Therapeutic Range 194
LMWH: Suggested Sampling Times and Effect on
    Therapeutic Range.................................. 195
LMWH: Pharmacodynamic Monitoring—
    Concentration-Related Efficacy..................... 195
LMWH: Pharmacodynamic Monitoring—
    Concentration-Related Toxicity 196
LMWH: Reversing the Effect of LMWHs 197
LMWH: Drug–Drug Interactions 197
LMWH: Drug–Disease State or Condition Interaction 197
Summary of LMWH Dosing and Monitoring 198
References 198

Chapter 11. Lidocaine *by* Paul E. Nolan, Jr. &
    Toby C. Trujillo 205
Usual Dosage Range in Absence of Clearance-Altering
    Factors 205
Dosage Form Availability 206
Bioavailability (*F*) of Dosage Forms 207
General Pharmacokinetic Information 207
  Distribution... 207
  Elimination 208
  Metabolism 208
  Protein binding... 209
Clearance (CL) 210

Volume of Distribution (V) 211
Half-Life and Time to Steady State 211
Therapeutic Range 212
Suggested Sampling Times and Effect on Therapeutic
    Range 212
Clinical Use 213
Pharmacodynamic Monitoring: Concentration-Related
    Efficacy and Toxicity 214
Drug–Drug Interactions 215
Drug–Disease State or Condition Interactions 216
    Congestive heart failure (CHF) 216
    Acute myocardial infarction (AMI) 217
    Hepatic disease 217
    Renal disease 218
    Morbid obesity 218
    Advanced age (elderly) 218
Pregnancy and Lactation 219
Dosing Strategies 219
    Explanation of Method 7: endotracheal administration .. 220
    Comparisons of dosing methods 223
References 224

Chapter 12. Lithium *by* Stanley W. Carson &
    Sarah H. Roberts 229
Usual Dosage Range in Absence of Clearance-Altering
    Factors 230
Dosage Form Availability 230
Bioavailability (*F*) of Dosage Forms 231
General Pharmacokinetic Information 231
    Distribution 231
    Elimination 232
Clearance (CL) 232
    Dosage prediction by a priori demographics 234
    *Dosage prediction by lithium renal clearance
        estimation* 234
    Dosage prediction by population pharmacokinetics ... 235
    Dosage prediction by Bayesian computer software 235
Volume of Distribution (*V*) 235
Half-Life and Time to Steady State 236
Therapeutic Range 236
Suggested Sampling Times and Effect on Therapeutic
    Range 236
Pharmacodynamic Monitoring—Concentration-Related
    Efficacy... 238

Pharmacodynamic Monitoring—"Follow-up"
  Concentrations 238
Pharmacodynamic Monitoring—Concentration-Related
  Toxicity 239
Drug–Drug Interactions................................ 239
Drug–Disease State or Condition Interactions 240
References 242

Chapter 13. Methotrexate *by* Mary E. Teresi &
  John N. McCormick 247
Usual Dosage Range in Absence of Clearance-Altering
  Factors 247
Dosage Form Availability 248
Bioavailability (*F*) of Dosage Forms 249
General Pharmacokinetic Information 250
  Protein binding 250
  Distribution.. 250
  Elimination 251
  Metabolism 252
Clearance (CL) 252
Volume of Distribution (*V*) 254
Half-Life and Time to Steady State 254
Therapeutic Range 255
Suggested Sampling Times and Effect on Therapeutic
  Range 256
Leucovorin Rescue..................................... 256
Pharmacodynamic Monitoring—Concentration-Related
  Efficacy... 257
  Psoriasis 258
  Rheumatoid arthritis 258
  Asthma 258
  Pregnancy termination 258
  Cancer 258
Pharmacodynamic Monitoring—Concentration-Related
  Toxicity 259
  Chronic LDMTX therapy 259
  HDMTX (follow protocol guidelines) 260
  Chronic liver toxicity (cirrhosis and fibrosis) 260
  Pulmonary fibrosis 261
  Myelosuppression 261
  GI toxicity... 261
  Acute hepatic toxicity 262
  Nephrotoxicity...................................... 262
  Leukoencephalopathy 262

Miscellaneous 262
Risk factors for LDMTX-induced hepatotoxicity 262
Risk factors for HDMTX toxicity 263
Drug–Drug Interactions 263
Cisplatin 263
Cytosine arabinoside (ARA-C) 264
Etretinate 264
5-Fluorouracil (5-FU) 264
Organic acids 264
Nonabsorbable antibiotics 264
Omeprazole 265
NSAIDs 265
Vincristine 265
VP-16 and VM-26 265
Miscellaneous 265
Drug–Disease State or Condition Interactions 265
References 266

Chapter 14. Phenobarbital *by* Douglas M. Anderson &
    Kimberly B. Tallian 271
Usual Dosage Range in Absence of Clearance-Altering
    Factors 271
Dosage Form Availability 272
Bioavailability (F) of Dosage Forms 273
General Pharmacokinetic Information 273
Clearance 273
Metabolism 274
Protein binding 274
Clearance (CL) 274
Volume of Distribution (V) 275
Half-Life and Time to Steady State 276
Therapeutic Range 276
Suggested Sampling Times and Effect on Therapeutic
    Range 278
Pharmacodynamic Monitoring—Concentration-Related
    Efficacy 279
Pharmacodynamic Monitoring—Concentration-Related
    Toxicity 279
Drug–Drug Interactions 280
Drug–Disease State or Condition Interactions 282
References 282

Chapter 15. Phenytoin and Fosphenytoin
    by Michael E. Winter 285

Usual Dosage Range in Absence of Clearance-Altering
    Factors 285
  Loading dose 285
  Maintenance dose 286
Dosage Form Availability 286
Bioavailability (F) of Dosage Forms 288
General Pharmacokinetic Information 289
Clearance (CL) 290
Volume of Distribution (V) 291
Half-Life and Time to Steady State 292
Therapeutic Range....................................... 293
Suggested Sampling Times 294
Pharmacodynamic Monitoring—Concentration-Related
    Efficacy 295
Pharmacodynamic Monitoring—Concentration-Related
    Toxicity 295
  Nystagmus 296
  CNS depression 296
  Nonconcentration-related side effects 297
Drug–Drug Interactions.................................. 297
Drug–Disease State or Condition Interactions 299
  Hepatic disease—cirrhosis 299
  Renal failure 299
  Obesity 299
  Malabsorption 300
  AIDS 300
  Pregnancy and lactation 300
References.. 301

Chapter 16. Procainamide *by* John A. Pieper 305
Usual Dosage Range in Absence of Clearance-Altering
    Factors 305
Dosage Form Availability................................ 307
Bioavailability (F) of Dosage Forms 308
General Pharmacokinetic Information 308
  Clearance 308
  Metabolism... 308
  Protein binding..................................... 308
Clearance (CL) 309
Volume of Distribution (V_{ss}).......................... 310
Half-Life and Time to Steady State 311
N-Acetylprocainamide (NAPA) Predictions 311
  NAPA production 311
  Clearance (CL) 312

Volume (V) 312
Half-life (t½) 312
Therapeutic Range 312
Suggested Sampling Times and Effect on Therapeutic
    Range 313
Pharmacodynamic Monitoring—Concentration-Related
    Efficacy 314
Pharmacodynamic Monitoring—Concentration-Related
    Toxicity 314
Important Drug–Drug Interactions 315
Drug–Disease State or Condition Interactions 316
References 317

Chapter 17. Quinidine *by* Paul E. Nolan, Jr. &
    Christy M. Evans 319
Usual Dosage Range in Absence of Clearance-Altering
    Factors 319
Bioavailability (*F*) of Dosage Forms 320
General Pharmacokinetic Information 321
    Absorption 322
    Distribution 323
    Elimination 323
    Metabolism 324
    Protein binding 324
Clearance (CL) 325
Volume of Distribution (*V*) 326
Half-Life and Time to Steady State 326
Therapeutic Range 326
Dosing Strategies 327
Suggested Sampling Times and Effect on Therapeutic
    Range 329
Pharmacodynamic Monitoring—Concentration-Related
    Efficacy 332
Pharmacodynamic Monitoring—Concentration-Related
    Toxicity 333
Drug–Drug Interactions 335
Pharmacodynamics Interactions 337
Drug–Disease State or Condition Interactions 337
References 338

Chapter 18. Theophylline *by* Edress H. Darsey 345
Usual Dosage Range in Absence of Clearance-Altering
    Factors 345
    Loading dose 345

Maintenance dose..........................346
Dosage Form Availability..............................347
Bioavailability (F) of Dosage Forms......................350
General Pharmacokinetic Information.....................351
Clearance and metabolism 351
Protein binding 351
Clearance (CL) 351
Volume of Distribution (V) 352
Half-Life and Time to Steady State 353
Therapeutic Range 353
Suggested Sampling Times and Effect on Therapeutic
 Range 354
Neonates 354
Infants, children, adults, and geriatrics 354
Pharmacodynamic Monitoring—Concentration-Related
 Efficacy..355
Asthma or COPD.....................................355
Apnea or bradycardia in neonates......................355
Pharmacodynamic Monitoring—Concentration-Related
 Toxicity 355
Drug–Drug Interactions 356
Drug–Disease State or Condition Interactions 357
References 359

Chapter 19. Valproic Acid *by* Barry E. Gidal &
 Nina M. Graves 361
Usual Dosage Range in Absence of Clearance-Altering
 Factors 361
Dosage Form Availability 362
Bioavailability (F) of Dosage Forms 362
General Pharmacokinetic Information 363
Clearance 363
Metabolism 363
Protein binding...364
Clearance (CL) 364
Volume of Distribution (V) 365
Half-Life and Time to Steady State 365
Therapeutic Range 365
Effect of age 367
Dosing..367
Suggested Sampling Times and Effect on Therapeutic
 Range 367
Timing of sample collections 367
Resampling guidelines 368

Initial monitoring guidelines 368
Dosage adjustment 368
Pharmacodynamic Monitoring—Concentration-Related
　Efficacy.. 369
Pharmacodynamic Monitoring—Concentration-Related
　Toxicity 369
Drug–Drug Interactions 369
Drug–Disease State or Condition Interactions 370
References 371

Chapter 20. Vancomycin *by* Reginald F. Frye & Gary R. Matzke 375

Usual Dosage Range in Absence of Clearance-Altering
　Factors 375
Dosage Form Availability 376
Bioavailability (*F*) of Dosage Forms 376
General Pharmacokinetic Information 376
　Disposition.. 376
　Elimination 377
　Protein binding... 377
Clearance (CL) 377
Volume of Distribution (*V*) 378
Half-Life and Time to Steady State 379
Therapeutic Range... 380
Suggested Sampling Times and Effect on Therapeutic
　Range 380
Pharmacodynamic Monitoring—Concentration-Related
　Efficacy.. 381
Pharmacodynamic Monitoring—Concentration-Related
　Toxicity.. 382
　Concentration-related toxicities 382
　Nonconcentration-related toxicities 382
Drug–Drug Interactions..................................... 383
Drug–Disease State Interactions 383
References... 385

Chapter 21. Warfarin *by* Douglas F. Covey 389

Usual Dosage Range in Absence of Clearance-Altering
　Factors 390
Dosage Form Availability................................... 391
General Pharmacokinetic Information 391
Pharmacodynamic Basis of Action......................... 394
　Prothrombin complex activity and half-life 394
　Time course of PT elevation 395

Therapeutic Range... 396
   Prothrombin time 396
   International normalized ration (INR).................. 396
Warfarin Dosing Strategies and Suggested Sampling
     Times 398
   Overlap with heparin therapy........................... 398
   Commencement of warfarin therapy 400
   Maintenance dose adjustment........................... 403
   Outpatient monitoring.................................. 403
Pharmacodynamic Monitoring 405
   Dosage adjustments based on INR values 406
   Safe practice recommendations for using vitamin K_1
     to reverse excessive warfarin anticoagulation 406
Drug–Drug Interactions..................................... 409
   Time course of drug interaction 410
   Specific drug interactions 410
Drug–Disease State or Condition Interactions 413
Summary... 414
References... 414

Chapter 22. Drug Dosing in the Neonate *by* Ana M.
    Lopez-Samblas, Philip R. Diaz & Kim H. Binion ... 419
General Pharmacokinetic Information 422
   Absorption 422
   Distribution.. 423
   Metabolism... 423
   Elimination 424
   Protein binding.. 425
Therapeutic Range.. 425
Factors Interfering with Therapeutic Monitoring 425
   Methods of intravenous drug administration 425
   Concentration measurements drawn from intravenous
     lines 432
   Medication errors 433
   Digoxin-like substances................................ 433
Factors Influencing Drug Disposition 433
   Asphyxia.. 433
   Exchange transfusion.................................. 434
   Extracorporeal membrane oxygenation (ECMO) 435
   Patent ductus arteriosus (PDA) 435
References.. 436

Chapter 23. Drug Dosing in Pediatric Patients
   by Vinita B. Pai & Milap C. Nahata 439

Absorption 440
   Intravenous 440
   Oral 441
   Intramuscular 442
   Percutaneous 443
   Rectal 443
Distribution 448
Metabolism 449
Elimination 453
Drug Disposition in Cystic Fibrosis 454
Therapeutic Drug Monitoring 460
References 460

Chapter 24. Therapeutic Drug Monitoring in the Geriatric Patient *by* Susan W. Miller 467
Physiologic Changes 468
   Absorption, distribution, metabolism, and excretion 468
   Binding proteins 471
   Increased free (unbound) fraction 471
   Lean body weight to fat ratio 472
Drug Elimination 474
Renal Clearance 475
Age-Related Pharmacodynamic Changes Influencing Drug Response 476
Summary of Changes 480
References 504

Chapter 25. Dosing Concepts in Renal Dysfunction *by* Sybelle Blakey 507
Renal Mechanisms of Drug Clearance 507
CrCl Limitations 508
Relationship of CrCl to Drug Elimination 510
Modifying Drug Dosages 511
Dialysis 513
Active or Toxic Metabolites 516
Clinical Considerations 516
Conclusion 527
References 528

Appendix A. Nomogram for Determining Body Surface Area of Adults from Height and Mass 531

Appendix B. Nomogram for Determining Body Surface Area of Children from Height and Mass 533

Appendix C. Therapeutic Ranges of Drugs in Traditional
and SI Units... 535

Appendix D. Nondrug Reference Ranges for Common
Laboratory Tests in Traditional and SI Units 537

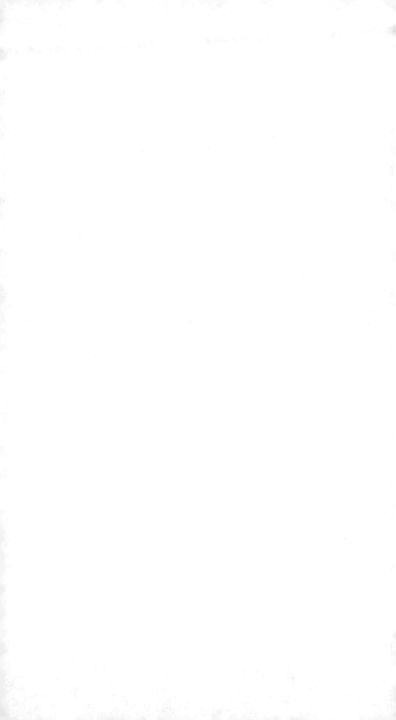

This second edition of the *Clinical Pharmacokinetics Pocket Reference* is dedicated in loving memory of

Brendan Michael Murphy (1985–2000), an exceptional young man and fine fisherman

The first edition of the *Clinical Pharmacokinetics Pocket Reference* is re-dedicated to

My students and residents, past and present, who inspired my interest in preparing this book

The pharmacists who helped make clinical pharmacokinetics and therapeutic drug monitoring a cornerstone of pharmacy practice, especially Earl and Martin

My family—Debbie, Elizabeth, Cullen, Patrick, Mom, Dad, Steve, and Kerry

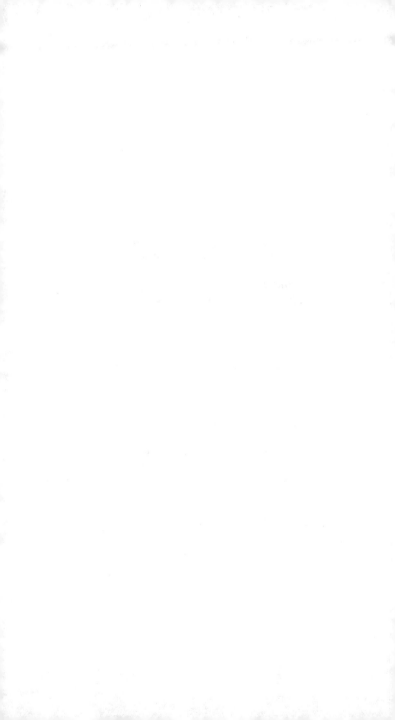

Preface

This *Pocket Reference* has been written for clinicians and students with experience in basic pharmacokinetic principles. It is intended to be used to initiate and monitor therapy in actual patients or to learn how to do so. It is intended as a textbook for teaching these principles to students and as a reference that can be easily accessed in clinical situations. It is not intended as a textbook for people interested in learning how to manipulate the pharmacokinetic formulae used in clinical pharmacokinetic monitoring. Hence, this knowledge is assumed.

Interest in writing the first edition of the *Pocket Reference* arose from the teaching of clinical pharmacokinetic principles to Doctor of Pharmacy candidates over the first 12 years of my career and from daily consultation on patients during 10 years as director of a pharmacokinetics service. I first developed a clerkship manual, including population values for many commonly monitored drugs, with the purpose of enhancing a student's ability to compare such values to actual patient results. That manual also aided me in keeping track of population values of drugs for which the pharmacokinetic service received consultation requests. Over the years, many pharmacists asked for a personal copy of this manual, demonstrating the need for such a reference.

In my pharmacokinetic practice, requests also were occasionally received for consultation on a drug that we did not routinely monitor. Invariably, such a request would come on the weekend when library facilities were closed, causing frustration in the initial dose and interval determination for the patient. I then realized that a more complete clerkship manual would be useful not only for our service but also for others in similar situations. Moreover, I wanted this new manual to fit easily in a laboratory jacket since larger texts with extensive discussions of population pharmacokinetic values are already available.

In reviewing other publications of a similar nature, it became evident that authors usually did not extensively examine a wide variety of patient populations for each drug. In addition, monitoring for pharmacodynamic response was not always discussed. For this *Pocket Reference,* the authors have attempted to gather information that should be useful in differentiating among many patients who will receive each drug to enhance the potential predictability of the resulting concentrations. The impact of drug interactions on pharmacokinetics and pharmacodynamics is also of great importance, so information has been gathered on these effects.

Users of this book should understand that the larger the number of confounding factors and interactions, the greater the likelihood that predictability will diminish since the patient will then belong to a population that has not been well studied. Also, many researchers have demonstrated the need for follow-up monitoring with drug concentration measurements in patients since predictability is often relatively poor. Thus the need for pharmacokinetic monitoring becomes evident.

Many new studies have published since the first edition of the *Pocket Reference*. The second edition takes advantage of these advances in understanding. Using the *Pocket Reference* as a textbook in my own teaching has also enhanced understanding of how these materials are accessed by individuals new to the processes of individualizing therapy based on population parameters and patient outcome.

As with the first edition, authors of the drug chapters were asked to evaluate the literature carefully and then put forth a method they would use to initiate and monitor therapy. Readers should understand that other authors might recommend different approaches based on their personal evaluation of the literature. Because decisions related to caring for patients are rarely completely black or white, this approach should not be unexpected. We urge all users of these approaches to compare them to other approaches. We are fairly confident that some will work better than others will at different times. Try them on all patients and adapt your thinking based on the results. Learn when a particular method works well and when it is not as useful. It is this learning that generally separates us from available computers and software—at least for now.

A full chapter on creatinine clearance estimations has been added, largely because many dose predictions depend on creatinine clearance, but also because I have been asked so many interesting questions about these predictions over the years. What to do when a patient has an amputation is a good example.

This book is obviously designed to help predict drug doses and drug concentrations for patients. Judicious use of drug concentration measurements is an important adjunct to verification of the predictions and for comparison to patient response. However, I generally believe that measurements are often not used effectively. For this reason, in addition to new chapters on individual drugs, a chapter with recommendations for appropriate use of drug concentration measurements has been added.

We have also included a table on international units along with conventional units for the drugs and laboratory tests. This inclusion should allow wider use of the *Pocket Reference* around the world.

I also gratefully acknowledge the chapter authors who volunteered a portion of their lives to turn the first and second editions of this book from concept to reality. All of them were already too busy with work but, like most pharmacists I know, they fortunately have not learned how to say no to a request. Thank you all for the sacrifices. I would also like to thank the secretaries of the authors for putting up with the many changes throughout this project.

The chapter reviewers also deserve a hearty thanks. They were very important to the quality and potential success of this book. They deserve much thanks for detailed and timely commentary.

Finally, many thanks to the best collaborators in the world—the ASHP staff and particularly Con Ann Ling—for all of their help in making both of these editions happen. They do much work and receive little credit. But I know their value and it is tremendous. Thanks.

John E. Murphy
September 2000

Contributors

Douglas M. Anderson, Pharm.D., BCPS
Senior Clinical Research and Education Manager
Amgen Incorporated
Thousand Oaks, California

Kim H. Binion, Pharm.D.
Clinical Pharmacist
Pediatric Clinical Pharmacy Services
Jackson Memorial Hospital
Miami, Florida
(at time of writing of first edition)

Sybelle A. Blakey, Pharm.D., BCPS
Clinical Assistant Professor
Mercer University Southern School of Pharmacy
Atlanta, Georgia

Glen Brown, Pharm.D.
Clinical Coordinator, Pharmacy
Department of Pharmacy
St. Paul's Hospital
Vancouver, British Columbia, Canada

Stanley W. Carson, Pharm.D., FCCP, BCPP
Associate Professor of Pharmacy
Research Associate Professor of Psychiatry
University of North Carolina at Chapel Hill
Chapel Hill, North Carolina

Douglas F. Covey, Pharm.D., MHA
Clinical Pharmacy Specialist for Ambulatory Care
James A. Haley Veterans Affairs Medical Center
Tampa, Florida

Clinical Associate Professor
Assistant Director Working Professional Doctor of Pharmacy Degree Program
University of Florida College of Pharmacy
Gainesville, Florida

Edress Darsey, Pharm.D.
Clinical Education Consultant, Pfizer, Inc.
Duluth, Georgia

Clinical Manager
Children's Healthcare of Atlanta
Atlanta, Georgia
(at time of writing)

C. Lindsay DeVane, Pharm.D.
Professor of Psychiatry and Behavioral Sciences
Department of Psychiatry and Behavioral Sciences
Medical University of South Carolina
Charleston, South Carolina

Philip R. Diaz, Pharm.D., BCPS
Associate Director
Pharmacy Education and Research
Greensboro AHEC
Moses H. Cone Memorial Hospital
Greensboro, North Carolina
Assistant Professor
School of Pharmacy, and Clinical Instructor
Department of Family Medicine
School of Medicine
University of North Carolina
Chapel Hill, North Carolina

Christy M. Evans, B.S., Pharm.D.
Cardiovascular Clinical Pharmacy Resident
Arizona Health Sciences Center
University of Arizona, College of Pharmacy
(at time of writing)

Reginald F. Frye, Pharm.D., Ph.D.
Assistant Professor, Department of Pharmaceutical Sciences and Member, Center for Clinical Pharmacology
University of Pittsburgh
School of Pharmacy
Pittsburgh, Pennsylvania

William R. Garnett, Pharm.D., FCCP
Professor of Pharmacy and Neurology

Virginia Commonwealth University
Medical College of Virginia
Richmond, Virginia

Barry E. Gidal, Pharm.D.
Associate Professor
School of Pharmacy and Department of Neurology
University of Wisconsin
Madison, Wisconsin

James B. Groce III, Pharm.D., CACP
Associate Professor of Pharmacy
Campbell University School of Pharmacy
Buies Creek, North Carolina
Clinical Assistant Professor of Medicine
UNC School of Medicine
Chapel Hill, North Carolina
Clinical Pharmacy Specialist–Anticoagulation
Moses Cone Health System
Greensboro, North Carolina

Martin L. Job, Pharm.D., M.A., BCPS, FASHP, FCCP
Manager Clinical Services
Abbott Laboratories
Abbott Park, Illinois

Janet Karlix, Pharm.D.
Associate Professor
College of Pharmacy
University of Florida
Gainesville, Florida

Ana M. Lopez-Samblas, Pharm.D.
Director of Pediatric Pharmacy Services
University of Miami/Jackson Memorial Medical Center
Assistant Adjunct Professor
University of Miami School of Medicine
Miami, Florida
Clinical Associate Professor
College of Pharmacy
NOVA Southeastern University
Ft. Lauderdale, Florida
Clinical Associate Profesor
College of Pharmacy
University of Florida
Gainesville, Florida

Gary R. Matzke, Pharm.D. FCP, FCCP
Professor of Pharmaceutical Sciences and Medicine

Director, Clinical Pharmaceutical Sciences Graduate Program
Co-Director, Clinical Research Training Program
Center for Clinical Pharmacology
Center for Research in Health Care
Schools of Pharmacy and Medicine
University of Pittsburgh
Pittsburgh, Pennsylvania

James P. McCormack, B.Sc. (Pharm), Pharm.D.
Associate Professor, Faculty of Pharmaceutical Sciences
University of British Columbia
Department of Pharmacy
St. Paul's Hospital
Vancouver, British Columbia, Canada

John N. McCormick, B.S., Pharm D.
Clinical Pharmacy Specialist
St. Jude Children's Research Hospital
Memphis, Tennessee

Susan W. Miller, Pharm.D, FASCP, CGP
Professor, Department of Pharmacy Practice
Mercer University Southern School of Pharmacy
Atlanta, Georgia

Milap C. Nahata, Pharm.D., FCCP, FASHP
Charles H. Kimberly Professor of Pharmacy
Professor of Pediatrics
Chair, Division of Pharmacy Practice and Administration
Colleges of Pharmacy and Medicine
The Ohio State University and Children's Hospital
Columbus, Ohio

Paul E. Nolan, Jr., Pharm.D.
Professor
Dept. of Pharmacy Practice and Science
College of Pharmacy
Clinical Scientist
Sarver Heart Center
University of Arizona
Tucson, Arizona

Robert E. Pachorek, Pharm.D., BCPS
Pharmacy Department
Scripps Mercy Hospital
San Diego, California

Vinita Pai, Pharm.D.
Assistant Professor of Pharmacy Practice
College of Pharmacy
Idaho State University and
St. Luke's Regional Medical Center
Boise, Idaho

John A. Pieper, Pharm.D., FCCP
Professor and Chariman
Division of Pharmacotherapy
School of Pharmacy
University of North Carolina
Chapel Hill, North Carolina

Kimberly B. Tallian, Pharm.D.
Clinical Coordinator of Pharmacy Services
Children's Hospital of San Diego
San Diego, California

Mary E. Teresi, Pharm.D.
Director, Pediatric Allergy/Pulmonary Clinical Trials
University of Iowa College of Medicine
Iowa City, Iowa

Toby C. Trujillo, Pharm.D.
Assistant Professor of Clinical Pharmacy
Massachusetts College of Pharmacy and Health Sciences
Boston, Massachusetts

Joe Walker, Pharm.D.
Clinical Pharmacologist
Orchid BioSciences, Inc.
Princeton, New Jersey

Fellow, Immunology/Transplantation
University of Florida
Gainesville, Florida
(at time of writing)

Michael E. Winter, Pharm.D.
Professor and Vice Chair
Department of Clinical Pharmacy
School of Pharmacy
University of California
San Francisco, California

Reviewers

The editor and ASHP gratefully acknowledge the following individuals, who donated their expertise in reviewing the chapters for this book:

Cara L. Alfaro, Pharm.D.
Rita R. Alloway, Pharm.D., BCPS
Amir Aminimanizani, Pharm.D.
Philip O. Anderson, Pharm.D.,
Paul Beringer, Pharm.D., BCPS
Maureen S. Boro, Pharm.D.
Bradley A. Boucher, Pharm.D.
Joseph C. Brooks, Pharm.D., BCPS
Marcia L. Buck, Pharm.D.
Lily K. Cheung, Pharm.D.
Melissa M. L. Choy, Pharm.D.
James W. Cooper, Jr., B.S. Pharm., Ph.D., BCPS, CGP
William R. Crom, Pharm.D.
Lorraine R. Deleon, Pharm.D.
Tamara J. Eide, Pharm.D., BCPS
Erika J. Ernst, Pharm.D.
Sandra G. Faucette, B.S. Pharm.
Vanessa L. Freitag, Pharm.D.
Peter Gal, Pharm.D., BCPS
Marie E. Gardner, Pharm.D. BCPP, CGP
Daniel E. Hilleman, Pharm.D.
Julie Hixson-Wallace, Pharm.D., BCPS
Holly L. Hoffman, Pharm.D.

Michael M. Hoppe, Pharm.D.
Julienne K. Kirk, Pharm.D.
Michael E. Klepser, Pharm.D.
Y. W. Francis Lam, Pharm.D.
Russell E. Lewis, Pharm.D.
Michael A. Marx, Pharm.D., BCPS
Charles Y. McCall, Pharm.D.
Howard Peckman, M.S., Pharm.D.
Keith A. Rodvold, Pharm.D., BCPS
Richard L. Slaughter, M.S.
Curtis L. Smith, Pharm.D. BCPS
William J. Spruill, Pharm.D.
Kevin M. Sowinski, Pharm.D.
James E. Tisdale, Pharm.D.
David F. Volles, Pharm.D. BCPS
William E. Wade, Pharm.D.
Jun Yan, Pharm.D.

John E. Murphy

Introduction

General Pharmacokinetic Principles

Initiating therapy

When therapy is initiated in a patient, a standard dose and interval may be used, or the dose and interval may be individualized by use of population means of volume of distribution, clearance, and half-life. These population pharmacokinetic parameters are useful for predicting drug concentrations based on an administered or planned dose and dosage schedule. To adjust therapy, these values then may be compared to actual drug concentration measurements and integrated with the patient's therapeutic outcome.

Using population mean values

Unfortunately, not all patients fit the population means, and some of these means were developed on small samples that do not represent the general population or the patient being monitored. For many drugs, population means with standard deviations will provide useful information on reasonable ranges of the values to expect.

In any case, a patient's actual pharmacokinetic values (i.e., clearance, volume of distribution, and half-life) may need to be determined to adjust therapy for a desired outcome.

Considering other factors in pharmacokinetic monitoring[1]

In addition to the problems with population pharmacokinetic means, unexpected drug concentration measurements can occur for various reasons. Some patients may be nonadherent with drug therapy, taking either more or less than was prescribed for them. In the institutional setting, administration errors can account for unexpected results; a patient may be administered the wrong dose of a drug, may be administered the drug at the wrong time, or may not receive the scheduled drug at all.

Errors on medication administration records also can occur, indicating that a drug was given at other than the actual time it was received by the patient. Furthermore, incomplete drug delivery due to patient problems (e.g., infiltration of an intravenous fluid or clogging of a nasal cannula) can influence drug concentration measurements.

Problems in sample collection can lead to unexpected drug concentration measurements. A blood sample may be drawn at the wrong time, or the wrong collection time may be reported. Samples can be taken from the wrong patient or obtained incorrectly (e.g., through a drug administration line that was inadequately flushed prior to sample withdrawal). In addition, samples may be improperly stored.

Finally, other things to consider include drug or disease state interactions, which may influence the prediction of drug concentration measurements, and the use of inaccurate assays.

Some reasons for drug concentration measurements that fall outside of the expected range of population estimates

- Patient truly does not well fit the population average values (i.e., falls outside of one standard deviation of the mean).
- The population values used for the predictions were determined in patients unlike the patient being monitored.
- Patient has been nonadherent with therapy (may have taken either more or less than prescribed).
- Nurse did not give the dose at the time prescribed (whether it has been signed off as given on time or not).
- Dose not given at all (whether it is signed off as given or not). Also doses are occasionally given but not signed off as such.
- Wrong dose given (either once or more often).
- Error made in dosing schedule on medication administration record (e.g., every 18-hr schedule is put on record such that patient is given doses 18 and 30 hr apart).
- The complete dose was not administered prior to sample withdrawal due to patient problems (e.g., infiltration of an intravenous line, clogging of nasal cannula).
- Phlebotomist drew blood at a time other than requested and:
  1. Reported that it was collected on time, or
  2. Did not report the time of collection and it is incorrectly assumed to have been drawn at the scheduled time.
- The sample was taken from the wrong patient.
- The sample was obtained incorrectly (e.g., through a drug administration line which has been improperly flushed prior to sample withdrawal).
- The sample was not stored properly, leading to artifactual results.
- Assay or assay instrument quality is not satisfactory and the report result is not accurate.

- A pharmacokinetic drug interaction has occurred which was not accounted for correctly in estimation of DCMs.
- An in vitro drug interaction occurred, resulting in artifactual results.
- Disease interaction occurred, such as reduced absorption rate due to poor blood flow.

Verifying drug concentration measurements

If measured values fall outside the range estimated using one standard deviation of the predicted clearance, volume of distribution, and/or half-life, one or more drug concentrations should be rechecked before the measured concentrations are accepted as valid. This step does not preclude changing the dose or interval if such a change would have been made empirically at the start of therapy. If the measured concentrations are far from those predicted, the clinician must determine whether the measured drug concentrations are reasonable (i.e., within reasonable expectation based on the range of population values) or whether one or more of the problems noted above occurred.

The occurrence of certain problems can be determined with detective work. For example, a patient can be questioned about compliance, past outpatient pharmacy records can be checked, and the nurse administering the drug or the phlebotomist drawing the blood sample can be interviewed. Unfortunately, the validity of the information gathered after the fact may be questionable.

Because of these potential problems, measured drug concentrations may not be a true reflection of the patient's actual drug distribution and elimination half-life. Therefore, a clinician can make an erroneous decision about the dosing needs of the patient. Accurate information is essential to quality therapeutic drug monitoring.

A well-coordinated system of communication is needed between those administering or taking a medication and those collecting blood (or other body fluid or tissue) for analysis. Such a system can prevent many of the problems associated with assessing the validity of reported drug concentrations and dose/sample collection timing. It also can reduce erroneous decision-making based on faulty data as well as the expense of repeating questionable drug concentration measurements. The lack of such a system should be considered a waste of resources and provides the potential for harming patients secondary to a high incidence of debatable data.

After as many causes of discrepancy as possible are eliminated, a decision must be made as to whether the difference between predicted and actual values is due to patient variability from population averages or to erroneous values. If the values are judged to be erroneous, drug concentrations probably should be remeasured, although the need for further evaluation should be as carefully considered as the original decision to monitor (see chapter 2, Rational Use of Drug Concentration Measurements).

Determining need for dosage adjustments

Once the drug concentration measurement and dosing information is determined to be as accurate as possible, dosage adjustments are assessed based on pharmacodynamic response and patient outcome. Usually, the need for dosage adjustment or the continuation of therapy should be based on patient response relative to measured drug concentration rather than on drug concentration alone.

This approach may not be proper, however, when the disease or symptoms are not continuous or easy to quantify. For example, keeping an anticonvulsant drug within the therapeutic range may be important since seizure activity may be infrequent. Without an adequate seizure history, the maintenance of a dosing schedule that produces drug concentration measurements above or below the normal accepted therapeutic range may not be prudent.

Deciding on monitoring frequency

How frequently a patient should be monitored for efficacy or side effects related to drug therapy varies with the drug, the intensity of the disease, the stability of body functions, and other factors. In general, the more severely compromised the patient, the more frequently the patient should be monitored.

Clinicians should be aware of the many factors that can alter a drug's pharmacokinetic and pharmacodynamic activities. Addition or deletion of other drug therapy (or diet) that may interact with the drug being monitored should signal the need for closer inspection. Changes in the function of the primary organs of drug elimination (e.g., liver and kidneys) or in cardiac function also should signal the need for closer monitoring.

Finally, patient (or caregiver) adherence must be assessed whenever a decision is based on a drug concentration measurement. Simply assuming appropriate adherence to the prescribed regimen can lead to grave errors in the worst case and a waste of resources in others.

A Basic Pharmacokinetic Glossary

As the science of pharmacokinetic evaluation of drug therapy has progressed, the terminology used has grown as well. Although terms such as half-life and volume of distribution are standardized in most pharmacokinetic texts, a wide variety of terminology is used to describe other basic concepts.

For this reason, an attempt was made to standardize the terminology used throughout this book. The wide collection of studies used to reference the chapters somewhat hindered this effort.

With that understanding, the following terminology is offered as a guideline to interpreting the values and terms in this book.

Selected pharmacokinetic terminology
   Actual body weight (ABW)—Patient's measured body weight.

*Css*_{av}—Concentration measured approximately halfway between the peak and trough for a drug administered long enough to be at steady state (except for some sustained-release preparations). Hence, for an intravenous bolus regimen on an every 6-hr interval, the Css_{av} would be at 3 hr after a dose. For a dose requiring absorption that peaks 2 hr after administration, the average would occur at approximately 4 hr on a 6-hr interval.

Ideal body weight (IBW)—Ideal weight for a patient based on insurance tables for longevity.

Lean body weight (LBW)—Patient's body weight minus fat weight. It is often used interchangeably with IBW.

Peak—Concentration of drug that occurs immediately after an intravenous bolus dose, at the end of an infusion, or at a particular time after dose administration for a drug requiring absorption. It is the highest or maximum concentration after any type of dosing method. However, occasionally the "peak" is the concentration measured within 30–60 min after the true peak time (e.g., 30 min after the end of a dose infusion for aminoglycosides); this peak might be considered a "therapeutic peak" for assessment of patient response rather than the actual peak. This time lag before collection in part acknowledges the fact that doses are not always given precisely on time and that blood samples are not always drawn precisely when scheduled for a true peak.

Steady state—Point in time reached after a drug has been given for approximately five elimination half-lives (97% of steady state has been achieved after five half-lives). At steady state, the rate of drug administration equals the rate of elimination; drug concentration–time curves found after each dose on an even schedule (e.g., every 8 hours) should be approximately superimposable.

Administration of a loading dose can affect the time to steady state if the loading and maintenance doses are matched correctly. If the loading dose provides exactly the amount needed to achieve the steady-state concentration that will be achieved by the maintenance dose, then steady state is achieved immediately. If the loading dose is too small or too large relative to attainment of the concentrations that will occur with maintenance doses, five half-lives will be required to achieve 97% of *the difference* between the loading dose concentrations and the final steady-state concentrations.

Therapeutic range—Range of concentrations where optimum outcome is expected, based on results of groups of individuals. In reality, each person has his or her own therapeutic range for each drug. Above the therapeutic range, the incidence of drug toxicity increases; below it, the probability of inadequate response increases. This range should be viewed only as an initial target, because patients may respond when below it and may not be toxic when above it. Furthermore, minor toxicity above a therapeutic range might be acceptable to a patient if efficacy increases. Serious toxicity is a definite upper limit to any individual's therapeutic range.

Trough—Concentration that occurs immediately before the next dose for drugs given intermittently but in a multiple-dose fashion. It is the lowest or minimum concentration after a dose given intermittently. However, quite often the "trough" is the concentration measured within 30–60 min of the next dose; this trough might be considered a "therapeutic trough" related to this time in pharmacokinetic and pharmacodynamic studies of the drug. This time period in advance of the true trough also acknowledges variance in compliance with precise dose administration time and phlebotomist arrival time.

Selected pharmacokinetic symbols

These symbols generally follow the nomenclature suggested by the Committee for Pharmacokinetic Nomenclature of the American College of Clinical Pharmacology.[2] An exception is volume of distribution (V versus V_z).

C	= plasma or serum concentration of drug
C_i	= initial plasma or serum concentration, the larger of two plasma or serum concentrations in an elimination portion of a concentration–time curve. For example, in Equation 1, C_i is the largest of two concentrations, C_i and C.
C_{max}	= maximum drug concentration
Css	= plasma or serum concentration at steady state
CL	= apparent total body clearance (either in units of volume per time, such as liters per hour, or in units of volume per time per body weight, such as liters per hour per kilogram). $CL = k \times V$.
CrCl	= clearance of creatinine (in units of milliliters per minute or liters per hour)
D	= dose (in amount, such as milligrams, or amount per patient body weight, such as milligrams per kilogram)
F	= bioavailability fraction of a dose (no units). It is the fraction or percent of a dose that reaches the systemic circulation.
k	= first-order elimination rate constant (in units of 1/time or time^{-1}). $k = 0.693/t\frac{1}{2}$.
k_a	= first-order absorption rate constant (in units of 1/time or time^{-1}). $k_a = 0.693/t\frac{1}{2}_a$.
K_m	= Michaelis–Menten constant (in units of concentration such as milligrams per liter). It is the concentration at which the system is one-half saturated.
R_0	= zero-order infusion rate (in amount per time such as milligrams per hour)
S	= fraction of a dose that is parent drug (i.e., the drug measured in plasma or serum). For example, aminophylline is 80% theophylline. Thus, $S = 0.8$ for aminophylline.
S_{Cr}	= serum creatinine
t	= elapsed time. For example, it is the time between two concentrations, known or estimated, in the

elimination phase of a drug following first-order elimination.

t' = time of an infusion (i.e., duration of infusion, usually in hours)

t_{max} = time to peak (maximum concentration) of a drug that requires absorption (e.g., oral, intramuscular, rectal, or buccal)

$t½$ = half-life of a drug (in units of time). It is the time needed to reduce the drug concentration or amount of drug in the body by one-half. $t½ = 0.693/k$.

$t½_a$ = absorption half-life of a drug product administered in a dosage form requiring absorption (in units of time). $t½_a = 0.693/k_a$.

T = time clapsed after the *end* of an infusion

Δt = change in time (or the time between two measured concentrations)

τ = dosage interval (in units of time, usually hours or days)

V = apparent volume of distribution (either in units of volume, such as liters, or in units of volume per body weight, such as liters per kilogram)

V_{max} = (V_m) maximum velocity of drug elimination for a drug following Michaelis–Menten (enzyme saturable) elimination. It is the amount of drug that can be biotransformed per unit of time (in units of amount per time such as milligrams per day).

General Estimating Equations

Like the above terms and symbols, several equations are frequently used in pharmacokinetic calculations and are considered to be standards. Frequently used equations for calculating ideal or lean body weight and body surface area are as follows. Creatinine clearance estimations are provided in chapter 1, Estimating Creatinine Clearance.

Calculating lean or ideal body weight (IBW) in adults[3]

$$\text{males} = 50 \text{ kg} + [(2.3)(HT - 60)] \text{ kg}$$
$$\text{females} = 45.5 \text{ kg} + [(2.3)(HT - 60)] \text{ kg}$$

where HT is a patient's height in inches.
Or,

$$\text{males} = 50 \text{ kg} + 0.9(HT - 152)$$
$$\text{females} = 45.5 \text{ kg} + 0.9(HT - 152)$$

where HT is height in centimeters.

Note: For patients who are less than 60 inches tall (152 cm), the weight should be decreased more conservatively than 2.3 kg/inch (2.3 kg/2.54 cm).

Calculating ideal body weight in children aged 1–18 years[4]
For children less than 5 feet (152 cm) tall

$$IBW = 2.05 e^{(0.02)(HT)}$$

where IBW is ideal body weight in kilograms and HT is height in centimeters.

For children 5 feet (152 cm) or taller

$$IBW \text{ (males)} = 39 + 2.27(HT - 60)$$
$$IBW \text{ (females)} = 42.2 + 2.27(HT - 60)$$

where HT is height in inches, IBW is ideal body weight in kilograms.
Or,

$$IBW \text{ (males)} = 39 + 0.9(HT - 152)$$
$$IBW \text{ (females)} = 42.2 + 0.9(HT - 152)$$

where HT is height in centimeters and IBW is ideal body weight in kilograms.

Calculating surface area (SA) in meters^2
For adults, children, and infants.[5]

$$SA = W^{0.5378} \times HT^{0.3964} \times 0.024265$$

where W equals weight in kilograms, and HT equals height in centimeters.

Note: Nomograms used to determine the surface areas for adults and children appear in Appendices A and B. The authors of the above formula found it to be a better predictor of surface area in infants than the nomogram in Appendix B.[6]

General Pharmacokinetic Equations

The following equations are used to determine concentration and other pharmacokinetic parameters.

These equations may be manipulated to determine volume of distribution from measured concentrations and the known times after a dose when the concentrations were determined. A dose also may be calculated from known or estimated CL, V, or k values by manipulating the applicable equations to solve for dose (D).

1. Concentration at any time t after some initial concentration (C_i):

$$C = C_i e^{-kt}$$

2. k from two known concentration–time points in the elimination phase:

$$k = \frac{\ln(C_i/C)}{\Delta t}$$

3. Concentration at any time t after a single intravenous bolus dose:

$$C = \frac{SD}{V} e^{-kt}$$

4. Concentration at any time t after an intravenous bolus dose given every τ hr (at steady state):

$$C = \frac{SD}{V} \frac{e^{-kt}}{(1 - e^{-k\tau})}$$

5. Concentration at any time t after the start of an intravenous infusion at rate R_0:

$$C = \frac{SR_0}{CL}(1 - e^{-kt})$$

6. Concentration at steady state of an intravenous infusion at rate R_0:

$$Css = \frac{SR_0}{CL}$$

7. Average steady-state concentration of a dose given intermittently (by all dosing methods):

$$Css_{av} = \frac{SFD}{CL}$$

or

$$Css_{av} = \frac{SFD}{kV\tau}$$

8. Concentration at any time t after a single dose requiring absorption:

$$C = \frac{SFDk_a}{V(k_a - k)}(e^{-kt} - e^{-k_a t})$$

9. Time to peak (maximum concentration) of a dose requiring absorption after a single dose:

$$t_{max} = \frac{\ln(k_a/k)}{(k_a - k)}$$

10. Concentration at any time t after a dose requiring absorption during steady-state conditions:

$$C = \frac{SFDk_a}{V(k_a - k)}\left[\frac{e^{-kt}}{(1 - e^{-k\tau})} - \frac{e^{-k_a t}}{(1 - e^{-k_a \tau})}\right]$$

11. Time to peak (maximum concentration) of a dose requiring absorption at steady state:

$$t_{max} = \frac{\ln[k_a(1 - e^{-k\tau})/k(1 - e^{-k_a \tau})]}{(k_a - k)}$$

12. Concentration at any time T after the end of a single short infusion lasting t' time:

$$C = \frac{SD}{kVt'}(1 - e^{-kt'})e^{-kT}$$

13. Concentration at any time T after the end of a short infusion lasting t' time given every τ hr:

$$C = \frac{SD}{kVt'}\frac{(1 - e^{-kt'})}{(1 - e^{-k\tau})}e^{-kT}$$

14. Average steady-state concentration of a drug that follows Michaelis–Menten elimination:

$$Css_{av} = \frac{SF(D/\tau) \times K_m}{V_m - SF(D/\tau)}$$

15. Dose to produce desired steady-state concentration for a drug that follows Michaelis–Menten elimination:

$$D = \frac{Css \times V_m \times \tau}{SF(Css + K_m)}$$

References

1. Murphy JE, Job ML, Ward ES. Rectifying incorrect dosage schedules. *Am J Hosp Pharm.* 1990; 47:2235–6.
2. Committee for Pharmacokinetic Nomenclature. Manual of symbols, equations, & definitions in pharmacokinetics. *J Clin Pharmacol.* 1982; 22: 1S–23S.
3. Devine BJ. Gentamicin therapy. *Drug Intell Clin Pharm.* 1974; 7:650–5.
4. Traub SL, Johnson CE. Comparison of methods of estimating creatinine clearance in children. *Am J Hosp Pharm.* 1980; 37:195–201.
5. Haycock GB, Schwartz GJ, Wisotsky DH. Geometric method for measuring body surface area: a height–weight formula validated in infants, children, and adults. *J Pediatr.* 1978; 93:62–6.

Chapter 1
Robert E. Pachorek

Estimating Creatinine Clearance

Estimating Glomerular Filtration Rate by Creatinine Clearance

The importance of accurate estimations of glomerular filtration rate (GFR), the principal measure of renal function, cannot be overemphasized. Many drugs or active metabolites are eliminated to some extent by renal excretion, creating the need for dosage adjustments as renal function deteriorates, particularly for drugs with a narrow therapeutic range. In general, decreases in the rate of elimination of renally excreted drugs are proportional to decreases in the GFR. The renal clearance of the endogenously produced amino acid, creatinine, is the most commonly used estimate of GFR in the hospitalized patient. Creatine, a product of protein metabolism, is primarily produced in the liver, pancreas, and kidneys and is actively transported into muscle tissue where it is stored. Creatinine, produced from creatine in muscle tissue proportionally to muscle mass, is released at a constant rate (approximately 1.5% of the total pool per day) into the general circulation and is distributed to total body water. Creatinine is passively filtered by the glomerulus proportionately to the GFR, although 10–40% of the total creatinine found in urine is a result of active renal tubular secretion.[1-3]

The creatinine clearance (CrCl), in milliliters per minute (ml/min), can be directly measured by a 24-hr urine collection and the following relationship:

$$CrCl = \frac{U_{Cr} \times V_{Cr}}{S_{Cr} \times t}$$

where U_{Cr} is the urine creatinine concentration (mg/dl), V_{Cr} is the urine volume (ml), S_{Cr} is serum creatinine (mg/dl) at the midpoint of the urine collection, and t is the time interval in minutes (1440 min for 24 hr).[1,2]

Because some creatinine found in the urine is due to secretion, the CrCl overestimates the GFR at all levels of renal function. Drugs such as amiloride, cimetidine, trimethoprim, salicylate, triamterene, and spironolactone that inhibit this secretory function may increase S_{Cr} and decrease the CrCl estimate without affecting the GFR.[2-4] As GFR declines, there is a progressive increase in creatinine tubular secretion and a progressive disparity between GFR and CrCl. Thus, when the true GFR is around 100 ml/min, the CrCl overestimates the GFR by about 20%; for a GFR of 60 ml/min, the CrCl would overestimate by about 60%; and for a GFR of 20 ml/min, the CrCl would overestimate by 100% or more.[2-4]

Disease states affecting muscle mass similarly affect creatinine production and turnover; however, the 24-hr CrCl is less likely to be affected than estimates using patient demographics and S_{Cr} to estimate CrCl. Drugs and exogenous or endogenous compounds that interact with the laboratory assays for creatinine may also affect the estimates of CrCl. The following compounds may negatively or positively affect the creatinine concentration by interfering with creatinine assays (dependent on the assay system/instrument used):

Jaffe-based assays
    Acetoacetate
    Acetohexamide
    Bilirubin
    Cefoxitin, cephalothin
    Other cephalosporins (supratherapeutic levels)
    Furosemide (supratherapeutic levels)
    Lactulose
    Methyldopa infusions

Enzymatic assay systems
    Flucytosine
    Lidocaine

These compounds all have the potential to interfere with the S_{Cr} assays but the extent of interference is dependent on the given instrument used. If a patient has a potential for a creatinine–lab assay interaction, the clinician should check with the laboratory for the specific interference with the instrument used. Judicious timing of the drawing of blood for serum creatinine determination (at minimal interfering drug concentration) or using an alternative assay method may be advised.[2-4]

Formulas to estimate creatinine clearance in adults

    Collecting urine for 24 hr for a urine creatinine measurement is tedious and must be done accurately (i.e., no missed collections and accurate measurement of urine volume) to properly measure the CrCl. Because this is difficult and time consuming, formulas have been derived that use the serum creatinine and patient demographics to estimate GFR.

    The numerous equations for rapid estimation of CrCl published over the last 25 years generally produce similar values. Two well-validated, commonly used steady-state equations for *adult* patients are the Cockcroft and Gault equation and the Jelliffe equation.[4–7]

Cockcroft and Gault equation:

$$\text{CrCl (males)(ml/min)} = \frac{(140 - \text{age})(W)}{(72)(S_{Cr})}$$

$$\text{CrCl (females)} = \text{CrCl (males)} \times 0.85$$

where S_{Cr} is in milligrams per deciliter (mg/dl) and W is weight (kg). The International Systems conversion is:

$$\text{CL}_{Cr} \text{ (males)} = \frac{1.23 \cdot (140 - \text{age}) \times BW}{S_{Cr}}$$

$$\text{CL}_{Cr} \text{ (females)} = \frac{1.04 \cdot (140 - \text{age}) \times BW}{S_{Cr}}$$

where S_{Cr} is in micromoles per liter (µM) and BW is body weight (kg).

Jelliffe equation:

$$\text{CrCl (males)(ml/min)/1.73 m}^2 \text{ BSA} = \frac{98 - [0.8(\text{age} - 20)]}{S_{Cr}}$$

$$\text{CrCl (females)} = \text{CrCl (males)} \times 0.9$$

where BSA is body surface area.

Weight in the Cockcroft and Gault equation is preferably ideal body weight (IBW) or actual body weight (ABW) if it is less than IBW. However, there are many important considerations in these generalizations (see section on body weight). The original authors used ABW in developing their equation, but other researchers have examined the impact of obesity on predictability. IBW is estimated by the following:[8]

$$\text{IBW (males) (kg)} = 50 + (2.3)(H - 60)$$
$$\text{IBW (females) (kg)} = 45.5 + (2.3)(H - 60)$$

where H is height in inches, or,

$$IBW\ (males)\ (kg) = 50 + 0.9(H - 152)$$
$$IBW\ (females)\ (kg) = 45.5 + 0.9(H - 152)$$

where H is patient's height in centimeters (cm).

In the Jelliffe equation, the CrCl is normalized to body surface area (BSA) by dividing the patient's BSA (calculated as follows) by 1.73 and multiplying this factor times the result.[9] BSA may be determined from the following equation or by a nomogram based on a different equation (see appendix A).

$$BSA\ (m^2) = W^{0.5378} \times H^{0.3964} \times 0.024265$$

where W is weight (kg) and H is height (cm).

The Cockcroft and Gault and Jelliffe equations work reasonably well for most adults with S_{Cr} at steady state because they allow for declining muscle mass (and creatinine production) often associated with reduced weight and advancing age and are adjusted for the average smaller muscle mass of females. The Cockcroft and Gault equation is the most commonly used and recommended equation for CrCl estimation and is discussed in greater detail in the following sections. The Jelliffe equation is still used by some clinicians and is reasonably accurate for use when height and weight are not available in average size patients.[7] However, the accuracy of these equations in predicting CrCl is often lacking in patients with many disease states or conditions. These include the elderly, the malnourished, the obese, patients with amputations or spinal cord injuries, those with chronic renal insufficiency, those with liver disease, critically ill patients, and pediatric patients.[1-3, 10-28] Other, possibly more accurate equations and methods for rapid prediction of CrCl will continue to evolve as more patients and larger subgroups are studied.[10,29]

Adjustments in the weight and/or creatinine variables based on a patient's clinical condition are commonly made in the Cockcroft and Gault equation to improve predictive performance. The clinician should carefully assess the patient's clinical status and may modify these variables or use another more suitable equation or a timed CrCl measurement. In general, the following subgroup reviews pertain to adult patients. (See section on pediatrics for CrCl estimation in children.)

Body weight

Creatinine production is dependent on muscle mass and the use of IBW in the Cockcroft and Gault equation appears to produce reliable results in patients whose ABW is not far from IBW. For patients who are malnourished or cachectic with an ABW less than their IBW, the ABW should be used.[1-3,8,11] For adult patients less than 1.52 m (60 inches) tall, use of the lesser of ABW or IBW (males = 50 kg, females = 45.5 kg) has been proposed.[12]

Obesity (defined as > 20% over IBW) is another factor that affects the Cockcroft and Gault CrCl estimation. Obese patients appear to have a larger muscle mass than would be predicted when using height in the IBW equation. Using IBW is still preferable to using ABW; however, using an adjusted body weight (BW_{adj}) between IBW and ABW may be more accurate. Use of a factor of 40 or 20% of the difference (ABW − BW) has been proposed.[3,10,12]

$$BW_{adj} = IBW + 0.4 (ABW - IBW)$$
$$BW_{adj} = IBW + 0.2 (ABW - IBW)$$

The notion of "correct" weight to use in the prediction equations is an interesting one. As mentioned earlier, Cockcroft and Gault used ABW to develop the equation. Numerous authors have suggested the use of IBW or BW_{adj} for patients who weigh more than their IBW. Intuitively such approaches seem reasonable since creatinine is produced in muscle, not fat tissue. One suggestion that might help in determining a reasonable weight is to avoid use of only standards and to visually examine the patient. For example, a 1.8-m (5'11") body builder who weighs 100 kg (220 lb) would clearly be expected to produce more creatinine daily than a sedentary individual of the same height and weight. Both patients would be considered to have the same IBW and both are considered obese by definition (>20% above IBW). One might anticipate that the former patient should have creatinine clearance estimated using ABW, since the additional weight will be creatinine producing, while the latter would be best estimated using BW_{adj} (or even IBW if they were extremely sedentary with little additional muscle mass associated with the adiposity). Finally, it should be expected that the more the patient differs from the patients used in the studies to develop the equations, the greater the potential that predictions might not match actual measured CrCl.

Another method of CrCl estimation may have better predictive ability in the obese patient (Salazar–Corcoran equation) but may be a bit more complicated to use.[3,10,13]

$$\mathrm{CrCl~(males)} = \frac{(137 - \mathrm{age}) \times [(0.285 \times W) + (12.1 \times H^2)]}{(51 \times S_{Cr})}$$

$$\mathrm{CrCl~(females)} = \frac{(146 - \mathrm{age}) \times [(0.287 \times W) + (9.74 \times H^2)]}{(60 \times S_{Cr})}$$

where W is weight (kg), H is height (cm), and S_{Cr} is measured in milligrams per deciliter.

Low serum creatinine/elderly patients

It is common practice for clinicians to round measured S_{Cr} concentrations that are less than 0.8 or 0.9 mg/dl to a higher value in adult patients before using these equations. The S_{Cr} is inversely proportional to CrCl and using an unrealistically low S_{Cr} value in an elderly or other patient with significantly decreased muscle mass or creatinine production may overestimate the CrCl. The use of a value of 1 mg/dl as the lower limit of S_{Cr} in these equations has been popular with clinicians; however, underprediction of CrCl may occur and using 0.8 or 0.7 (or less) as the lower limit of S_{Cr} may be more appropriate.[10,14–17] Intuitively, it would seem to make sense that a patient's muscle mass would give some guide to how much "fudging" should be done in setting a lower limit of S_{Cr}. That is, in a patient with obviously limited muscle mass it might be more reasonable to adjust the S_{Cr} upward than in a patient with average muscle mass. Also, it seems reasonable to assume that the larger the degree of "fudging" of the S_{Cr} upward to some minimum value, the greater the likelihood of poor prediction. That is, changing a measured S_{Cr} from 0.3 to 0.7 might result in a poorer prediction of actual CrCl than changing from 0.6 to 0.7.

Amputations

Estimation of CrCl in patients with amputated limbs poses a dilemma for IBW calculation. A reasonable approach would be to determine the height-based IBW before the amputation, then subtract the percent of the missing limb based on data from a body segment percentage table.[18] The weight used would be the lesser of this adjusted IBW or the ABW. The average weight of body segments of a 68-kg (150-lb) man are: upper limb, 4.9%; entire lower limb, 15.6%; thigh, 9.7%; leg, 4.5%; foot, 1.4%. This method for IBW calculation in amputees has not been validated for accuracy.

Spinal cord injury

CrCl estimation in patients with spinal cord injury appears to be largely unpredictable because of the changes in muscle mass that occur over time after the injury. The 24-hr CrCl measurement should be used in these patients if accuracy is necessary.[19]

Chronic renal insufficiency

As already noted, with declining renal function, S_{Cr} may become a less accurate indicator of renal function because of the increasing percentage of tubular secretion of creatinine in relation to the total urinary excretion. That is, as renal function decreases, tubular secretion becomes a larger part of creatinine elimination. In addition, there appears to be an extrarenal route of creatinine elimination via the GI tract in uremic patients. These patients in general may have a poor dietary intake and reduced muscle mass.[2,10] Use of cimetidine (up to 1200 mg as a single dose) to inhibit tubular secretion of creatinine prior to urine collection or S_{Cr} measurement has been advocated to improve estimation of GFR.[20]

Dialysis

Estimating creatinine clearance in patients receiving dialysis is problematic and not recommended. A patient without functioning kidneys has no glomerular filtration. Thus, the S_{Cr} concentration becomes primarily a function of the dialysis procedure rather than the patient's kidney function. Because no urine output indicates no renal function, monitoring residual urine output gives some idea whether the patient's kidneys have any potential role in drug elimination.

Liver disease

Another dilemma is the estimation of renal function in patients with cirrhosis. Estimates of GFR using CrCl estimations (Cockcroft and Gault) and 24-hr CrCl measurements are unreliable as shown by inulin clearance tests (considered the gold standard for estimating GFR). These patients should have their drug therapy closely monitored. For drugs with a narrow therapeutic index, drug concentration monitoring is recommended whenever possible.[21-24]

Pediatrics

Creatinine clearance in children has been shown to accurately predict the GFR. Because a measured 24-hr CrCl is as difficult and time consuming as in adults, equations have been developed for rapid estimation based on a patient's height and weight. These estimates appear most accurate for patients of average weights for their size. The equations use S_{Cr} and height (body length) to estimate the normalized CrCl (as if BSA was 1.73 m²). The correlation of a child's muscle mass with their height helps factor in the relationship between muscle mass and creatinine production. However, these estimations may be less accurate for children who are significantly under- or overweight for their height and in the first week of life when the infant serum creatinine still reflects the maternal serum creatinine and renal function is immature.[26] The most commonly used equation for *children 1–18 years of age* is the Traub equation:[25]

$$\text{CrCl (ml/min/1.73 m}^2\text{ BSA)} = \frac{(0.48)(H)}{S_{Cr}}$$

For *neonates and infants less than 1 year of age*, the following equation has been used:[26]

$$\text{CrCl (ml/min/1.73 m}^2\text{ BSA)} = \frac{(0.45)(H)}{S_{Cr}}$$

where H is height (cm).

Both of these equations provide values that are automatically normalized to 1.73 m². To calculate the actual CrCl, this result is multiplied by the patient's BSA (calculated as follows) and divided by 1.73.[9]

$$\text{BSA (m}^2\text{)} = W^{0.5378} \times H^{0.3964} \times 0.024265$$

where W is weight (kg) and H is height (cm).

A nomogram to determine BSA in children based on a different equation appears in appendix B.

Patients with unstable renal function

The discussed equations for CrCl estimation are based on patients with stable renal function with S_{Cr} at steady state. In patients with changing renal function, S_{Cr} may not reflect the current function for several days. Using a value of S_{Cr} that is not at steady state to calculate a CrCl may significantly over- or underestimate the patient's renal function and result in inappropriate drug dosing.

Time to Steady-State Serum Creatinine Concentration

The time to a steady-state S_{Cr} value increases as the patient's renal function declines. The time to 95% of steady state has been estimated to be 0.92, 1.85, and 4.5 days as a patient's renal function declines to 50, 25, and 10% of normal, respectively. It is estimated that if the S_{Cr} changes by more than 0.2 mg/dl in 12 hr, steady state probably has not been reached.[27]

Determining a rough estimate of the half-life of creatinine in a specific adult patient may be made by assuming that the Cockcroft and Gault equation is accurate in estimating CrCl and that the patient's volume of distribution (V) of creatinine is approximately 0.6 L/kg[27,28] and doing the following calculations:

1. Estimate the patient's CrCl (ml/min) based on the Cockcroft and Gault equation.
2. Convert the patient's CrCl in milliliters per minute (ml/min) to liters per hour (L/hr) by multiplying by 0.06 (because of the following conversion):

$$\frac{60 \text{ min}}{1 \text{ hr}} \times \frac{1 \text{ L}}{1000 \text{ ml}} = 0.06 \text{ (units will cancel appropriately below)}$$

Thus, ml/min × 0.06 = L/hr

3. Use the relationship $CL = K \times V$ or $K = CL/V$ to calculate K, the elimination rate constant, where CL is the creatinine clearance in liters per hour (L/hr), and V is the volume of distribution of creatinine in liters (0.6 L/kg × IBW[27,28]).

4. Use $t\frac{1}{2} = 0.693/K$ to determine the half-life.
5. Approximately 4 times the half-life equals time to steady state.

Creatinine Clearance Estimation in Unstable Renal Function

Several equations for use in patients with unstable renal function are available and may be useful for initial drug dosing; however, estimating CrCl in a patient with changing renal function is problematic and drug concentration monitoring is recommended for drugs with a narrow therapeutic index.[1-3,27,28] For 24-hr CrCl measurements in patients with changing renal function, use the midpoint (12th hr) S_{Cr} or the average of the S_{Cr} at the beginning and the end of the 24-hr urine collection.[28] The following equation has been used to estimate CrCl in patients with unstable renal function:[30]

$$\text{CrCl (males)(ml/min)} = \frac{[293 - 2.03(\text{age})] \times 1.035 - 0.01685(S_{Cr1} + S_{Cr2})] + 49(S_{Cr1} - S_{Cr2})/\Delta t}{S_{Cr1} \times S_{Cr2}}$$

$$\text{CrCl (females)} = \text{CrCl (males)} \times 0.86$$

where Δt is the change in time in number of days between measurement of S_{Cr1} and S_{Cr2}.

References

1. Lam YW, Banerji S, Hatfield C, et al. Principles of drug administration in renal insufficiency. *Clin Pharmacokinet*. 1997; 32:30–57.
2. Duarte CG, Preuss HG. Assessment of renal function—glomerular and tubular. *Clin Lab Med*. 1993; 13(1):33–52.
3. Robert S, Zarowitz BJ. Is there a reliable index of glomerular filtration rate in critically ill patients? *DICP Ann Pharmacother*. 1991; 25:169–78.
4. Ducharme MP, Smythe M, Strohs G. Drug-induced alterations in serum creatinine concentrations. *Ann Pharmacother*. 1993; 27:622–33.
5. Cockcroft DW, Gault MH. Prediction of creatinine clearance from serum creatinine. *Nephron*. 1976; 16:31–41.
6. Lott RS, Hayton WL. Estimation of creatinine clearance from serum creatinine concentration—a review. *Drug Intell Clin Pharm*. 1978; 12:140–50.

7. Jelliffe RW. Creatinine clearance: a bedside estimate. *Ann Intern Med*. 1973; 79:604–5.
8. Devine BJ. Gentamicin therapy. *Drug Intell Clin Pharm*. 1974; 7:650–5.
9. Haycock GB, Schwartz GJ, Wisotsky DH. Geometric method for measuring body surface area: a height-weight formula validated in infants, children, and adults. *J Pediatr*. 1978; 93:62–6.
10. Spinler SA, Nawarskas JJ, Boyce EG, et al. Predictive performance of ten equations for estimating creatinine clearance in cardiac patients. Iohexol Cooperative Study Group. *Ann Pharmacother*. 1998; 32:1275–83.
11. Boyce EG, Dickerson RN, Cooney GF, et al. Creatinine clearance estimation in protein-malnourished patients. *Clin Pharm*. 1989; 8:721–6.
12. Sawyer WT, Canaday BR, Poe TE, et al. Variables affecting creatinine clearance prediction. *Am J Hosp Pharm*. 1983; 40:2175–80.
13. Salazar DE, Corcoran GB. Predicting creatinine clearance and renal drug clearance in obese patients from estimated fat-free body mass. *Am J Med*. 1988; 84:1053–60.
14. Reichley RM, Ritchie DJ, Bailey TC. Analysis of various creatinine clearance formulas in predicting gentamicin elimination in patients with low serum creatinine. *Pharmacother*. 1995; 15:625–30.
15. Smythe M, Hoffman J, Kizy K, et al. Estimating creatinine clearance in elderly patients with low serum creatinine concentrations. *Am J Hosp Pharm*. 1994; 51:198–204.
16. O'Connell MB, Dwinell AM, Bannick-Mohrland SD. Predictive performance of equations to estimate creatinine clearance in hospitalized elderly patients. *Ann Pharmacother*. 1992; 26:627–35.
17. Bertino JS Jr. Measured versus estimated creatinine clearance in patients with low serum creatinine values. *Ann Pharmacother*. 1993; 27:1439–42.
18. Brunnstrom S. Clinical kinesiology. 4th ed. Philadelphia, PA: F.A. Davis Co; 1983:56.
19. Mohler JL, Ellison MF, Flanigan RC. Creatinine clearance prediction in spinal cord injury patients: comparison of 6 prediction equations. *J Urol*. 1988; 139:706–9.
20. Walser M. Assessing renal function from creatinine measurements in adults with chronic renal failure. *Am J Kidney Dis*. 1998; 32:23–31.
21. DeSanto NG, Anastasio P, Loguercio C, et al. Creatinine clearance: an inadequate marker of renal filtration in patients with early posthepatitic cirrhosis (Child A) without fluid retention and muscle wasting. *Nephron*. 1995; 70:421–4.
22. Papadakis MA, Arieff AI. Unpredictability of clinical evaluation of renal function in cirrhosis. *Am J Med*. 1987; 82:945–52.
23. Hull JH, Hak LJ, Koch GG, et al. Influence of range of renal function and liver disease on predictability of creatinine clearance. *Clin Pharmacol Ther*. 1981; 29:516–21.
24. Pachorek RE, Wood F. Vancomycin half-life in a patient with hepatic and renal dysfunction. *Clin Pharm*. 1991; 10:297–300.
25. Traub SL, Johnson CE. Comparison of methods of estimating creatinine clearance in children. *Am J Hosp Pharm*. 1980; 37:195–201.

26. Schwartz GJ, Feld LG, Langford DJ. A simple estimate of glomerular filtration rate in full-term infants during the first year of life. *J Pediatr*. 1984; 104:849–54.

27. Winter ME. Creatinine clearance. In: Winter ME. Basic Clinical Pharmacokinetics, 3rd ed. Vancouver, WA: Applied Therapeutics; 1994:93–103.

28. Chow MS, Schweizer R. Estimation of renal creatinine clearance in patients with unstable serum creatinine concentrations: comparison of multiple methods. *Drug Intell Clin Pharm*. 1985; 19:385–90.

29. Levey AS, Bosch JP, Lewis JB, et al. A more accurate method to estimate glomerular filtration rate from serum creatinine: a new prediction equation. *Ann Intern Med*. 1999; 130:461–70.

30. Brater DC. Drug use in renal disease. Balgowlah, Australia: ADIS Health Science Press; 1983:22–56.

Chapter 2
James P. McCormack & Glen Brown

Rational Use of Drug Concentration Measurements

For the vast majority of medications, drug concentration monitoring is unnecessary. The value of such monitoring in achieving desired therapeutic outcomes and patient well-being for those drugs where concentration monitoring is generally considered useful is often debated. Some suggest that concentration monitoring is excessive and, when concentrations are measured, they are frequently used inappropriately. Others consider it a routine part of outcome assessment for a number of important drugs with narrow therapeutic ranges. Clinicians who use drug concentration monitoring should always ask themselves if the pharmacodynamics (potential efficacy or toxicity) of a particular drug are better predicted by measuring drug concentrations or evaluating the clinical response. They must also carefully determine whether a patient is responding appropriately and without toxicity using pharmacodynamic assessment (i.e., establish goals of therapy and monitor whether or not they are achieved) even when drug concentrations are used as an adjunct to regimen evaluation.

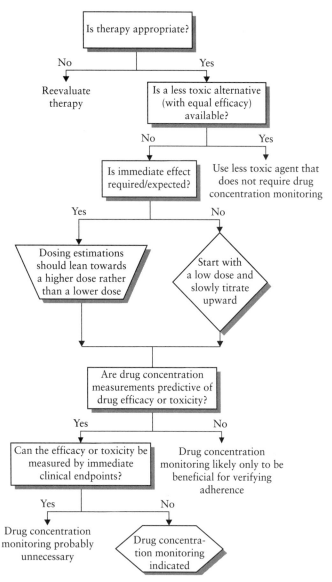

FIGURE 1. Decision-making process for using drug concentration measurements.

For drugs where concentration monitoring is fairly routine, but the desired effect of the drug can be easily and quickly measured clinically—the value of measuring its concentration is limited or even potentially harmful if one spends time measuring concentrations at the expense of proper clinical assessment. Where the signs and symptoms of benefit and toxicity can be assessed easily and quickly (within hours or in some case days), appropriate dosage adjustments can usually be based on the clinical response of the patient rather than on drug concentrations. When drug concentration monitoring adds to the predictability of response over monitoring the patient clinically, a number of key issues should be considered before ordering a drug concentration measurement. Figure 1 is a graphic representation of the decision-making process involved in considering those issues.

Evaluating the Need for a Drug Concentration Measurement

Drug selection

Before ever considering the need for drug concentration monitoring, the appropriateness of the selected drug for obtaining the desired outcome in the specific patient should be determined. The clinician should ensure that there is reasonable scientific evidence suggesting that the selected medication will be effective in the patient. Next, the clinician should determine if the drug selected is the drug-of-choice or whether there are potentially equally effective, less toxic, and less expensive alternatives that should be considered (e.g., cephalosporins instead of aminoglycosides for nonlife-threatening infections; valproic acid instead of phenytoin for certain types of epilepsy). After this important assessment, the need for concentration monitoring as an adjunct to overall outcome monitoring can be considered.

Efficacy issues

When therapeutic and toxic end points cannot be readily and quickly determined clinically, drug concentration measurements may be useful if they are predictive of therapeutic or toxic effect. For instance, in a patient started on an antiepileptic medication for relatively infrequent (every 2–3 months) seizures, improved seizure control may not become apparent for several weeks or even months. Ensuring that the patient's concentrations are in the generally accepted population therapeutic range may be the only guide to determine an appropriate dose and schedule.

Clinicians should always ask themselves whether pharmacodynamic effects are better predicted by the population-based "therapeutic range" or by the individual clinical response. If the clinically important event occurs infrequently (e.g., seizures or arrhythmias) or if the beneficial effect of the drug may be delayed (e.g., resolution of depression), the drug concentration found to be effective in similar patients can be used as an initial goal. However, population-based therapeutic ranges can be weak predictors of therapeutic success because the concentration-effect relationship is variable between individuals. Thus, dosage adjustments may still be needed based on the clinical response.

For many patients, there likely exists a specific threshold concentration (assuming the drug will be effective at some point) above which a desired effect or toxicities can be seen. Some clinicians have recommended measuring the drug concentration associated with therapeutic success to serve as a benchmark for subsequent therapy and that subsequent failure of therapy could be evaluated based on the maintenance of drug concentrations above this established benchmark. This approach assumes that the threshold for efficacy does not change with time. Because physiologic and pathophysiologic conditions can change with time, this assumption may not be valid in all cases.

Toxicity issues

When patients exhibit signs or symptoms of toxicity, the practitioner should first determine if the dosage could be decreased empirically without loss of benefit. If the patient is at risk for toxicity or develops toxicity that is likely caused by the drug, the dose should be empirically decreased or the drug stopped. If this cannot be done because of concerns over the loss of therapeutic benefit, a drug concentration measurement may help to determine if the drug is the likely cause. This situation is only appropriate if the drug concentrations have been shown to predict toxicity.

Drug concentration measurements may also be useful in patients who develop dysfunction in the primary organ of clearance for the drug (e.g., liver or kidney) or in whom an interacting drug was started after the patient was stabilized on the initial drug. Measurements are not required if empiric reduction or increase in the drug dosage (depending on whether the interaction increases or decreases drug concentrations) is possible.

Adherence issues

Lack of adherence by patients to medication regimens is a frequently occurring problem. When a patient is suspected of not adhering to his or her medication regimen, drug concentration monitoring may be a useful tool, along with evaluation of pharmacy records or the medication administration record, to help establish whether or not it is the case.

Approaches to Dosing with Limited Need for Drug Concentration Measurements

Immediate effect required or expected

If a patient requires treatment for an immediate life-threatening process, the initial dosage should be selected based on avoidance of underdosing, not overdosing. The largest dose usually associated with efficacy and acceptable toxicities should be chosen to ensure the greatest chance of a positive outcome. When concentrations are not measured, concern for toxicity, if it occurs acutely, may be assessed clinically (if possible) and evaluated on the basis of the benefits versus risks of continued therapy at the selected dosage.

For drugs such as the aminoglycosides, vancomycin, and phenytoin that may be used for life-threatening illness, severe toxicity, if it occurs, usually does not develop until after at least a few days of therapy (e.g., renal/ototoxicity from aminoglycosides/vancomycin) or the acute toxicities are minor (nystagmus, or ataxia with phenytoin). The acute treatment of life-threatening infections with aminoglycosides or vancomycin should utilize dosages known to produce effective clinical results, while concerns over possible toxicity should be relevant but secondary. The initial dosage selected for the life-threatening infection does not have to be the dosage used for continued therapy. Dosage adjustment can be guided by drug concentration measurements, when appropriate, based on all other considerations.

Immediate effect not required or expected

For the vast majority of conditions treated with medications, an immediate response is not needed. In these cases the dosing can be approached in one of two ways.

Titrating the dose up

In conditions that do not require an immediate response, it may be possible to gradually titrate the dose up to the usual recommended starting dose with the understanding that the medicines that can extend or improve a patient's quality of life can also produce a number of side effects. To avoid the chance of adverse effects from the onset and to end up treating the patient with the lowest effective dose, it is reasonable to consider starting off with the smallest available dose and titrating the dose upward as needed. This dose may be as little as ¼ to ½ of the recommended starting dose in the product monographs (which might require cutting tablets in pieces, a cost-saving approach in many cases). This dose titration approach may require more time for the clinician to monitor patient outcomes as well as more time for clinician-patient discussion, as the patient often needs to be made aware of how to monitor efficacy and toxicity. Patients should be told that the dose titration process takes time and that an immediate effect is not necessarily expected, nor is it necessary, based on selection of this approach. The patient should be made to understand that the time spent in determining the appropriate dose may save him or her from unnecessary adverse effects and may reduce drug product expense.

Taking this approach may be justified from the perspective that many clinical trials begin with fairly aggressive doses to establish efficacy. Studies are not conducted on lower doses until after the product has been on the market for a considerable length of time.

Titrating the dose down

A second approach that may be used to determine the lowest effective dose is to begin therapy with the product monograph recommended dose (empirically adjusted on the basis of kidney and liver function), assess response, and gradually reduce the dose according to the response of the patient (weighing beneficial and toxic effects). The advantage of this approach is that an effect will likely be seen more quickly than by titrating upward. Titrating down may not lead to finding the lowest effective dose because clinicians and patients may be unwilling to decrease the dose once benefits are being achieved. However, it is important to remember that higher than necessary doses increase the chance of adverse effects, may increase the frequency of dosing and thereby compromise adherence, and usually increase the cost of therapy. Even in the face of drug efficacy without signs of toxicity, there may be value in tapering to the lowest effective dose. Sometimes this turns out to be no drug at all. Such an outcome may be the result of incorrect diagnosis, fluctuating disease state, or effective nondrug therapy such as lifestyle changes.

This approach applies to many medical conditions for which clinical end points are frequent and easily measurable (e.g., asthma and hypertension). However, when the clinical end points are infrequent (e.g., seizures) or life threatening (e.g., arrhythmias), this approach may be of less value.

Conclusion

Drug concentration monitoring should be considered as a tool to supplement clinical assessment of patient response. Consideration of appropriate drug selection and dosage along with the clinical monitoring of response are the most crucial components of pharmacotherapy.

Chapter 3
John E. Murphy

Aminoglycosides
(AHFS 8:12.02)

Aminoglycoside antibiotics have been available for the treatment of infections for more than 50 years. Agents currently available or in clinical trials include amikacin, arbekacin, dibekacin, gentamicin, isepamicin, kanamycin, neomycin, netilmicin, sisomicin, spectinomycin, streptomycin, trospectomycin, and tobramycin. Usage and pharmacokinetic monitoring have generally been focused on amikacin, gentamicin, and tobramycin which are therefore emphasized in this chapter. Netilmicin is also discussed briefly.

Usual Dosage Range in Absence of Clearance-Altering Factors

Aminoglycoside dosage regimens vary widely because of interpatient (and occasionally intrapatient) variation in pharmacokinetics. Average gentamicin and tobramycin doses of 80 mg/8 hr produce low peak concentrations in many patients.[1,2] Dosing schedules where the entire daily dose is given at one time or a large dose is given every 24–48 hr (or even at longer intervals) are used more frequently now and are generally considered at least equally effective to traditional dosing as well as less toxic when used appropriately. This large dose-extended interval (LDEI) dosing approach is the standard method for many patients and further study should focus on the situations where traditional (every 8–12 hr) dosing might be more beneficial. A consensus on who should *not be candidates* is needed for LDEI.[3] At this time, LDEI is not generally recommended for patients who are pregnant or those with renal failure, osteomyelitis, meningitis, endocarditis, or extensive burns.

Since the kidneys eliminate aminoglycosides, decreased renal function affects the dosage interval used, but it has less effect on the size of individual doses.

Loading dose

The following traditional loading doses are for gentamicin and tobramycin. Amikacin and netilmicin doses are approximately 3–4 and 1.3 times these amounts, respectively. Loading doses are not administered in the LDEI approach since it is generally expected (and likely should be ensured) that the concentration reaches zero before the next dose is given. No accumulation therefore occurs, negating the need for a loading dose.

Age	Traditional Loading Dose, mg/kg
Neonates (≤4 weeks)[4–6]	2.5–4
Infants (>4 weeks–1 year)[5]	2.5–3
Children (>1–≤13 years)[7]	2–2.5
Adolescents (>13 years), adults, and geriatrics[7,8]	1.5–2

In neonates, a first dose of 2.5 mg/kg generally produces a peak of less than 6 mg/L. The therapeutic implications of a low first-dose peak in this population, particularly early in life for "presumed" infections, are not clearly established. In adults, treatment failures may occur secondary to a low first-dose peak. Generally speaking, there is minimal accumulation with traditional aminoglycoside dosing regimes due to the use of intervals of three or more times the half-life. Thus, the usual reason for loading doses—rapid achievement of steady-state concentrations in situations where accumulation is extensive—does not hold. Rather, loading doses are given to ensure achievement of a higher first-dose peak concentration to enhance the potential for therapeutic success due to the concentration-dependent killing of organisms by aminoglycosides.

Maintenance dose

The following traditional and LDEI maintenance doses are for gentamicin and tobramycin. (Amikacin and netilmicin doses are approximately 3–4 and 1.3 times these amounts, respectively.)

Age	Traditional Dosage	LDEI Dosage
Neonates (≤4 weeks)	2–2.5 mg/kg/12–24 hr	3.5–5 mg/kg/24–48 hr[a]
Infants (>4 weeks–1 year)	2–2.5 mg/kg/8–12 hr	4–5 mg/kg/24–48 hr
Children (>1–≤13 years)	2–2.5 mg/kg/8 hr	4–7.5 mg/kg/24–48 hr[b]
Adolescents (>13–≤18 years)	1.5–2.5 mg/kg/8 hr	4–7.5 mg/kg/24–48 hr[b]
Adults (>18–≤60 years)	1–1.7 mg/kg/8 hr[c]	3.5–7 mg/kg/24–48 hr[b]
Younger geriatrics (>60–≤75 years)	1–1.7 mg/kg/8–12 hr	4–5 mg/kg/24–48 hr
Older geriatrics (>75 years)	1–1.7 mg/kg/12–24 hr	4–5 mg/kg/24–48 hr[d]

[a]Data extrapolated from one study of neonates 24–42 weeks gestation given gentamicin indicated that 4 mg/kg/24 hr resulted in 13% with troughs ≥2 mg/L [primarily (10%) those with gestational ages ≤36 weeks] and 30% with troughs of 1–<2 mg/L. A dose of 4 mg/kg/36 hr led to no troughs above 2 mg/L, only 5% with troughs ≥ 1 mg/L, and 75% with troughs <0.5 mg/L. With 4 mg/kg every 48 hr all but 5% had troughs <0.5 mg/L.[9]
[b]15 mg/kg of tobramycin[10,11] and 35 mg/kg of amikacin[12] have been used in patients with cystic fibrosis.
[c]Every 8 or 12 hr initially for amikacin and netilmicin.
[d]Although larger doses have been used, reduced renal function with aging and the potential for therapy with other toxins should probably lead to a more conservative approach.[13,14]

For LDEI, amikacin doses have tended to be 15 mg/kg for adults and 20 mg/kg in neonates. Uncomplicated urinary tract infections may respond to lower doses. Reduced renal function necessitates increases in the dosing interval, in some cases beyond the usual recommendation given. Some clinicians use the higher end of the range for more severe infections and vice versa. However, others use target concentrations or the usual averages.

The average *traditional* doses frequently produce concentrations outside of the accepted traditional therapeutic range.[1,2,15–17] In adults and geriatrics, 1-mg/kg doses often result in steady-state peaks of less than 6 mg/L. Use of larger doses reduces the incidence of low peaks but can also increase the incidence of elevated troughs if intervals are not simultaneously lengthened. Individualized dosing using Sawchuk–Zaske[18] or Bayesian dosing methods produce desired concentrations more reliably.[19]

LDEI dosing initially was not used in certain populations (ascites, total body surface area burns >20%, pregnancy, enterococcal endocarditis, end-stage renal disease including dialysis, granulocytopenia, or cystic fibrosis).[20,21] Increasingly, studies are examining its safety and efficacy in more patient types.[12–14, 22–27] However, several populations are still not routinely recommended to receive this dosing. These include endocarditis, pregnancy, burns, renal failure, meningitis, and osteomyelitis.[3] A simulation study suggested that many burn patients are not candidates for once-daily LDEI because of pronounced variability in the length of the aminoglycoside free period (i.e., the time when concentrations are essentially zero). The authors suggested monitoring aminoglycoside concentrations if LDEI is used in burn patients to ensure that the aminoglycoside free period is not extensive.[28]

For newborns when traditional doses of 2.5 mg/kg are used, dosing intervals may be based on birth weight: 1000 g or less, interval of 24 hr; 1001–2000 g, interval of 18 hr; and over 2000 g, initial interval of 12 hr.[29] Another approach uses 2.5 mg/kg with intervals of 24 hr if the newborn is ≤34 weeks of gestation and <1000 g, 18 hr if ≤34 weeks of gestation and >1000 g, and 12 hr if ≥35 weeks of gestation.[6]

Dosing interval determination–traditional dosing

The dosing interval should be approximately two to three times the half-life (see half-life and time to steady state section). Obviously, this value must be rounded off to a logical time (e.g., 6, 8, 12, 16, 18, 24, 36, or 48 hr). Clinicians generally do not use less than 8-hr dosing intervals for aminoglycosides, even in patients with excellent elimination, although some have used 6-hr intervals in patients with very high clearance (e.g., burn patients).[18]

If a calculated interval is rounded down to less than two times the half-life, the trough and peak will be slightly higher than if the interval is rounded up (i.e., if an interval greater than two times the half-life is chosen, the trough and peak will be slightly lower than would occur with the shorter interval). Intervals such as 16, 18, and 36 hr can cause confusion in scheduling and the correctness of dosing times should be verified when these schedules are ordered.[30]

Dosing and dosing intervals–(LDEI) dosing

There are essentially four recommended approaches to LDEI dosing.

1. The first, and most common in studies, is to give the usual total daily dose (e.g., 80 mg or 1.5 mg/kg/8 hr for gentamicin and tobramycin) as a single dose once daily (e.g., 240 mg or 4.5 mg/kg/24 hr) and perhaps adjust the dose or interval based on measured concentrations.[31]
2. The second approach is to give a large dose (e.g., 7 mg/kg of gentamicin or tobramycin) designed to produce a certain peak to minimum inhibitory concentration (MIC) ratio (e.g., 10:1) or simply a high concentration. The initial dosing interval is then determined based on the

patient's estimated or actual renal function (either by using CrCl for adults and children or by gestational age in neonates) and can be 24, 36, or 48 hr or, in some protocols, even longer. In some cases the interval is adjusted based on measured concentrations.
3. The third approach is to adjust the LDEI dose that would be used in patients with normal renal function downward based on estimated or actual CrCl.
4. The fourth approach is individualized dosing that targets desired peak and trough concentrations (similar to traditional approaches except that peaks are higher and troughs lower).

For *adults*, there are many examples of the first approach (i.e., the total daily dose given as a single dose) in the literature.[31] Studies of these methods generally show equal efficacy and reduced toxicity to multiple daily dosing. In some cases a trough concentration might be monitored and the interval extended if not below 2 mg/L. Another suggested method simply decreases the starting dose by half if the trough is above 1 mg/L.[32]

The authors of the "Hartford" method (an example of the second approach) suggest the initial use of 7 mg/kg of gentamicin or tobramycin (or 15 mg/kg of amikacin) given every 24 hr if CrCl is ≥60 ml/min, every 36 hr if CrCl is 40–59 ml/min, and every 48 hr if CrCl is 20–39 ml/min.[20] The dosing weight is the patient's actual weight unless >20% above IBW (ABW/IBW ratio is >1.2) where the weight would be determined as in step 4 in the section on volume of distribution. In 2184 patients treated with this approach, 77% were dosed every 24 hr, 15% every 36 hr, 6% every 48 hr, and 2% >48 hr.[20] This method has been examined in a number of studies. The monitoring for this approach is described in the section on monitoring aminoglycoside patients.

Two examples of the third approach—keeping the dosing once daily and simply adjusting the dose downward based on renal function—are shown here:

CrCl, ml/min, estimated	Example I[33] Dose, mg/kg[a]	Example II[34] Dose, mg/kg[b]
≥80	5.1	4.0
61–80	3.9	3.25
51–60	3.6	3.25
30–50	3.0	2.5
<30	Not used	2.0

[a]*Doses are based on ABW unless ABW/IBW ratio is ≥1.35, then an adjusted body weight (BW_{adj}) is used (see volume of distribution section for determination of BW_{adj}).*
[b]*Doses based on ABW.*

An example of the fourth approach—individualized dosing—is found in a study by Rybak and colleagues.[35] Target peak concentrations were 16–20 mg/L for gentamicin and tobramycin for patients with respiratory infections (60–80 mg/L for amikacin) and 10–12 mg/L for patients with other infections (40–60 mg/L for amikacin). Target trough concentrations were <1 mg/L.

For *neonates*, pharmacokinetic data generated from studies of gentamicin and tobramycin dosing in more than 600 neonates were used to generate[36] and confirm[9] the following LDEI dosing recommendations. A dose of 4 mg/kg is given every 48 hr for gestational age <32 weeks; every 36 hr for gestational age of 32–37 weeks; and every 24 hr for gestational age >37 weeks.

These recommendations were extrapolated from the two studies to produce peaks greater than 5 mg/L in more than 96% of the neonates. Troughs above 2 mg/L would be very rare (<2%) and less than 1 mg/L in the great majority (more than 85%). These results and the patient outcome from the different dosing approaches have not been confirmed prospectively.

Dosage Form Availability[7]

Pharmacokinetic monitoring of the aminoglycosides is generally reserved for intramuscular and intravenous dosage forms. Although these drugs are distributed as the sulfate salts, the manufacturers express the doses in terms of drug equivalence; thus, $S = 1$ for calculations.

The injectable forms used in irrigations have resulted in nephrotoxicity and ototoxicity. Size of dose used, site, contact time, and degree of denuding present are all factors that affect the amount absorbed. Caution should be exercised.

Topical dosage forms (creams, ointments, and solutions) of gentamicin and tobramycin do not appear to require pharmacokinetic monitoring, although toxicity has been reported.

Inhalation dosing of aminoglycosides, particularly tobramycin, is used in patients with cystic fibrosis. Studies have shown differences in delivery and bioavailability depending on the devices and concentrations used.[37-39]

Since gentamicin, tobramycin, and amikacin are available in different concentrations, care must be taken to avoid dosing confusion. Neonates have received overdoses when the dose volume for the 10–mg/ml dosage form was inadvertently used with a 40-mg/ml vial.[40]

Drug	Dosage Form	Product
Amikacin	Intravenous and intramuscular injection: 50, 62.5, and 250 mg/ml	Amikin Pediatric
Gentamicin	Intravenous and intramuscular Injection: 10 mg/ml	Garamycin Pediatric
	40 mg/ml	
	Intrathecal injection: 2 mg/ml	Garamycin
	Premixed in normal saline (NS): 40, 60, 70, 80, and 100 mg in 50 ml 60, 80, 90, and 100 mg in 100 ml	

Netilmicin	Intravenous and intramuscular injection: 100 mg/ml	Netromycin
Tobramycin	Intravenous and intramuscular injection: 10 and 40 mg/ml	Nebcin Pediatric
	Premixed in normal saline: 60 and 80 mg in 50 ml 80 mg in 100 ml	
	Powder for injection: 60 and 80 mg and 1.2 g	Nebcin

For intramuscular injection of amikacin, gentamicin, and tobramycin, the most concentrated forms are recommended. Intravenous bolus and short, intravenous infusions (0.5–1 hr) yield pharmacokinetic profiles similar to intramuscular administration.[41]

Bioavailability (F) of Dosage Forms

Dosage Form	Bioavailability Comments
Intravenous	100%
Intramuscular[7,42,43]	Assumed complete (100%), although absorption rate may vary with diminished muscle mass and poor circulation (peak at 30–90 min after dosing)
Oral[44]	≤5% with absorption usually being ≤1%; diseases of the bowel (e.g., ulcers and inflammatory bowel disease) may lead to enhanced absorption
Intraperitoneal[45,46]	55% with absorption being variable; duration of exposure and inflamed peritoneum may affect bioavailability
Intrathecal	Assumed complete (100%); passes into systemic circulation
Irrigations[7]	Significant with absorption dependent on site and degree of denuding present (e.g., burns, wounds, and ulcers)

Inhalations[36,47,48]	Negligible, but may lead to absorption of 30% of a dose (concentrations can average 1 mg/L)
Polymethylmeth-acrylate beads[49] and collagen-gentamicin implants[50]	High concentration at site with minimal effect on serum/plasma concentration
Hypodermoclysis[51]	100% with time to peak approximately 1.5 hr, peak decreased

General Pharmacokinetic Information

Protein binding

Amikacin, gentamicin, netilmicin, and tobramycin are essentially unbound to plasma proteins.

Clearance (CL)

The aminoglycosides are eliminated by glomerular filtration in the kidney. Studies indicating some nonrenal elimination were affected by tissue accumulation of drug and described the pharmacokinetics assuming one-compartment distribution. Aminoglycoside clearance correlates reasonably well with glomerular filtration rate.

Numerous studies have evaluated population values and dosage prediction techniques for the aminoglycosides. One review concluded that individualized dosing using Sawchuk–Zaske techniques or Bayesian analysis after monitoring of drug concentrations (particularly with parameters based on the patient population being monitored) provided the best predictive performance.[19]

The following clearance values are based on the approximate average renal function for each age group. Reduced renal function in any age group results in decreased clearance.

In newborns, renal function increases rapidly; the glomerular filtration rate tends to double during the first 14 days of life. In premature or low birth weight infants, clearance is decreased compared to normal gestation and weight newborns. For this group, the value given minus one standard deviation may be used initially.

Age	Clearance (mean ± SD)[a]
Neonates (≤4 weeks)[4,9,52,53]	0.05 ± 0.01 L/hr/kg
Infants (>4 weeks–1 year)[54]	0.10 ± 0.05 L/hr/kg
Children (>1–≤13 years)[54–58]	0.13 ± 0.03 L/hr/kg
Adolescents (>13–≤18 years)[55–58]	0.11 ± 0.03 L/hr/kg
Adults (>18–≤60 years)[59]	0.08 ± 0.03 L/hr/kg
Geriatrics (>60 years)[59,60]	0.06 ± 0.03 L/hr/kg

[a]*These values have been rounded off and approximate those found in the original studies.*

Many methods for estimating the clearance of aminoglycosides have been evaluated. They relate the aminoglycoside clearance (CL_{ag}) to the patient's estimated or actual creatinine clearance (CrCl) and utilize one-compartment approaches to dosing.[19] Two problems that can occur in comparing studies of the prediction of CL_{ag} are the different CrCl prediction methods used and the weight used to estimate CrCl in the methods.

The following equation has been used to relate CL_{ag} to CrCl:[7,61]

$$CL_{ag} = CrCl$$

Volume of Distribution (V)

The aminoglycosides demonstrate three-compartment distribution when given by intravenous bolus.[44] The central compartment volume is quite small (approximately one-third to one-half of the volumes used for general dosing with one-compartment approaches). The first distribution phase, during the first hour, is generally not detected due to its masking by the infusion time (0.5–1 hr) and peak-sampling schedule (0.5 hr after a 0.5-hr infusion, at the end of a 1-hr infusion, or 0.5–1 hr after intravenous bolus).

The late distribution phase involves slow distribution into and redistribution from tissues. This phase has been associated with nephrotoxicity. The final phase half-life, approximately 150 hr, is generally not detected without urine collection and analysis during therapy and for a week or more after therapy is completed.

The volume of distribution values for the aminoglycosides are based on population studies. Although some researchers have found subtle differences among the aminoglycosides, the same volume estimate is suggested for each drug. Amikacin, gentamicin, netilmicin, and tobramycin are generally considered to distribute into the extracellular fluid volume. Dehydration, overhydration, and ascites affect the volume of distribution. Seriously ill adult patients are reported to have larger volumes of distribution per body weight.

Age	Volume (mean ± SD)[a,b]
Neonates (≤4 weeks)[6,9,53,62,63]	0.45 ± 0.1 L/kg
Infants (>4 weeks–1 year)[64]	0.40 ± 0.1 L/kg
Children (>1–≤13 years)[55–56]	0.35 ± 0.15 L/kg
Adolescents (>13–≤18 years)[55–56]	0.30 ± 0.1 L/kg
Adults (>18 years) and geriatrics[14, 65–67]	0.30 ± 0.13 L/kg[c]

[a]*Due to the variability in the ages studied, some of these age ranges and values are extrapolated or rounded off from those given in the original studies.*
[b]*Studies are inconsistent in the reporting of volume of distribution relative to body weight. Volume may be related to actual, ideal, or an adjusted "dosing" weight. Many studies have patients both above and below ideal weight. See Steps 5 and 6 to estimate a patient's volume of distribution.*
[c]*A value of 0.25 L/kg has been suggested frequently in the past. Many studies are now finding larger volumes, perhaps due to differences in assays, collection times, or modeling.[68] This larger volume is now suggested and believed to be reasonable because larger doses and higher peaks appear to be safe and effective while lower peaks may pose a danger of lack of efficacy.*

Premature neonates tend to have larger volumes of distribution[5,6] (nearer 0.50–0.55 L/kg), while full-term neonates tend to have smaller values (nearer 0.40–0.45 L/kg).[4,5,9]

To determine the volume of distribution for neonates and infants, actual body weight (ABW) should be used. For children and adolescents, ideal body weight (IBW) is suggested, although one study found that an adjusted body weight (BW_{adj}) might need to be used in obese children[69] (see Step 4).

For adults and geriatrics (and perhaps older children), the following algorithm should be followed to determine dosing weight and appropriate population volume of distribution. To determine dosing weight:

Step 1. Patient's ABW in kilograms is determined.

Step 2. Patient's IBW in kilograms is determined (see introduction).

Step 3. ABW is compared to IBW:

(a) For a patient whose ABW/IBW ratio is 0.9–<1.2, use of the ABW is suggested (Step 4 is not used).

(b) For a patient whose ABW/IBW ratio is ≥1.2, Step 4 is followed.

(c) For a patient whose ABW/IBW ratio is >0.75–<0.9, IBW is used[70] (Step 4 is not used).

(d) For a patient whose ABW/IBW ratio is <0.75 (emaciated), the ABW is multiplied by 1.13 (Step 4 is not used).[66]

Step 4. Adjusted body weight (BW_{adj}) is determined for obese patients:[66,71]

$$BW_{adj} (kg) = IBW + 0.4 (ABW - IBW)$$

And then to estimate volume (in liters):

Step 5. The volume of distribution is determined for all patients *except* emaciated and severely ill or trauma patients using:

$$V = 0.30 \text{ L/kg} \times \text{dosing weight (kg)}$$

Step 6. The volume of distribution is determined for emaciated, severely ill, and trauma patients:[66,72–75]

$V = 0.35$ L/kg × dosing weight (kg) (emaciated patients)

$V = 0.40$ L/kg × dosing weight (kg) [severely ill and trauma patients (some studies show even larger V in this group)]

Patients who are dehydrated may have smaller actual volumes while edematous patients may have larger volumes than predicted. The values used in these equations for volumes approximate those in the original studies but are rounded off.

Half-Life and Time to Steady State

The following half-lives are associated with one-compartment dosing. The half-life of aminoglycosides may increase by 10–20% as therapy continues, although in newborns it may decrease due to the natural rapid maturation of renal function in the first few weeks of life.

Age or Condition	Half-Life (mean ± SD)	Time to Steady State
Neonates (≤4 weeks)[9,29,44,53]	6 ± 2 hr	20–40 hr
Infants (>4 weeks–1 year)[a,64]	4 ± 1 hr	15–25 hr
Children (>1–≤13 years)[a,55,57,58,76]	1.5 ± 1 hr	3–12 hr
Adolescents (>13–≤18 years)[57,58,77]	1.5 ± 1 hr	3–12 hr
Adults (>18–≤60 years)[59]	2 ± 1 hr	5–15 hr
Younger geriatrics (>60–≤75 years)[59]	3.5 ± 2 hr	8–27 hr
Older geriatrics (>75 years)[59,60]	4 ± 2 hr	10–30 hr
Renal failure[78]	40–60 hr	8–12 days
During peritoneal dialysis[79,80]	10–20 hr	
During hemodialysis[79,80]	5–8 hr	

[a] *In infants and children, half-life tends to decrease with advancing age. Premature neonates would tend to have $t\frac{1}{2}$ = mean + 1 SD (8 hr).*[9]

These times to steady state (approximately five half-lives ± 1 SD) occur without a loading dose. With an appropriate loading dose, steady state may be achieved immediately. With an inappropriate loading dose (under- or overloading), the time to reach steady state is similar to that achieved when no loading dose is given, although the concentration difference may be less.

During peritoneal dialysis, efficiency can be affected by various solutes in the dialysis solution and by the integrity of the peritoneal membrane. During hemodialysis, drug removal is affected by numerous variables including dialysate and blood flow rates, efficiency of dialyzer, positive and negative pressures, and length of dialysis.

Aminoglycoside concentrations demonstrate a rebound phenomenon after hemodialysis; concentrations increase due to redistribution from tissue. Therefore, sampling should be delayed approximately 2 hr after dialysis to improve the accuracy of dosing and avoid the possibility of dosing errors based on this phenomenon.[78]

Many methods for estimating the half-life of aminoglycosides have been evaluated. There are two main approaches. Both relate the patient's actual or estimated creatinine clearance (CrCl) to the parameter being considered [e.g., the aminoglycoside clearance (CL_{ag}) or the elimination rate constant (K)] and utilize one-compartment approaches to dosing.[19] When CrCl is related to CL_{ag}, the following approach is taken.

First, estimate CL_{ag} using[7,61]

$$CL_{ag} = CrCl$$

Then, K is determined by

$$K = CL_{ag}/V$$

where CL_{ag} and CrCl are in liters per hours (L/hr), K in hours^{-1} and V in liters (L). CrCl is converted from milliliters per minute to liters per hour by multiplying by 0.06.

$$CrCl\ (L/hr) = CrCl\ (ml/min) \times 0.06$$

The following equation has been used to relate K to CrCl:[8]

$$K = 0.0024 \times CrCl + 0.01$$

where K is in units of hours^{-1} and CrCl in milliliters per minute.

Half-life (in hours) in both approaches is then estimated by:

$$t\frac{1}{2} = 0.693/K$$

Therapeutic Range

SI units have been reported for several aminoglycosides but their use worldwide is rare. Thus, all blood (serum or plasma) concentrations are expressed in milligrams per liter.

With *traditional dosing* approaches for the treatment of *pneumonia*, peak concentrations of gentamicin or tobramycin—drawn approximately 0.5 hr after a 0.5-hr infusion or at the end of a 1-hr infusion—should be greater than 7 mg/L.[81] Trough concentrations—drawn approximately 0.5 hr or less before the next dose—should be 1–2 mg/L.[1,44] With amikacin, peak concentrations should be greater than 28 mg/L,[81] and trough levels should be 4–8 mg/L.[1,44]

For *other infections*, gentamicin and tobramycin peak concentrations of greater than 5 mg/L[82] and trough concentrations between 0.5 and 2 mg/L are recommended.[83]

With *LDEI dosing* approaches, the peak concentration desired varies. Doses recommended in adults range from 4 to 7 mg/kg, which would produce peak concentrations of approximately 13–23 mg/L in average patients. Patients with cystic fibrosis have received 15-mg/kg doses that produce peaks as high as 40 mg/L.[10]

The desired trough concentration varies depending on the approach. The Hartford protocol assumes that the concentration drops to zero 4 hr or more before the next dose.[20] Others suggest less than 1 mg/L.[35] For neonates receiving LDEI doses of 3.5–5 mg/kg of gentamicin and tobramycin (or 6 mg/kg of netilmicin) every 24 hr, the trough may not go below 1 mg/L for many patients.[9,36,84,85] It is unknown whether this presents a greater risk of toxicity, although at least one study shows no apparent increase in toxicity.[86] However, the often brief duration of therapy for neonates and adults (5 days or less) may obscure the potential for toxicity that could occur if these doses are continued for a longer period. Greater caution should always be used in patients who will receive aminoglycosides longer than 5 days, so it is prudent to ensure the lowest possible trough concentrations.

In traditional dosing approaches, patients of very advanced age (and consequent reduced renal function) and those with diminished renal function may have received once daily-dosing of traditional aminoglycoside doses to keep peaks of 5–8 mg/L and troughs of <2 mg/L. If these same patients are given LDEI and their interval is not extended beyond 24 hr, the risk of toxicity increases.[14] This issue is critical with LDEI dosing approaches. The advantages seen with LDEI in terms of decreased toxicity are likely due to having very low to nonexistent troughs.[87] Extrapolating the benefits of LDEI on a once-daily dosing basis to those who would have received traditional doses at extended intervals should not be done.

It has been suggested for traditional dosing approaches that the peak aminoglycoside concentration to MIC ratio should be greater than 4:1[88] and preferably greater than 8:1.[88,89] The likelihood of success appears to increase with higher values since the aminoglycosides demonstrate concentration-dependent killing. When a favorable peak to MIC ratio cannot be attained, synergistic agents or another antibiotic with good organism sensitivity should be used.

The Hartford LDEI dosing approach using 7 mg/kg for gentamicin and tobramycin was based on the assumption of need for a 10:1 peak to MIC ratio for best results and assumes an MIC of 2 mg/L for organisms.[20] The success of other LDEI approaches using lower doses and the fact that some organisms have lower MICs should lead researchers to consider regimens that take advantage of knowledge of the actual MIC to adjust dose size. Since organisms sometimes demonstrate different levels of susceptibility to the various aminoglycosides, it is also conceivable that using the aminoglycoside to which the organism is most susceptible could allow for use of lower doses.

Since total dose exposure appears to relate to toxicity, use of the lowest effective dose is desirable.

Suggested Sampling Times and Effect on Therapeutic Range

For consistency of evaluation among patients, sites, and studies, *peak* aminoglycoside concentrations usually should be drawn 0.5-hr after a 0.5 hr infusion or less than 15 min after a 1-hr infusion. The true peak occurs precisely at the end of the infusion. However, to avoid possible predistribution values and unrelated delays in blood drawing, these recommendations have been generally adopted. The *British National Formulary* suggests that peak concentrations be drawn 1 hr after a bolus injection.

Trough aminoglycoside concentrations are usually scheduled for 30 min or less before a dose. The true trough occurs precisely before the next infusion or bolus begins. Again, unrelated delays in sample collection and the need for consistency in the evaluation of efficacy and toxicity lead to the recommendation to check the trough approximately 30 minutes before the next dose.

Serial collection refers to multiple sampling within a dosage interval, along with a sample predose if the sampling interval is not after the first dose. Drug concentration measurements should be collected approximately one half-life apart for improved accuracy (to reduce the impact of assay error). A number of studies have examined the accuracy of using four versus three versus two versus one concentration measurement.[90–92] Recommendations vary (three versus two versus one) and cost considerations are obviously important. For traditional dosing at least two concentrations continue to predominate monitoring suggestions, while for LDEI many recommendations are for one measurement. Others suggest traditional approaches where a "peak" is drawn at some point in the hour or so after a dose (fairly similar to traditional "peak" measurements) with a second concentration measured approximately two estimated half-lives later (usually 6–12 hr). Doses and intervals may then be individualized to ensure achievement of a trough concentration of zero or near zero. Others are recommending that no concentration measurements are needed in patients with normal renal function who do not have confounding factors. Bayesian approaches tend to enhance the accuracy when fewer concentrations are measured. However, inaccurate information about dose and sample collection timing can make any concentration report problematic.

Varying definitions of when peak concentrations are to be drawn will affect the desired concentrations. These times must be standardized to ensure appropriate and consistent dosing within and among various institutions.

Monitoring Aminoglycoside Patients

Aminoglycoside concentration measurements

Monitoring of aminoglycoside concentrations helps to ensure therapeutic peak concentrations, enhance the likelihood of clinical response, and reduce the possibility of toxicity. It has been argued that aminoglycoside concentrations are monitored too soon and too often based on the number of patients who have short-term therapy (4 days or less), who do not exhibit toxicity despite elevated aminoglycoside concentrations, and who survive despite "subtherapeutic" concentrations.[93] Many authors still support the value of measurements, while some deny the value, and others suggest reducing the number of measurements around a dose or the total frequency of measurement.[20,94-96]

Certain patients may not derive benefit from having aminoglycoside concentrations measured, and clinicians should evaluate the cost to benefit for each patient.[95,97,98] In a patient whose risk of death from infection is significant or the risk of toxicity high, the assurance of adequate concentrations would appear to be worthwhile.

Assay issues

Although assay quality for aminoglycosides is good,[99] some variation exists between methods and laboratory quality and should be evaluated. Other factors can affect assay results. One study showed differences in peak (but not trough) concentrations of gentamicin and tobramycin when serum concentrations were compared to samples collected with sodium citrate (12% decrease primarily due to dilution), edetate (EDTA) (5% decrease), and heparin (17–22% depending on heparin concentration).[100] These interactions might even be more important in LDEI situations.

Initial concentration measurement

If a course of traditional dosing aminoglycoside therapy is planned (3 or more days), peak and trough concentration determinations can enhance the potential for adequate therapy. These measurements should be obtained by the second day of treatment to ensure adequate peak concentrations or to allow for early dosage adjustment to achieve target concentrations. Unless a patient has considerably reduced renal function or their intervals are shorter than 8 hr, steady-state conditions are usually in place by the second dose. A study of burn patients demonstrated rapid achievement of therapeutic steady-state concentrations when first dose measurements were used to guide therapy.[101] Patients also had fewer dosing changes than with conventional dosing. Thus, early assessment has utility if it is known that a full course of therapy is fairly certain.

Recommendations for initial monitoring of LDEI dosing generally suggest measurements on the first or second day of treatment. It has also been suggested that no monitoring is necessary if the patient has normal renal function, no confounding factors, and therapy will be for 5 days or less.

Follow-up concentration measurements
The need to recheck aminoglycoside concentrations depends on several factors.

- The duration of therapy is extended.
- Serum creatinine rises or falls considerably.
- More aggressive dosing (e.g., shorter intervals with higher troughs or very high peaks) is used or when initial troughs do not reach zero on LDEI. Rechecking of the trough (at least) would be necessitated by a small rise in creatinine in these cases. However, if the targeted trough based on initial serum concentrations were approximately 1 mg/L or less for traditional dosing, small changes in creatinine would not usually indicate significant increases in the trough concentration so dosage adjustment would not be as likely.
- Unexpected values result. In health systems without well-developed procedures for ensuring the correct timing of peak and trough concentration measurements, the potential for error is high, particularly if the dose times and collection times are not reported to the clinician. Peaks that are drawn late will be lower than anticipated, and troughs drawn early will be higher. The times of dose administration and blood sampling are important. When unexpected results are obtained and the need to know the concentrations is considered to be high, concentrations should be redrawn with strict instructions as to the time of dose, duration of infusion, and sampling times for both the peak and trough. If only one concentration appears inaccurate, it should be the one to be repeated. As a rule, all orders for peak and trough serum concentrations should be written with strict timing instructions unless a scheduling service is provided for ordered drug concentrations.

LDEI dosing

A single concentration measured between 6 and 14 hr after a dose is plotted on Figure 1 below for the Hartford method.[20] The result suggests adjustments to therapy if the place the concentration lies does not represent the current dosing interval. The initial dosage interval determinations for this method are explained in the maintenance dose section. The authors suggested discontinuation of monitoring concentrations in their institution for "patients: (a) receiving 24 hr dosing regimens, (b) without concurrently administered nephrotoxic agents (e.g., amphotericin, cyclosporine, vancomycin), (c) without exposure to contrast media, (d) not quadriplegic or amputee, (e) not in the intensive care unit, and (f) >60 years old."[102] The adoption of these suggestions at their institution yielded extrapolated savings of >$100,000/year for their 600-bed

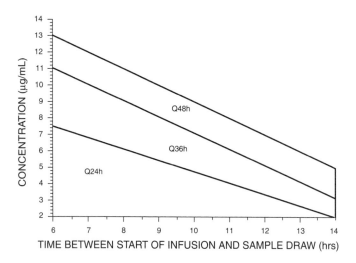

FIGURE 1. ODA nomogram for gentamicin and tobramycin at 7 mg/kg. Time represents time between infusion and sample draw.

Reproduced, with permission, from Nicolau DP, Freeman CD, Belliveau PP, et al. Experience with a once-daily aminoglycoside program administered to 2,184 adult patients. *Antimicrob Agents Chemother.* 1995; 39(3):650–5.

tertiary-care hospital and did not demonstrate an increase in nephrotoxicity (ototoxicity was not evaluated).

Approach to monitoring

It seems reasonable to assume that patients who are treated appropriately (i.e., their interval is appropriately adjusted for their renal function) with either larger traditional doses or LDEI approaches will have sufficiently high aminoglycoside peak concentrations to improve the chance of therapeutic success, unless the organism is resistant. This assumption should reduce the need to monitor peak concentrations. Thus, suggestions to avoid measuring concentrations early in therapy for such patients who have normal renal function seem appropriate. However, serum creatinine should be followed in such a setting. For therapy that will be extended beyond 5 days an aminoglycoside concentration measurement is suggested. Furthermore, confounding factors such as concomitant nephrotoxins, impaired physiology (e.g., ascites, burns, advanced age, or early age), or changing serum creatinine should signal the need for more aggressive monitoring.

Renal function

Serum creatinine should be monitored at the beginning of therapy and routinely throughout treatment. The frequency of monitoring varies according to the patient's stability. Litigation associated with aminoglycoside therapy may be prevented by the monitoring of serum creatinine and aminoglycoside concentrations and by dosage adjustment to provide target serum concentrations in the accepted therapeutic range. Even more important, patients may have a greater likelihood of successful treatment without toxicity.

In general, serum creatinine should be monitored daily in any aminoglycoside patient whose serum creatinine varies by 20% or more between measurements. For patients with stable measurements, serum creatinine may be monitored approximately every 3 days. Renal dysfunction associated with aminoglycosides takes several days to manifest as rising serum creatinine; therefore, it may be useful to check serum creatinine 2–3 days after treatment is completed. In the presence of other factors that may affect renal function (e.g., treatment with other nephrotoxins or hypotensive episodes), it is suggested that serum creatinine should be monitored frequently (daily) until stable.

Urine tests and BUN also can be used to monitor renal function. Urine can be tested for decreasing specific gravity (indicating reduced ability to concentrate urine), excretion of protein, cells, and casts. Although an increase in BUN may indicate decreasing renal function, it can also be caused by other factors. Diminished urine output over time relative to intake of fluid may also be a sign of decreasing renal function.

Pharmacodynamic Monitoring—Concentration-Related Efficacy

Moore and colleagues determined that patients with bacteremia responded better when peak gentamicin or tobramycin concentrations were above 5 mg/L and when peak amikacin concentrations were above 20 mg/L.[82] They also found that peaks of all three agents needed to be higher for patients with gram-negative pneumonia (7 mg/L for gentamicin and tobramycin and 28 mg/L for amikacin).[81] Binder and colleagues found a 71% response rate in febrile immunocompromised patients with hematologic malignancies whose gentamicin or tobramycin peak was 4.8 mg/L but only 30% response if the peak was ≤4.8 mg/L.[103]

Deziel-Evans and colleagues showed that peak to MIC ratios might be a better predictor of success.[88] Ratios of 4:1 or more dramatically improved survival rate. Others have shown improvement if the ratio is at least 3:1 for infections with gram-negative organisms.[104]

Moore and colleagues also observed a graded dose–response effect with peak to MIC ratios and showed that the likelihood of success increased as the peak to MIC ratio increased.[89] With a ratio of less than 2:1 as unity, the relative odds of clinical response were 4.35 times higher at a peak to MIC ratio of 6–8:1 and 8.41 times higher at a ratio of 10:1 or more. These results are supported by a recent study of patients with nosocomial pneumonia where a 10:1 ratio in the first 2 days of treatment predicted a 90% probability of temperature and leukocyte reduction.[105]

It has been suggested that organisms should be considered resistant at gentamicin and tobramycin MICs of 4 mg/L or higher and amikacin MICs of 16 mg/L or higher.[88,89] These values are one-half of the National Committee for Clinical Laboratory Standards values for susceptibility. However, if a peak to MIC ratio of at least 4:1 is desired, gentamicin and tobramycin peak concentrations of 16 mg/L would be required for an organism with an MIC of 4 mg/L. Prior to LDEI dosing, clinicians would have been hesitant to use aminoglycosides doses that could produce such concentrations. However, the goal of some LDEI methods is a 10:1 ratio. To achieve this would require a peak of 40 mg/L, a value beyond the majority of LDEI dosing approaches. The use of additional antibiotics with synergistic effect may enhance the potential for successful outcome when organisms are relatively resistant to aminoglycosides.

All of the cited studies were traditional dosing methods. While it is attractive to assume even better results with LDEI approaches, this assumption should not be made without confirmation.

Pharmacodynamic Monitoring—Concentration-Related Toxicity

Aminoglycosides cause nephrotoxicity and ototoxicity (vestibular and cochlear). Neuromuscular toxicity also has occurred; aminoglycosides should be used with caution in patients receiving neuromuscular blocking agents and in patients with muscular disorders such as myasthenia gravis and parkinsonism.

Nephrotoxicity has been related to a number of factors, including excessive trough concentrations and prolonged drug exposure.[44] The exact relationship has been debated, but it is generally accepted that troughs of gentamicin and tobramycin should be as low as possible (<2 mg/L) and that troughs of amikacin should be <8 mg/L, if possible. With LDEI dosing, the goal is to have the trough reach zero for several hours before the next dose is given.[20] Renal function must be monitored in patients receiving aminoglycosides. Factors such as decreased renal function and concomitant treatment with other nephrotoxins increase the incidence of nephrotoxicity. Minor nephrotoxicity often resolves after therapy is discontinued.

One study of LDEI dosing showed timing of dosing as an independent risk factor for nephrotoxicity.[21] Patients receiving their dose during midnight to 7:30 am had a higher incidence of nephrotoxicity. This finding might suggest some value in adjusting the timing after the first dose for patients started in this period, although further study would be necessary to determine the utility of such an approach. There is evidence that liver disease and biliary obstruction are associated with increased potential for nephrotoxicity.[106,107]

Ototoxicity has been related to prolonged drug exposure[108] and can be monitored by vestibular and auditory tests. However, these tests are notoriously difficult to use in many hospital settings. Symptoms of ototoxicity include dizziness, vertigo, tinnitus, roaring in the ears, and hearing loss. Patients should be questioned regarding such symptoms periodically. Deafness may evolve after therapy is concluded. Deafness is usually irreversible.

It has been suggested that the choice of aminoglycoside plays the greatest role in the risk of ototoxicity.

Prolonged duration of therapy is a frequently cited factor. Also, older age, bacteremia, poor physical condition, fever, liver and renal impairment, and the combination with another ototoxic agent are reported often,[13,22,109] and genetic predisposition may even play a role.[110] Iron chelators and radical scavengers have prevented ototoxicity in guinea pigs and may be on the horizon of human use.[111]

Other symptoms of toxicity that occur to a minor extent (less than 3% incidence) include hypersensitivity, headache, nausea and vomiting, and abnormal liver function tests. Some brands of aminoglycosides may contain sodium bisulfite, which may cause allergic reactions including anaphylaxis in certain individuals. A syndrome of endotoxin-like reactions has been reported with the use of gentamicin for LDEI dosing.[112,113] One product apparently contained enough endotoxin that the large dose led to pyrogenic adverse consequence for patients. The products of two companies, American Pharmaceutical Partners (40-mg/ml dosage forms) and ESI Lederle (20 lots only) have been voluntarily withdrawn but clinicians should watch for similar reactions when LDEI approaches are used.

Drug–Drug Interactions[7,44,83]

In vitro studies have found that the administration of *beta-lactams, extended-spectrum penicillins,* or *vancomycin* with an aminoglycoside can have a synergistic effect, improving the response to therapy. However, in vitro studies also have shown that concomitant administration of *carbenicillin, mezlocillin,* and *ticarcillin* decreases aminoglycoside concentrations. In vitro studies also have indicated that a precipitate may form when aminoglycosides are administered concomitantly with *cefoperazone* and *cephalothin*. These agents should not be mixed together and the time between collection of blood and concentration determination should be as short as possible. Samples should be refrigerated until analyzed. A study of piperacillin-tazobactam and gentamicin showed no interaction.[114]

In vivo studies indicated that concomitant administration of *beta-lactams* or *extended-spectrum penicillins* may decrease the half-life and increase clearance of the aminoglycosides, especially in patients with renal failure. Although an interaction has been suggested to be more likely in patients with reduced renal function, it appears that there is no need to consider separating gentamicin and ampicillin dosing times.[115] In vivo studies also have found an increase in aminoglycoside toxicity when administered concomitantly with *amphotericin, carboplatin, cisplatin, furosemide, ethacrynic acid, vancomycin,* and possibly, *some cephalosporins.*

Drug–Disease State or Condition Interactions

The following disease states or conditions influence certain aspects of aminoglycoside pharmacokinetics.

- *Ascites*[116,117] and *pancreatitis*[118]—The volume of distribution may increase by as much as 25%.
- *Intensive care setting/severely ill patients*—Patients may have a volume of distribution 25–50% higher than normal and increased clearance.[43,74,75,119]
- *Postpartum*[120]—The volume of distribution increases; 1.5 times the IBW should be used in calculations. A recent study showed that use of BW_{adj} (similar to use in obese patients) provided good prediction of volume.[121] The first approach is more aggressive.
- *Postoperative, mechanical ventilation*[122]—The volume of distribution increases.
- *Burns*[123,124]—Clearance increases and/or half-life decreases.
- *Obesity*[71] (see volume of distribution section, Step 4)—The volume of distribution decreases relative to total body weight.

- *Cystic fibrosis*[10,11,125]—The volume of distribution or clearance may increase.
- *Hemodialysis, peritoneal dialysis*[80,126,127]—Clearance increases and half-life decreases compared to values obtained when patient is not on dialysis. Studies of the use of a once-daily dose of aminoglycosides intraperitoneally differ on whether it provides appropriate coverage.[128–130]
- *Patent ductus arteriosus*[131]—This decreases clearance 11% and increases volume 13%.
- *Cirrhosis*[132]—Critically ill patients with cirrhosis and sepsis may have 40% larger volume (L/kg) and 38% lower clearance than similar patients without cirrhosis.
- *Pregnancy*—Aminoglycosides can cause fetal harm (e.g., streptomycin- and kanamycin-induced ototoxicity) when administered during pregnancy.[83] It is not known whether amikacin, gentamicin, netilmicin, and tobramycin cause fetal harm or whether LDEI approaches would increase risk. As always, the benefits should outweigh the risks, and patients should be warned of the potential hazard to the fetus.

Summary

- LDEI dosing approaches are now generally considered the standard for all but a few patient categories. A consensus of the types of patients who should not be given this type of dosing is warranted. Generally, LDEI is not recommended in patients who are pregnant or those with renal failure, osteomyelitis, meningitis, endocarditis, or extensive burns.
- All patients must have their renal function monitored.
- All patients should be queried about signs and symptoms of ototoxicity.
- The duration of dosing should be kept as limited as possible because total exposure seems to be an important

factor in toxicity, although some patients may become toxic from limited doses.[22] Use of larger doses should allow for a shorter duration of treatment due to more rapid elimination of the organism. This approach should lead to less toxicity compared with traditional dosing approaches.
- It appears that less monitoring (i.e., one concentration versus two or none at all) is possible with the larger doses as long as the interval is adjusted appropriately, the patient has normal renal function, there are no contraindicating factors, and treatment will not be extended.
- Extrapolation of results from traditional dosing studies to LDEI and vice versa should be avoided.

References

1. Murphy JE. Aminoglycosides: another look at current and future roles in antimicrobial therapy. *Pharmacother.* 1990; 10:217–23.
2. Hurley SC, Hegman G. Attainment of adequate serum aminoglycoside concentrations. Proceedings of American Society of Hospital Pharmacists 45th Annual Meeting. San Francisco, CA; June 1988.
3. Rodvold KA, Danziger LH, Quinn JP. Single daily doses of aminoglycosides. *Lancet.* 1997; 350:1412.
4. Waterberg Kl, Kelly HW, Angelus P, et al. The need for a loading dose of gentamicin in neonates. *Ther Drug Monit.* 1989; 11:16–20.
5. Semchuk W, Borgmann J, Bowman L. Determination of a gentamicin loading dose in neonates and infants. *Ther Drug Monit.* 1993; 15:47–51.
6. Isemann BT, Kotagal UR, Mashni SM, et al. Optimal gentamicin therapy in preterm neonates includes loading doses and early monitoring. *Ther Drug Monit.* 1996; 18:549–55.
7. Physician's desk reference, 54th ed. Montvale, NJ: *Med Econ.* 2000:1018–20, 1628–31, 2803–5, 2820–3.
8. Sarubbi FA, Hull HH. Amikacin serum concentrations: prediction of levels and dosage guidelines. *Ann Intern Med.* 1978; 89:612–8.
9. Murphy JE, Austin ML, Frye RF. Evaluation of gentamicin pharmacokinetics and dosing protocols in 195 neonates. *Am J Health-Syst Pharm.* 1998; 55:2280–8.
10. Bragonier R, Brown NM. The pharmacokinetics and toxicity of once-daily tobramycin therapy in children with cystic fibrosis. *J Antimicrob Chemother.* 1998; 42:103–6.
11. Bates RD, Nahata MC, Jones JW, et al. Pharmacokinetics and safety of tobramycin after once-daily administration in patients with cystic fibrosis. *Chest.* 1997; 112:1208–13.

12. Canis F, Huson MO, Turck D, et al. Pharmacokinetics and bronchial diffusion of single daily dose amikacin in cystic fibrosis patients. *J Antimicrob Chemother.* 1997; 39:431–3.
13. Paterson DL, Robson JMB, Wagener MM. Risk factors for toxicity in elderly patients given aminoglycosides once daily. *J Ger Intern Med.* 1998; 13:735–9.
14. Koo J, Tight R, Rajkumar V, et al. Comparison of once-daily versus pharmacokinetic dosing of aminoglycosides in elderly patients. *Am J Med.* 1996; 101:177–83.
15. Ismail R, Haw AHSM, Azman M, et al. Therapeutic drug monitoring of gentamicin: a 6-year follow-up audit. *J Clin Pharm Ther.* 1997; 22:21–5.
16. Eltahawy AT, Bahnassy AA. Aminoglycoside prescription, therapeutic monitoring and nephrotoxicity at a university hospital in Saudi Arabia. *J Chemother.* 1996; 8:278–83.
17. Saunders NJ, Adams DJ, Lynn WA. Antimicrobial practice: a prospective laboratory-based audit of gentamicin use and therapeutic monitoring. *J Antimicrob Chemother.* 1995; 36:729–36.
18. Sawchuk RJ, Zaske DE. Pharmacokinetics of dosing regimens which utilize multiple intravenous infusions: gentamicin in burn patients. *J Pharmacokinet Biopharm.* 1976; 4:183–95.
19. Erdman SM, Rodvold KA, Pryka RD. An updated comparison of drug dosing methods, part III: aminoglycoside antibiotics. *Clin Pharmacokinet.* 1991; 20:374–88.
20. Nicolau DP, Freeman CD, Belliveau PP, et al. Experience with a once-daily aminoglycoside program administered to 2184 adult patients. *Antimicrob Agents Chemother.* 1995; 34:650–5.
21. Prins JM, Weverling GJ, van Ketel RJ, et al. Circadian variations in serum levels and the renal toxicity of aminoglycosides in patients. *Clin Pharmacol Ther.* 1997; 62:106–11.
22. El Bakri F, Pallett A, Smith AG, et al. Ototoxicity induced by once-daily gentamicin. *Lancet.* 1998; 351:1407–8.
23. Postovsky S, Ben Arush MW, Kassis E, et al. Pharmacokinetic analysis of gentamicin thrice and single daily dosage in pediatric cancer patients. *Pediatr Hematology Oncol.* 1997; 14:547–54.
24. Mitra AG, Whitten MK, Laurent SL, et al. A randomized, prospective study comparing once-daily gentamicin versus thrice-daily gentamicin in the treatment of puerperal infection. *Am J Obstet Gynecol.* 1997; 177:786–92.
25. Tod M, Lortholary O, Seytre D, et al. Population pharmacokinetic study of amikacin administered once or twice daily to febrile, severely neutropenic adults. *Antimicrob Agents Chemother.* 1998; 42:849–56.
26. Pession A, Prete A, Paolucci G. Cost-effectiveness of ceftriaxone and amikacin as single daily dose for the empirical management of febrile granulocytopenic children with cancer. *Chemother.* 1997; 43:358–66.
27. Finnell DL, Davis GA, Cropp CD, et al. Validation of the Hartford nomogram in trauma surgery patients. *Ann Pharmacother.* 1998; 32:417–21.

28. Loey LL, Tschida SJ, Rotschafer JC, et al. Wide variation in single, daily-dose aminoglycoside pharmacokinetics in patients with burn injuries. *J Burn Care Rehabil.* 1997; 18:116–24.
29. Charlton CK, Needelman H, Thomas RW, et al. Gentamicin dosage recommendations for neonates based on half-life predictions from birthweight. *Am J Perinatol.* 1986; 3:28–32.
30. Murphy JE, Job Ml, Ward ES. Rectifying incorrect dosage schedules. *Am J Hosp Pharm.* 1990; 47:2235–6.
31. Preston S, Briceland L. Single daily dosing of aminoglycosides. *Pharmacother.* 1995; 15(3):297–316.
32. Cooke RPD, Grace RJ, Gover PA. Audit of once-daily dosing gentamicin therapy in neutropenic fever. *Int J Clin Pract.* 1997; 51:229–31.
33. Gilbert DN, Lee BL, Dworkin RJ, et al. A randomized comparison of the safety and efficacy of once-daily gentamicin or thrice-daily gentamicin in combination with ticarcillin-clavulanate. *Am J Med.* 1998; 105:182–91.
34. Prins JM, Weverling GJ, de Blok K, et al. Validation and nephrotoxicity of a simplified once-daily aminoglycoside dosing schedule and guidelines for monitoring therapy. *J Antimicrob Chemother.* 1996; 40:2494–9.
35. Rybak MJ, Abate BJ, Kang SL, et al. Prospective evaluation of the effect of an aminoglycoside dosing regimen on rates of observed nephrotoxicity and ototoxicity. *Antimicrob Agents Chemother.* 1999; 43:1549–55.
36. de Hoog M, Schoemaker RC, Mouton JW, et al. Tobramycin population pharmacokinetics in neonates. *Clin Pharmacol Ther.* 1997; 62:392–9.
37. Touw DJ, Jacobs FAH, Brimicombe RW, et al. Pharmacokinetics of aerosolized tobramycin in adult patients with cystic fibrosis. *Antimicrob Agents Chemother.* 1997; 41:184–7.
38. Coates AL, MacNeish CF, Lands LC, et al. A comparison of the availability of tobramycin for inhalation from vented vs unvented nebulizers. *Chest.* 1998; 113:951–6.
39. Touw DJ, Vinks ATMM, Mouton JW, et al. Pharmacokinetic optimisation of antibacterial treatment in patients with cystic fibrosis. *Clin Pharmacokinet.* 1998; 35:437–59.
40. Murphy JE, Job ML, Ward ES. Dosing error due to use of adult concentration of gentamicin injection rather than the pediatric concentration. *Hosp Pharm.* 1996; 31:219–20, 230.
41. Meunier F, Van der Auwera P, Schmit H, et al. Pharmacokinetics of gentamicin after iv infusion or iv bolus. *J Antimicrob Chemother.* 1987; 19:225–31.
42. Pechere JC, Dugal R. Clinical pharmacokinetics of aminoglycoside antibiotics. *Clin Pharmacokinet.* 1979; 4:170–99.
43. Mayer PR, Brown CH, Carter RA, et al. Intramuscular tobramycin pharmacokinetics in geriatric patients. *Drug Intell Clin Pharm.* 1986; 20:611–5.
44. Zaske DE. Aminoglycosides. In: Evans WE, Schentag JJ, Jusko WJ, eds. Applied pharmacokinetics: principles of therapeutic drug monitoring, 3rd ed. Vancouver, WA: Applied Therapeutics; 1992:14-1–14-47.

45. Smeltzer BD, Schwartzman MS, Bertino JS. Amikacin pharmacokinetics during continuous ambulatory peritoneal dialysis. *Antimicrob Agents Chemother.* 1988; 32:236–40.
46. Low CL, Bailie GR, Evans A. Pharmacokinetics of once-daily IP gentamicin in CAPD patients. *Peritoneal Dialysis Int.* 1996; 16:379–84.
47. Crosby SS, Edwards WAD, Brennan C, et al. Systemic absorption of aminoglycosides instilled through the endotracheal tubes of ten hospitalized patients. *Drug Intell Clin Pharm* 1987; 21:19A.
48. McCall CY, Spruill WJ, Wade WE. The use of aerosolized tobramycin in the treatment of a resistant pseudomonal pneumonitis. *Ther Drug Monit.* 1989; 11:692–5.
49. Walenkamp GHIM, Vree TB, Van Rens TJG. Gentamicin-PMMA beads: pharmacokinetic and nephrotoxicological study. *Clin Orthop.* 1986; 205:171–83.
50. Gomez GGV, Guerrero TS, Llack MC, et al. Effectiveness of collagen-gentamicin implant for treatment of "dirty" abdominal wounds. *World J Surg.* 1999; 23:123–7.
51. Champoux N, DuSouch P, Ravaoarinoro M, et al. Single-dose pharmacokinetics of ampicillin and tobramycin administered by hypodermoclysis in young and older healthy volunteers. *Br J Clin Pharmacol.* 1996; 42:325–31.
52. Faura CC, Feret MA, Horga JF. Monitoring serum levels of gentamicin to develop a new regimen for gentamicin dosage in newborns. *Ther Drug Monit.* 1991; 13:268–76.
53. Botha JH, du Preez MJ, Miller R, et al. Determination of population pharmacokinetic parameters for amikacin in neonates using mixed-effect models. *Eur J Clin Pharmacol.* 1998; 53:337–41.
54. Kelman AW, Thomson AH, Whiting B, et al. Estimation of gentamicin clearance and volume of distribution in neonates and young children. *Br J Clin Pharmacol.* 1984; 18:685–92.
55. Shevchuk YM, Taylor DM. Aminoglycoside volume of distribution in pediatric patients. *DICP Ann Pharmacother.* 1990; 24:273–6.
56. Jacobson PA, West NJ, Price J, et al. Gentamicin and tobramycin pharmacokinetics in pediatric bone marrow transplant patients. *Ann Pharmacother.* 1997; 31:1127–31.
57. Bass KD, Larkin SE, Paap C, et al. Pharmacokinetics of once-daily gentamicin dosing in pediatric patients. *J Pediatric Surg.* 1998; 33:1104–7.
58. Ho KK, Bryson SM, Thiessen JJ, et al. The effects of age and chemotherapy on gentamicin pharmacokinetics and dosing in pediatric oncology patients. *Pharmacother.* 1995; 15:754–64.
59. Zaske DE, Cipolle RJ, Rotschafer JC, et al. Gentamicin pharmacokinetics in 1,640 patients: method of control of serum concentrations. *Antimicrob Agents Chemother.* 1982; 21:407–11.
60. Zaske DE, Irvine P, Strand LM, et al. Wide interpatient variations in gentamicin dose requirements for geriatric patients. *JAMA.* 1982; 248:3122–6.
61. Winter ME. Aminoglycoside antibiotics. In: Winter ME. Basic clinical pharmacokinetics, 3rd ed. Vancouver, WA: Applied Therapeutics; 1994:128–38.

62. Carlstedt BC, Uaamnulchal M, Day RB, et al. Aminoglycoside dosing in pediatric patients. *Ther Drug Monit.* 1989; 11:38–43.

63. Bloome MR, Warren AJ, Ringer I, et al. Evaluation of an empirical dosing schedule for gentamicin in neonates. *Drug Intell Clin Pharm.* 1988; 22:618–22.

64. Gennrich JL, Nitake M. Devising an aminoglycoside dosage regimen for neonates seven to ninety days chronological age. *Neonatal Pharmacol Q.* 1992; 1:45–50.

65. Ristuccia AM, Cunha BA. The aminoglycosides. *Med Clin North Am.* 1982; 66:303–12.

66. Traynor AM, Nafziger AN, Bertino JS. Aminoglycoside dosing weight correction factors for patients of various body sizes. *Antimicrob Agents Chemother.* 1995; 39:545–8.

67. Debord J, Charmes JP, Marquet P, et al. Population pharmacokinetics of amikacin in geriatric patient studies with the NPEM-2 algorithm. *Int J Clin Pharmacol Ther.* 1997; 35:24–7.

68. Dager W. Aminoglycoside pharmacokinetics: volume of distribution in specific adult patient subgroups. *Ann Pharmacother.* 1994; 28:944–51.

69. Koshida R, Nakashima E, Taniguchi N, et al. Prediction of the distribution volumes of cefazolin and tobramycin in obese children based on physiological pharmacokinetic concepts. *Pharm Res.* 1989; 6:486–91.

70. Tointon MM, Job ML, Peltier TT, et al. Alterations in aminoglycoside volume of distribution in patients below ideal body weight. *Clin Pharm.* 1987; 6:160–2.

71. Bauer LA, Blouin RA, Griffen WO, et al. Amikacin pharmacokinetics in morbidly obese patients. *Am J Hosp Pharm.* 1980; 37:519–22.

72. Hassan E, Ober JD. Predicted and measured aminoglycoside pharmacokinetic parameters in critically ill patients. *Antimicrob Agents Chemother.* 1987; 11:1855–8.

73. Townsend PL, Fink MP, Stein KL, et al. Aminoglycoside pharmacokinetics: dosage requirements and nephrotoxicity in trauma patients. *Crit Care Med.* 1989; 17:154–7.

74. Romano S, Gonzalez P, Tejada P, et al. Influence of diagnostic and treatment factors in the population pharmacokinetics of gentamicin. *J Clin Pharm Ther.* 1998; 23:141–8.

75. Lugo G, Castaneda-Hernandez G. Relationship between hemodynamic and vital support measures and pharmacokinetic variability of amikacin in critically ill patients with sepsis. *Crit Care Med.* 1997; 25:806–11.

76. Lanao JM, Dominguez-Gil A, Malaga S, et al. Modification in the pharmacokinetics of amikacin during development. *Eur J Clin Pharmacol.* 1982; 23:155–60.

77. Hoecker Jl, Pickering LK, Swaney J, et al. Clinical pharmacology of tobramycin in children. *J Infect Dis.* 1978; 137:592–6.

78. Halstenson CE, Berkseth RO, Mann HJ, et al. Aminoglycoside redistribution phenomenon after hemodialysis: netilmicin and tobramycin. *Int J Clin Pharmacol Ther Toxicol.* 1987; 25:50–5.

79. Reguer L, Colding H, Jensen H, et al. Pharmacokinetics of amikacin during hemodialysis and peritoneal dialysis. *Antimicrob Agents Chemother.* 1977; 11:214–8.
80. Kaojarern S, Arkaravichien W, Indraprasit S, et al. Dosing regimen of gentamicin during intermittent peritoneal dialysis. *J Clin Pharmacol.* 1989; 29:140–3.
81. Moore RD, Smith CR, Lietman PS. Association of aminoglycoside plasma levels with therapeutic outcome in gram-negative pneumonia. *Am J Med.* 1984; 77:657–62.
82. Moore RD, Smith CR, Leitman PS. The association of aminoglycoside plasma levels with mortality in gram-negative bacteremia. *J Infect Dis.* 1984; 149:443–8.
83. Zaske DE, Shikuma LR, Tholl DA. Aminoglycosides. In: Taylor WJ, Caviness MHD, eds. A textbook for the clinical application of therapeutic drug monitoring. Irving, TX: Abbott Laboratories; 1986:285–320.
84. Hayani KC, Hatzopoulos FK, Frank AL, et al. Pharmacokinetics of once-daily dosing of gentamicin in neonates. *J Pediatr.* 1997; 131:76–80.
85. Ettlinger JJ, Bedford KA, Lovering AM, et al. Pharmacokinetics of once-a-day netilmicin (6mg/kg) in neonates. *J Antimicrob Chemother.* 1996; 38:499–505.
86. Langhendries JP, Battisti O, Bertrand JM, et al. Adaptation in neonatology of the once-daily concept of aminoglycoside administration: evaluation of a dosing chart for amikacin in an intensive care unit. *Biol Neonate.* 1998; 74:351–62.
87. Barclay ML, Kirkpatrick CMJ, Begg EJ. Once daily aminoglycoside therapy. Is it less toxic than multiple daily doses and how should it be monitored? *Clin Pharmacokinet.* 1999; 36:89–98.
88. Deziel-Evans LM, Murphy JE, Job ML. Correlation of pharmacokinetic indices with therapeutic outcome in patients receiving aminoglycosides. *Clin Pharm.* 1986; 5:319–24.
89. Moore RD, Lietman PS, Smith CR. Clinical response to aminoglycoside therapy: importance of the ratio of peak concentration to minimal inhibitory concentration. *J Infect Dis.* 1987; 155:93–9.
90. Mann HJ, Wittgrodt ET, Baghaie AA, et al. Effect of pharmacokinetic sampling methods on aminoglycoside dosing in critically ill surgery patients. *Pharmacother.* 1998; 18:371–8.
91. Jameson JP, Lewis JA. Three-point versus two-point method for early individualization of aminoglycoside doses. *DICP.* 1991; 25:635–7.
92. Matthews J, Chow MSS. Simpler approaches to aminoglycoside monitoring. *Am J Hosp Pharm.* 1994; 51:2847–8.
93. Averbuch M, Weintraub M, Nolte F. Gentamicin blood levels: ordered too soon and too often. *Hosp Form.* 1989; 24:598–612.
94. Begg EJ, Barclay ML, Kirkpatrick CJM. The therapeutic monitoring of antimicrobial agents. *Clin Pharmacol.* 1999; 47:23–30.
95. Logsdon BA, Phelps SJ. Routine monitoring of gentamicin serum concentrations in pediatric patients with normal renal function is unnecessary. *Ann Pharmacother.* 1997; 31:1514–8.
96. MacGowan A, Reeves D. Serum aminoglycoside concentrations: the case for routine monitoring. *J Antimicrob Chemother.* 1994; 34:829–37.

97. Massey KL, Hendeles L, Neims A. Identification of children for whom routine monitoring of aminoglycoside serum concentrations is not co-effective. *J Pediatr.* 1986; 109:897–901.

98. Robinson D. Gentamicin monitoring in pediatric patients. *Ann Pharmacother.* 1997; 31:1539–40.

99. Blaser J, Konig C, Fatio R, et al. Multicenter quality control study of amikacin assay for monitoring once-daily dosing regimens. *Ther Drug Monit.* 1995; 17:133–136.

100. Rodriguez-Mendizabal M, Lucena MI, Cabello MR, et al. Variations in blood levels of aminoglycosides related to in vitro anticoagulant usage. *Ther Drug Monit.* 1998; 20:88–91.

101. Hollingsed TC, Harper DF, Jennings JP, et al. Aminoglycoside dosing in burn patients using first-dose pharmacokinetics. *J Trauma.* 1993; 35:394–8.

102. Nicolau DP, Wu AHB, Finocchiaro S, et al. Once-daily aminoglycoside dosing: impact on requests and costs for therapeutic drug monitoring. *Ther Drug Monit.* 1996; 18:263–6.

103. Binder L, Schiel X, Binder C, et al. Clinical outcome and economic impact of aminoglycoside peak concentrations in febrile immunocompromised patients with hematologic malignancies. *Clin Chem.* 1998; 44:408–14.

104. Bezirtzoglou E, Golegou S, Savvaidis I. A relationship between serum gentamicin concentrations and minimal inhibitory concentration. *Drugs Exptl Clin Res.* 1996; 2:57–60.

105. Kashuba ADM, Nafziger AN, Drusano GL, et al. Optimizing aminoglycoside therapy for nosocomial pneumonia caused by gram-negative bacteria. *Antimicrob Agents Chemother.* 1999; 43:623–9.

106. Sawyers CL, Moore RD, Lerner SA, et al. A model for predicting nephrotoxicity in patients treated with aminoglycosides. *J Infect Dis.* 1986; 153:1062–8.

107. Desai TK, Tsang TK. Aminoglycoside nephrotoxicity in obstructive jaundice. *Am J Med.* 1998; 85:47–50.

108. Beaubien AR, Desjardins S, Ormsby E, et al. Incidence of amikacin ototoxicity: a sigmoid function of total drug exposure independent of plasma levels. *Am J Otolaryngol.* 1989; 10:234–43.

109. Barclay ML, Begg EJ. Aminoglycoside toxicity and relation to dose regimen. *Adverse Drug React Toxicol Rev.* 1994; 13:207–34.

110. Hamasaki K, Rando RR. Specific binding of aminoglycosides to a human rRNA construct based on a DNA polymorphism which causes aminoglycoside-induced deafness. *Biochem.* 1997; 40:12323–8.

111. Schacht J. Aminoglycoside ototoxicity: prevention in sight? *Otolaryngology-Head & Neck Surg.* 1998; 118:674–7.

112. Anonymous. Endotoxin-like reactions associated with intravenous gentamicin—California, 1998. *Morbidity Mortality Weekly Rep.* 1998; 47:877–80.

113. Lucas KH, Schliesser SH, O'Neill MG. Shaking, chills, and rigors with once-daily gentamicin. *Pharmacother.* 1999; 19:1102–4.

114. Hitt CM, Patel KB, Nicolau DP, et al. Influence of piperacillin-tazobactam on pharmacokinetics of gentamicin given once daily. *Am J*

Health-Syst Pharm. 1997; 54:2704–8.
115. Daly JS, Dodge RA, Glew RH, et al. Effect of time and temperature on inactivation of aminoglycosides by ampicillin at neonatal dosages. *J Perinatol.* 1997; 17:42–5.
116. Sampliner R, Perrier D, Powell R, et al. Influence of ascites on tobramycin pharmacokinetics. *J Clin Pharmacol.* 1984; 24:43–6.
117. Gill MA, Kern JW. Altered gentamicin distribution in ascitic patients. *Am J Hosp Pharm.* 1979; 36:1704–6.
118. Carr MR, Dick SP, Bordley J, et al. Gentamicin dosing requirement in patients with acute pancreatitis. *Surgery.* 1988; 103:533–7.
119. Mann HJ, Fuhs DW, Awang R, et al. Altered aminoglycoside pharmacokinetics in critically ill patients with sepsis. *Clin Pharm.* 1987; 6:148–53.
120. Briggs GG, Ambrose P, Nageotte MP. Gentamicin dosing in postpartum women with endometritis. *Am J Obstet Gynecol.* 1989; 160:309–13.
121. Cropp CD, Davis GA, Ensom MHH. Evaluation of aminoglycoside pharmacokinetics in postpartum patients using Bayesian forecasting. *Ther Drug Monit.* 1998; 20:68–72.
122. Triginer C, Fernandez R, Izquirdo I, et al. Gentamicin pharmacokinetic changes related to mechanical ventilation. *DICP Ann Pharmacother.* 1989; 23:923–4.
123. Zaske DE, Sawchuk RJ, Gerding DN, et al. Increased dosage requirements of gentamicin in burn patients. *J Trauma.* 1976; 16:824–8.
124. Loirat P, Rohan J, Baillet A, et al. Increased glomerular filtration rate in patients with major burns and its effect on the pharmacokinetics of tobramycin. *N Engl J Med.* 1978; 299:915–9.
125. Delage G. Desautels L, Legault S, et al. Individualized aminoglycoside dosage regimens in patients with cystic fibrosis. *Drug Intell Clin Pharm.* 1988; 22:386–9.
126. Indraprasit S, Ukaravichien V, Pummangura C, et al. Gentamicin removal during intermittent peritoneal dialysis. *Nephron.* 1986; 44:18–21.
127. Goetz DR, Pancorbo S, Hosg S, et al. Prediction of serum gentamicin concentrations in patients undergoing hemodialysis. *Am J Hosp Pharm.* 1980; 37:1077–83.
128. Low CL, Bailie GR, Evans A, et al. Pharmacokinetics of once-daily IP gentamicin in CAPD patients. *Peritoneal Dialysis Int.* 1996; 16:379–84.
129. Lai, M, Kao M, Chen C, et al. Intraperitoneal once-daily dose of cefazolin and gentamicin for treating CAPD peritonitis. *PDI.* 1997; 17:87–9.
130. Anding K, Krume B, Pelz K, et al. Pharmacokinetics and bactericidal activity of a single daily dose of netilmicin in the treatment of CAPD-associated peritonitis. *Int J Clin Pharm Ther.* 1996; 34:465–9.
131. Williams BS, Ransom JL, Gal P, et al. Gentamicin pharmacokinetics in neonates with patent ductus arteriosus. *Crit Care Med.* 1997; 25:273–5.
132. Lugo G, Castaneda-Hernandez G. Amikacin Bayesian forecasting in critically ill patients with sepsis and cirrhosis. *Ther Drug Monit.* 1997; 19:271–6.

Chapter 4
William R. Garnett

Newer Antiepileptic Drugs

Five new antiepileptic drugs have been approved by the FDA since 1994 with several more in development and pending approval. These drugs differ in structure and mechanism of action from the older or first generation drugs. While limited animal and clinical studies suggest that some of these drugs will have efficacy in a variety of seizure types, the primary indication for approval has been the treatment of patients with partial seizures refractory to traditional therapy, e.g. carbamazepine, phenytoin, and valproic acid.

In the International League Against Epilepsy's "Guidelines for therapeutic monitoring of antiepileptic drugs," the League stated: "Use of blood levels to adjust dosage so that numbers fall within the "therapeutic range" is a waste of time and money and may even be dangerous if effective and well-tolerated therapy is changed simply because levels are not in the published ranges. It is better to develop a target range for each patient based on severity of epilepsy and tolerance of side effects."[1] No target concentration ranges have been established for the new antiepileptic drugs. Therapy is generally started at a low dose and titrated to patient response. High initial doses and rapid titration have been shown to significantly increase the incidence of side effects with lamotrigine, tiagabine, and topiramate.

Dosage Forms of Newer Antiepileptic Drugs

Felbamate (Felbatol)	Suspension: 600 mg/5 ml Tablets 400 and 600 mg
Gabapentin (Neurontin)	100- and 300-mg capsules 400-, 600-, and 800-mg tablets
Lamotrigine	25-, 100-, 150-, and 200-mg tablets 5- and 25-mg chewable, dispersible tablets (which may be swallowed, chewed, or diluted with 5 ml of water or fruit juice and taken immediately)
Topiramate (Topamax)	15 and 25-mg capsules 25-, 100-, and 200-mg tablets 15- and 25-mg sprinkle capsules (swallowed whole but not chewed)
Tiagabine (Gabitril)	4-, 12-, 16-, and 20-mg tablets

Felbamate (Felbatol)

Felbamate blocks the glycine receptor on the N-methyl-D-aspartate (NMDA) complex, thereby inhibiting the response to NMDA neuronal excitation. Felbamate may also prevent seizure propagation by blocking voltage-dependent sodium channels, blocking calcium channels, blocking bursting from kainic acid, and affecting the γ-aminobutyric acid (GABA) system. It is structurally related to meprobamate but dependency does not develop and there are no withdrawal problems.[2] Felbamate is approved for use in patients with refractory partial seizures and in patients with Lennox-Gastaut syndrome. The range of effective serum concentrations reported with felbamate is 40–100 mg/L.[3,4]

Felbamate displays linear pharmacokinetics and available oral products are rapidly absorbed, reaching a peak concentration in 1–4 hr. Food does not affect the absorption of felbamate from the tablet dosage form. The apparent bioavailability is estimated at 100%. The volume of distribution of felbamate is 0.7–0.8 L/kg, and protein binding is only 25–35%.[5] It is eliminated equally by hepatic metabolism, involving hydroxylation and subsequent conjugation and renal elimination. There may be conjugation of the parent molecule. The half-life in drug-naive individuals is around 20 hr. However, the half-life is decreased in patients taking enzyme-inducing drugs such as carbamazepine and phenytoin. The concentration of felbamate in children is less than the concentration in adults receiving a comparable dose (milligram per kilogram), suggesting a more rapid elimination.[5,6] Elderly subjects require a lower initial dose and slower rates of titration.[7] Gender does not affect the pharmacokinetics of felbamate,[8] and neither do race, renal function and liver function.[6]

Felbamate is an enzyme inhibitor and increases the half-life and decreases the clearance of phenobarbital, phenytoin, and valproic acid. Interestingly, felbamate decreases the concentration of carbamazepine but increases the concentration of the active 10,11-di-epoxide metabolite. The doses of phenobarbital, phenytoin, carbamazepine and valproic acid should be decreased by 30–50% when felbamate is added. The FDA has approved felbamate doses of up to 3.6 g/day. In contrast to other antiepileptic drugs, felbamate is associated with CNS stimulation, and insomnia and decreased appetite with weight loss are side effects.[9,10] The use of felbamate is associated with aplastic anemia and hepatic failure. Since the approval of the drug, 31 cases of aplastic anemia and 16 cases of hepatic failure have been reported. Aplastic anemia may be the result of the formation of an uncommon but toxic metabolite.[10] Patients taking felbamate should have frequent CBCs and liver function tests.[11] The FDA currently limits the use of felbamate to patients who are refractory to other antiepileptics and places the following restrictions: 1. Full hematologic evaluations should be performed before felbamate therapy, frequently during felbamate therapy, and for a significant time after discontinuing felbamate therapy, and 2. Liver function tests (AST, ALT, and bilirubin) should be done before felbamate therapy is started and at 1- to 2-week intervals while the patient is taking felbamate.

Pharmacokinetics Summary Table

Bioavailability (F)	100%
T_{max}	1–4 hr
V	0.7–0.8 L/kg
Protein binding	25–35 %
Elimination	50% renal, 50% hepatic
$t½$	20 hr 11–16 hr (enzyme-inducing antiepileptics)
Usual dose	Initiate at 1200 mg/day and titrate up to 3600 mg/day

Gabapentin (Neurontin)

Although gabapentin was designed to potentiate GABA penetration through the blood-brain barrier, it does not work at either $GABA_A$ or $GABA_B$ receptors. Gabapentin does cause a dose-proportional increase in GABA in the brain, possibly by enhancing the rate of synthesis from glutamate or by binding to a novel amino acid site. Gabapentin may also decrease the concentration of glutamate, and it inhibits the sodium channel by mechanisms different from phenytoin and carbamazepine. Gabapentin is indicated for patients with partial seizures refractory to traditional therapy.[12] It is widely used in the treatment of pain and is also used for anxiety, panic attacks, migraine headaches, and other central nervous system disorders. The reported range of effective serum concentrations with gabapentin is 4–16 mg/L.

Following oral administration, gabapentin binds to an L-amino acid transport system in the gut. This system facilitates transport across the gut into the bloodstream and across the blood-brain barrier to the site of activity in the brain. However, binding to the L-amino acid transport system becomes saturated, and the bioavailability of gabapentin decreases with an increase in dose.[13] At doses of 300–400 mg, the apparent bioavailability is 60%. The bioavailability of a 1.6-g dose was 35%. Because of the dose-proportional bioavailability, the achieved concentrations are not proportional to dose. The absorption of gabapentin is rapid with peak concentrations occurring 2–4 hr after an oral dose. Bioavailability may be increased by giving the drug more frequently, e.g., four times a day rather than three.[14] Food does not affect the absorption rate,[15] but, a high-protein meal will increase gabapentin absorption.[16] The bioavailability of gabapentin given orally in a capsule and in a solution is comparable. Gabapentin is not absorbed after rectal administration.[17] The volume of distribution is 0.6–0.8 L/kg, and the protein binding is less than 10%. It does not undergo any liver metabolism and is excreted unchanged in the urine with a half-life of 5–9 hr.[18] The clearance of gabapentin is proportional to the creatinine clearance, and the dose should be deceased in patients with renal impairment.[19] Age-related decreases in renal function decrease gabapentin clearance. Gabapentin is removed by hemodialysis, and a replacement dose of 200–300 mg for each 4 hr of dialysis was suggested.[20]

Doses may be adjusted according to renal function as follows:

If CrCl is			
	>60 ml/min	400 mg three times a day	1200 mg/day
	30–60 ml/min	300 mg twice a day	600 mg/day
	15–30 ml/min	300 mg every day	
	<15 ml/min	300 mg every other day	

If the patient is anephric and on dialysis, give 200–300 mg after each 4-hr hemodialysis. The guidelines above were established before there was significant experience with large doses (e.g., 5–10 g). The ultimate guide to dosing is a patient's response. The dose may be increased in patients with renal dysfunction if clinical benefit based on the guidelines above was limited and no side effects occur.

Because gabapentin does not undergo liver metabolism and is poorly protein bound, it is not associated with significant drug interactions. Concurrent administration with antacids may decrease absorption by 20%, and cimetidine may decrease clearance by 10% by competing for tubular secretion.[20] Dosage adjustments are usually not necessary.

Gabapentin is generally well tolerated. Some CNS effects may be noted at the onset of therapy; however, as tolerance develops, the CNS side effects seem to plateau. Other side effects are weight gain, edema, and behavioral abnormalities. The consequences of overdose appear to be minimal. Gabapentin has a bitter taste when put into solution. The initial dose of gabapentin is 900 mg which is usually titrated upward over three days; then the dose is titrated to the patient's response.[21] The initially approved dose of 3.6 g for gabapentin is inadequate for some patients. Many patients require larger doses, and doses up to 10 g have been reported. Because the CNS side effects do not seem to correlate with dose, the dose of gabapentin can be rapidly titrated to response.

Pharmacokinetics Summary Table

Absorption	Actively absorbed; bioavailability decreases with an increase in dose
T_{max}	2–4 hr
V	0.7–1.0 L/kg
Protein binding	<10%

Elimination	Almost 100% renal
$t\frac{1}{2}$	5–7 hr
Usual dose	Initiate at 900 mg/day and titrate up to 3600 mg/day. Doses of 5–10 g have been well tolerated.
Dosing in renal dysfunction (CrCl)	>60 ml/min 400 mg three times a day 1200 mg/day
	30–60 ml/min 300 mg twice a day 600 mg/day
	15–30 ml/min 300 mg every day
	<15 ml/min 300 mg every other day
Anephric	200–300 mg after each hemodialysis

Lamotrigine (Lamictal)

Although lamotrigine was originally synthesized as a folate antagonist, it is a very weak folate antagonist. It is currently believed that lamotrigine works by blockade of use-dependent sodium currents, slow binding of inactivated sodium channels, blockade of voltage-activated calcium currents, inhibition of presynaptic N-type calcium channels, and inhibition of glutamate release.[22] Lamotrigine is approved for patients with partial seizures refractory to traditional therapy and for patients with Lennox-Gastaut syndrome.[23] The range of effective concentrations reported with lamotrigine is 2–20 mg/L.

The pharmacokinetics of lamotrigine appear to be linear. Lamotrigine is rapidly absorbed, reaching a peak concentration in 2–4 hr. Bioavailability is believed to be 100%. Lamotrigine is about 55% bound to plasma proteins and is eliminated predominately by glucuronidation in the liver.[24,25] The volume of distribution is 1.4 L/kg, and the clearance is 0.076 L/hr/kg.[26] A 25% decrease in elimination half-life at steady state has been reported, suggesting that lamotrigine induces its own metabolism.[27] Its metabolites are inactive. The half-life in a drug-naive individual is about 24 hr. However, the half-life of lamotrigine is affected by enzyme inducers and inhibitors.[24,25] The clearance of lamotrigine is unaffected by body weight, age, gender, oral contraceptive use, or dose.[27] Clearance has been reported to be reduced by 25% in nonwhites.[28] Children have a higher weight-normalized clearance of lamotrigine than healthy adults,[29] and the elderly have decreased clearance. The metabolic clearance of lamotrigine is not affected by hepatic impairment.[30]

The half-life in patients taking enzyme inducers is 12–14 hr, and the half life in patients taking enzyme inhibitors (valproic acid) exceeds 60 hr. The interaction between lamotrigine and valproate is believed to result from competition during glucuronidation. Acetaminophen, in doses of 900 mg in healthy volunteers, increased the total body clearance of lamotrigine by 15%.[31] Lamotrigine does not affect the metabolism of other drugs,[28] and it does not affect the concentration of carbamazepine or the active 10, 11-di-epoxide metabolite of carbamazepine.[32,33] Side effects increase in patients taking carbamazepine when lamotrigine is added, suggesting that there is a pharmacodynamic interaction at the receptor site.[34]

The most common side effects of lamotrigine are somnolence, dizziness, sedation, and diplopia. The incidence of CNS effects is increased in patients taking carbamazepine concurrently. The most troublesome side effect of lamotrigine is skin rash, which generally occurs in the first 3–4 weeks of therapy. The initial rash is usually a generalized, erythematous, morbilliform rash but may progress to a Stevens-Johnson reaction or toxic epidermis necrolysis (TEN).[23] The rash occurs more frequently in children than in adults. High starting doses, rapid dosage titration, and concurrent valproic acid therapy increase the incidence of skin rash. Therefore, the dose of lamotrigine should be started low and gradually titrated to the patient's response. Titration over several months is common. Doses up to 700 mg/day have been well tolerated.[35]

Pharmacokinetics Summary Table

Bioavailability	1.0
T_{max}	2–4 hr
V	0.9–1.3 L/kg
Protein binding	55%
Elimination	Liver by glucoronidation
$t\frac{1}{2}$	24 hr 15 hr (enzyme-inducing antiepileptics) >59 hr (valproic acid)
Usual dose	300–500 mg/day in patients taking enzyme-inducing antiepileptics; doses up to 700 mg/day have been well tolerated 150–200 mg/day in patients taking valproic acid

Tiagabine (Gabitril)

Tiagabine was specifically designed to block the reuptake of GABA into presynaptic terminals. This antiepileptic drug blocks one GABA uptake transporter, which makes more GABA available at the presynaptic cleft. Chronic administration increases $GABA_A$ sites and decreases $GABA_B$ sites. Tiagabine also prolongs inhibitory post synaptic potentials (IPSP). It is approved for use in patients with refractory partial seizures. The reported range of serum concentrations is 5–70 µg/L.[36]

Tiagabine exhibits linear absorption.[37] Food delays the absorption with peak concentrations occurring within 45 min in the fasting state and 2.5 hr in the nonfasting state. Bioavailability is reported to be 90%. Tiagabine is 96% protein bound, and valproic acid increases the percentage unbound to 40%. Tiagabine is extensively metabolized by CYP3A4 and by glucuronidation, with only 2% being excreted as the parent drug. The half-life in healthy volunteers ranges from 5.4 to 8.0 hr.[38] It is reduced in patients taking enzyme-inducing drugs, e.g., phenytoin and carbamazepine, and prolonged in patients taking enzyme-inhibiting drugs, e.g., valproic acid.[39] The T_{max}, dose-adjusted C_{max}, and AUC are independent of the administered dose, indicating linear pharmacokinetics. The pharmacokinetics of tiagabine are not affected by increasing age,[40] smoking, race,[41] or renal impairment.[42] Impaired liver function has been shown to decrease tiagabine elimination.[43]

Tiagabine does not interact with drug-metabolizing enzymes to any clinically significant extent.[10,44–46] The primary side effects of tiagabine are CNS related. Adverse reactions reported with tiagabine include amblyopia, incoordination, tremors, speech disorders, nervousness, paresthesia, abnormal thinking, somnolence, and dizziness. The incidence of CNS side effects with tiagabine may be reduced by slow dosage titration.[36]

Pharmacokinetics Summary Table

Bioavailability	90%
T_{max}	45 min fasting 2.5 hr fed
V	1.1 to 1.3 L/kg
Protein binding	96% (valproic acid increases the unbound percentage up to 40%)
Elimination	Extensively metabolized by the liver
$t\frac{1}{2}$	5–13 hr
	3.2 hr (enzyme-inducing antiepilpetics)
	5.7 hr (valproic acid)
Usual dose	Initiate therapy at 4 mg/day and titrate at weekly intervals up to 56 mg/day, if needed

Topiramate (Topamax)

Topiramate is a weak inhibitor of carbonic anhydrase. More importantly, it decreases the firing of neurons via action on the sodium channel, inhibits the D-amino-3-hydroxy-5-methyl isoxazole-4-propionic acid (AMPA) subtype of the glutamate receptor and the release of glutamate, and has effects on GABA systems.[47] Topiramate is approved for patients with refractory partial seizures, and may be useful in pediatric patients with a variety of seizure types.[48] The range of effective concentrations reported with topiramate is 2–25 mg/L.

Topiramate has linear pharmacokinetics. It is rapidly absorbed reaching peak concentrations in 2–4 hr.[49] Administration of topiramate with food delays the rate of absorption but does not change the extent of absorption. The absolute bioavailability is 100% in rats. The plasma protein binding of topiramate is only 13–17%. The volume of distribution was reported to be 58.0 L after a 100-mg dose and 38.5 L after a 1.2-g dose.[49] This change in volume of distribution may reflect saturation of low-capacity binding sites on or in erythrocytes. Topiramate is eliminated unchanged in the urine and, to a lesser extent, by hepatic metabolism. Unchanged topiramate represents 85.4% of the total dose. The half-life of topiramate is 18–23 hr. There is no change in plasma half-life with multiple dosing. The clearance of topiramate was reported to be 36.1 ml/min following a 100-mg dose and 22.5 ml/min following a 1.2-g dose.[50] Weight-adjusted clearance in children appears to be higher than in adults. For the same milligram-per-kilogram dose, the resulting concentrations are 33% lower in children. No age effect *per se* has been reported in older patients. However, if older patients have decreased renal function as a function of age, they will have a decreased clearance of topiramate.

The clearance of topiramate is decreased by 42% in patients with moderate renal impairment (CrCl 30–69 ml/min) and by 54% in patients with severe impairment (CrCl <30 ml/min). It is recommended that one half of the usual dose be used to initiate therapy and that the time between dosage adjustments be increased in patients with reduced renal function. Hemodialysis increases the clearance of topiramate four- to six-fold. The recommendations for supplemental doses after dialysis are that a supplemental dose may be required, taking into account the duration of dialysis, the clearance rate of the dialysis system, and the patient's effective renal clearance. In patients with hepatic impairment, there may be a reduced clearance of topiramate.[37,50-53]

Phenytoin and carbamazepine induce the metabolism of topiramate and decrease concentrations by 48 and 40%, respectively.[54,55] Valproate acid causes a 14% decrease in topiramate concentrations. These interactions are especially important if concurrent antiepileptic drugs are withdrawn after dosage stabilization with topiramate.[56] Topiramate may increase the clearance of oral contraceptives, and patients should report changes in menstrual patterns.[57] A 12% decrease in digoxin concentrations has been reported with topiramate. Because topiramate depresses CNS function, it may have an additive effect with other CNS depressants. The concurrent use of other carbonic anhydrase inhibitors may increase the incidence of renal stones.

The most common side effects seen with topiramate are CNS related. These side effects include psychomotor slowing, trouble concentrating, speech and language difficulties, somnolence, and fatigue. Anorexia and weight loss have been reported. There is a 1.5% increase in kidney stones in patients taking topiramate; the incidence is higher in men. Paraesthesias have also been reported. Both kidney stones and paraesthesia have been reported with other carbonic anhydrase inhibitors.[49,58]

The incidence of CNS side effects with topiramate increases with high initial doses and with high-maintenance doses. Therefore, the dose of topiramate should start low and be titrated to the patient's response.[51] The package insert suggests an initial starting dose of 50 mg with dosage increments of 50 mg/week in adults. Some clinicians choose to start at a lower dose and titrate more slowly. Patients taking topiramate should be encouraged to maintain adequate fluid intake to reduce the incidence of renal stones.

Pharmacokinetics Summary Table

Bioavailability	~80%
T_{max}	2 hr
V	0.6–0.8 L/kg
Protein binding	13–17%
Elimination	Predominately renal with some hepatic
$t\frac{1}{2}$	18–23 hr
Usual dose	Initiate therapy at 25–50 mg/day and increase at weekly intervals up to 400 mg/day in two doses. Renal dysfunction: use half of the usual dose and increase the interval between dosing adjustments.

Use of the New Antiepileptic Drugs

Currently the "second generation" antiepileptic drugs are approved for partial seizures refractory to conventional therapy. However, trials are ongoing to determine efficacy as monotherapy and in various types of generalized seizures.

The availability of newer drugs with different mechanisms of action increases the options for treating patients with epilepsy. No patient with epilepsy should be considered refractory until several different combinations of antiepileptic drugs have been tried. However, therapy should begin with the antiepileptic drug that is most efficacious for the patient's seizure type. This drug dose should be increased gradually until the patient becomes seizure free or to the maximum dose tolerated by the patient. Then a second drug with a different mechanism of action should be selected that is appropriate for the seizure type. This approach is referred to as "rational polytherapy." In selecting the second drug, consideration should also be given to avoiding potential drug interactions and to overlapping drug side effects, if possible. It is not always possible to avoid drug interactions, and drug interactions do not necessarily contraindicate the use of interacting drugs. Drug interactions do mandate closer patient monitoring. The two drugs should be given in adequate doses and for an adequate time to assess the frequency of seizures. One estimate is that the trial period at full dosage should encompass the period normally encompassing five seizures. Thus, the less frequent the seizures the more difficult it is to determine if the combination therapy is effective. If the patient has a positive response to the second drug or becomes seizure free, consideration should be given to withdrawing the first drug. The ultimate goal of antiepileptic drug therapy is to make the patient seizure free with minimal or no side effects.

References

1. Commission on antiepileptic drugs, International League Against Epilepsy. Guidelines for therapeutic monitoring of antiepileptic drugs. *Epilepsia* 1993; 34:585–7.
2. Sofia RD. Felbamate: mechanism of action. In: Levy RH, Mattson RH, Meldrum BS, editors. *Antiepileptic Drugs*. 5th ed. New York: Raven Press; 1995. p 791–7.
3. Graves NM. Ferlbamate. *Ann Pharmacother*. 1993; 27:1073–81.
4. Palmer KJ, McTavish D. Felbamate: A review of its pharmacodynamic and pharmacokinetic properties, and therapeutic efficacy in epilepsy. *Drugs*. 1993; 45:1041–65.
5. Sachdeo R, Narang-Sachdeo SK, Shumaker RC, et al. Tolerability and pharmacokinetics of monotherapy felbamate doses of 1,200–6,000 mg/day in subjects with epilepsy. *Epilepsia*. 1997; 38:887–92.

6. Perhach JL, Shumaker RC. Felbamate: absorption, distribution, and excretion. In: Levy RH, Mattson RH, Meldrum BS, editors. *Antiepileptic Drugs*, 4th ed. New York: Raven Press; 1995. p. 807–12.
7. Richens A, Banfield CR, Salfi M, et al. Single and multiple dose pharmacokinetics of felbamate in the elderly. *Br J Clin Pharmacol*. 1997; 44:129–34.
8. Chang SI, McAuley JW. Pharmacotherapeutic issues for women of childbearing age with epilepsy. *Ann Pharmacother*. 1998; 32:794–801.
9. Glue P, Banfield CR, Perhach JL, et al. Pharmacokinetic interactions with felbamate. In vitro-in vivo correlation. *Clin Pharmacokinet* 1997; 33:214–24.
10. Riva R, Albani F, Contin M, et al. Pharmacokinetic interactions between antiepileptic drugs. Clinical considerations. *Clin Pharmacokinet*; 1996; 6:470–93.
11. Natsch S, Hekster YA, Keyser A, et al. Newer anticonvulsant drugs: role of pharmacology, drug interactions and adverse reactions in drug choice. *Drug Safety* 1997; 17:228–40.
12. Taylor CP. Gabapentin: mechanism of action. In: Levy RH, Mattson RH, Meldrum BS, editors. *Antiepileptic Drugs*, 4th ed. New York: Raven Press; 1995. p. 829–41.
13. Stewart BH, Kugler AR, Thomson RR, et al. A saturable transport mechanism in the intestinal absorption of gabapentin is the underlying cause of the lack of proportionality between increasing dose and drug levels in plasma. *Pharm Res*. 1993; 10:276–81.
14. Gidal BE, DeCerce J, Bockbrader HN, et al. Gabapentin bioavailability: effect of dose and frequency of administration in adult patients with epilepsy. *Epilepsy Res*. 1998; 31:91–9.
15. Gidal BE, Maly MM, Kowalski JW, et al. Gabapentin absorption: effect of mixing with foods of varying macronutrient composition. *Ann Pharmacother*. 1998; 32:405–9.
16. Gidal BE, Maly MM, Budde J, et al. Effect of a high protein meal on gabapentin pharmacokinetics. *Epilepsy Res*. 1996; 23:71–6.
17. Kriel RL, Birnbaum AK, Cloyd JC, et al. Failure of absorption of gabapentin after rectal administration. *Epilepsia*. 1997; 38:1242–4.
18. McLean MJ. Clinical pharmacokinetics of gabapentin. *Neurology*. 1994; 44(Suppl 5):S17–22.
19. Blum RA, Comstock TJ, Sica DA, et al. Pharmacokinetics of gabapentin in subjects with various degrees of renal function. *Clin Pharmacol Ther*. 1994; 56:154–9.
20. Andrews CO, Fischer JH. Gabapentin: a new agent for the management of epilepsy. *Ann Pharmacother*. 1994; 28:1188–96.
21. Beydoun A, Uthman BM, Sachellares JC. Gabapentin: pharmacokinetics, efficacy, and safety. *Clin Neuropharmacol*. 1995; 18:469–81.
22. Meldrum BS. Lamotrigine—a novel approach. *Seizure*. 1994; 3(Suppl A):41–5.
23. Gilman JT. Lamotrigine: an antiepileptic agent for the treatment of partial seizures. *Ann Pharmacother*. 1995; 29:144–51.
24. Rambeck B, Wolf P. Lamotrigine clinical pharmacokinetics. *Clin Pharmacokinet*. 1993; 25:433–43.

25. Peck AW. Clinical pharmacology of lamotrigine. *Epilepsia*. 1991; 32(Suppl 2):S9–12.
26. Ramsay RE, Pellock JM, Garnett WR, et al. Pharmacokinetics and safety of lamotrigine (Lamictal) in patients with epilepsy. *Epilepsy Res*. 1991; 10:191–200.
27. Hussein Z, Posner J. Population pharmacokinetics of lamotrigine monotherapy in patients with epilepsy: retrospective analysis of routine monitoring data. *Br J Clin Pharmacol*. 1997; 43:457–65.
28. Grasela TH, Fiedler KJ, Cox E, et al. Population pharmacokinetics of lamotrigine adjunctive therapy in adults with epilepsy. *J Clin Pharmacol*. 1999; 39:373–84.
29. Chen C, Casale EJ, Duncan B, et al. Pharmacokinetics of lamotrigine in children in the absence of other antiepileptic drugs. *Pharmacother*. 1999; 19:437–41.
30. Furlan V, Demirdjian S, Bourdon O, et al. Glucuronidation of drugs by hepatic microsomes derived from healthy and cirrhotic human livers. *J Pharmacol Exp Ther*. 1999; 289:1169–75.
31. Garnett WR. Lamotrigine: pharmacokinetics. *J Child Neurol* 1997;12 (Supp 1):S10–S15.
32. Eriksson AS, Boreus LO. No increase in carbamazepine-10,11-epoxide during addition of lamotrigine treatment in children. *Ther Drug Monit* 1997; 19:499–501.
33. Gidal BE, Rutecki P, Shaw R, et al. Effect of lamotrigine on carbamazepine epoxide/carbamazepine serum concentration ratios in adult patients with epilepsy. *Epilepsy Res*. 1997; 28:207–11.
34. Besag FM, Berry DJ, Pool F, et al. Carbamazepine toxicity with lamotrigine: pharmacokinetic or pharmacodynamic interaction? *Epilepsia*. 1998; 39:183–7.
35. Matsuo F, Gay P, Madsen J, et al. Lamotrigine high-dose tolerability and safety in patients with epilepsy: a double-blind, placebo-controlled, eleven-week study. *Epilepsia*. 1996; 37:857–62.
36. Rosenfeld WE. Topiramate: a review of preclinical, pharmacokinetic, and clinical data. *Clin Ther*. 1997; 19:1294–308.
37. Samara EE, Gustavson LE, El-Shourbagy T, et al. Population analysis of the pharmacokinetics of tiagabine in patients with epilepsy. *Epilepsia*. 1998; 39:868–73.
38. Doose DR, Walker SA, Gisclon LG, et al. Single-dose pharmacokinetics and effect of food on the bioavailability of topiramate, a novel antiepileptic drug. *J Clin Pharmacol*. 1996; 36:884–91.
39. Langtry HD, Gillis JC, Davis R. Topiramate. A review of its pharmacodynamic and pharmacokinetic properties and clinical efficacy in the management of epilepsy. *Drugs*. 1997; 54:752–73.
40. Perucca E. Pharmacokinetic profile of topiramate in comparison with other new antiepileptic drugs. *Epilepsia*. 1996; 37(Suppl 2):S8–13.
41. Walker MC, Patsalow PN. Clinical pharmacokinetics of new antiepileptic drugs. *Pharmacol Ther*. 1995; 67:351–84.
42. Bourgeois BF. Drug interaction profile of topiramate. *Epilepsia*. 1996; 37(Suppl 2):S14–17.
43. Johannessen SI. Pharmacokinetics and interaction profile of

topiramate: review and comparison with other newer antiepileptic drugs. *Epilepsia*. 1997; 38(Suppl 1):S18–23.

44. Rosenfeld WE, Liao S, Kramer LD, et al. Comparison of the steady-state pharmacokinetics of topiramate and valproate in patients with epilepsy during monotherapy and concomitant therapy. *Epilepsia*. 1997; 38:324–33.

45. Rosenfeld WE, Doose DR, Walker SA, et al. Effect of topiramate on the pharmacokinetics of an oral contraceptive containing norethindrone and ethinyl estradiol in patients with epilepsy. *Epilepsia* 1997; 38:317–23.

46. Sachdeo RC. Topiramate: Clinical profile in epilepsy. *Clin Pharmacokinet*. 1998; 34:335–46.

47. Adkins JC, Noble S. Tiagabine. A review of its pharmacodynamic and pharmacokinetic properties and therapeutic potential in the management of epilepsy. *Drugs*. 1998; 55:437–60.

48. Perucca E, Bialer M. The clinical pharmacokinetics of the newer antiepileptic drugs. Focus on topiramate, zonisamide and tiagabine. *Clin Pharmacokinet*. 1996; 31:29–46.

49. Gustavson LE, Mengel HB. Pharmacokinetics of tiagabine, a gamma-aminobutyric acid-uptake inhibitor, in healthy subjects after single and multiple doses *Epilepsia*. 1995; 36:605–11.

50. So EL, Wolff D, Graves NM, et al. Pharmacokinetics of tiagabine as add on therapy in patients taking enzyme inducing antiepilepsy drugs. *Epilepsy Res*. 1995; 22:221–6.

51. Snel S, Jansen JA, Mengel HB, et al. The pharmacokinetics of tiagabine in healthy elderly volunteers and elderly patients with epilepsy. *J Clin Pharmacol*. 1997; 37:1015–20.

52. Cato A, Gustavson LE, Qian J, et al. Effect of renal impairment of the pharmacokinetics and tolerability to tiagabine. *Epilepsia*. 1998; 39:43–7.

53. Lau AH, Gustavson LE, Sperelakis R, et al. Pharmacokinetics and safety of tiagabine in subjects with various degrees of hepatic function. *Epilepsia*. 1997; 38:445–51.

54. Richens A, Marshall RW, Dirach J, et al. Absence of interaction between tiagabine, a new antiepileptic drug, and the benzodiazepine triazolam. *Drug Metabol Drug Interact*. 1998; 14:159–77.

55. Thomsen MS, Groes L, Agerso H, et al. Lack of pharmacokinetic interaction between tiagabine and erythromycin. *J Clin Pharmacol*. 1998; 38:1051–6.

56. Snel S, Jansen JA, Pedersen PC, et al. Tiagabine, a novel antiepileptic agent: lack of pharmacokinetic interaction with digoxin. *Eur J Clin Pharmacol*. 1998; 54:355–7.

57. Schneiderman JH. Topiramate: pharmacokinetics and pharmacodynamics. *Can J Neurol Sci*. 1998; 25:S3–5.

58. Glauser TA. Preliminary observations on topiramate in pediatric epilepsies. *Epilepsia*. 1997; 38(Suppl 1):S37–41.

Chapter 5
Janet Karlix & Joe Walker

Antirejection Agents
(AHFS 92:00)

Cyclosporine: Usual Dosage Range in Absence of Clearance-Altering Factors[1-3]

Cyclosporine is a large lipophilic cyclic polypeptide that is the cornerstone of transplant immunosuppression. The improvements in transplant outcomes provided by cyclosporine have allowed extrarenal (liver, heart, lung, and pancreas) solid organ transplantation to become routine. The following dosing recommendations are based on average pharmacokinetic parameters. However, due to the wide inter- and intrapatient pharmacokinetic variability, individual monitoring is absolutely necessary.

Three oral cyclosporine products are available. Sandimmune is the original formulation. It is highly dependent on bile salts for consistent absorption and displays significant intra- and interpatient variability in bioavailability. Neoral is a microemulsion formulation of cyclosporine that is only minimally dependent on bile salts. Intra- and interpatient variability in bioavailability is reduced with Neoral compared to Sandimmune.

Currently, there are two A/B rated generic cyclosporine microemulsions available that produce bioavailabilities similar to Neoral. For purposes of this chapter, the information relating to the microemulsion formulation will be referred to as Neoral.

Cyclosporine is most commonly administered every 12 hr; however, pediatric patients may require every 8-hr dosing.[4] Dosing intervals should be titrated to obtain the desired cyclosporine concentrations.

Dosage Form[1-3]	Initial Dosage	Maintenance Dosage
Intravenous	1–3 mg/kg (IBW) over 6–12 hr, some centers administer preoperatively	1–3 mg/kg (IBW) over 2–6 hr
Oral	4–8 mg/kg (IBW)	4–15 mg/kg (IBW) twice daily

Wide dosing range due to inter- and intrapatient variability. Recommend starting and titrating up based on target concentrations and toxicity.

Cyclosporine: Dosage Form Availability

Dosage Form	Product
Intravenous (concentrate for infusion): 50 mg/ml (5-ml ampul)	Sandimmune
Oral capsules Microemulsion: 25, 50, and 100 mg Microemulsion capsule, modified: 25, 50, and 100 mg	Neoral Abbot Laboratories (GENGRAF) Eon Labs Manufacturing Inc.
Liquid-filled capsule: 25 and 100 mg	Sandimmune
Oral liquid Oral solution: 100 mg/ml Microemulsion: 100 mg/ml	Sandimmune Neoral

Cyclosporine: Bioavailability (F) of Dosage Forms[1-3]

Dosage Form	Bioavailability Comments
Intravenous	100%
Oral (capsules and liquid)	average = 30%; range = 19–95%;

bioavailability increases over time, resulting in dose reduction. Sandimmune has larger intra- and interpatient variability than other forms.

Conversion between parenteral and oral routes of administration is usually in a 1:3 ratio. The oral solution and liquid capsules are bioequivalent.[1-3] Absorption of the microemulsion is more consistent over time in transplant patients, with less intrapatient variability.[5] Patients requiring intravenous administration of cyclosporine should have test samples drawn from a site other than the administration site because cyclosporine binds to plastics.

Cyclosporine: General Pharmacokinetic Information

Absorption

Cyclosporine has widely variable pharmacokinetics. The erratic absorption is impacted by first-pass metabolism, gastric motility, mode of administration, and drug–food interactions.

Time to peak concentration is different with Neoral (1–2 hr) compared to Sandimmune (2–3 hr). Sandimmune has a bimodal concentration curve with a second lower peak occurring between 8 and 18 hr. The second peak is thought to be due to enterohepatic recirculation.

Due to the highly lipophilic nature of cyclosporine, bile salts and fatty foods enhance absorption. Patients with impaired hepatic function may require higher doses if bile production is compromised. Following liver transplantation, patients also require lower doses after the biliary drain (t-tube) is closed. As patients increase dietary fat intake, cyclosporine concentrations increase due to enhanced absorption. Grapefruit juice and other inhibitors of P-glycoprotein may increase cyclosporine concentrations by increasing absorption. Cyclosporine absorption is also affected by intestinal cytochrome P450 activity.[6–10]

Binding
Cyclosporine is highly bound to erythrocytes, lipoproteins, and albumin.[11]

Metabolism
Cyclosporine is highly metabolized by hepatic biotransformation primarily by CYP450-3A4 into more than 25 metabolites.[2]

There are four metabolites postulated to possess activity: M1, M17, M18, and M21. Metabolite 17 is thought to exert the greatest activity for immunosuppression and nephrotoxicity. The clinical relevance of these potentially active metabolites is unknown.

Elimination
Cyclosporine is eliminated by metabolism and through the biliary pathway. Dosing adjustments are not necessary in renal failure or hemodialysis.[1–3]

Cyclosporine: Clearance (CL)

Cyclosporine and its metabolites are eliminated principally through the bile and feces.[3]

Cyclosporine: Volume of Distribution (V)

Cyclosporine has a large volume of distribution, 13 L/kg. It crosses the placenta and is found in breast milk.

Cyclosporine is 90% bound to proteins (primarily lipoproteins), and approximately 50% of the drug in the blood is bound to erythrocytes.[1–3] The fluid sampled for therapeutic drug monitorig (e.g., whole blood, plasma, or serum) impacts the target cyclosporine concentration.

Cyclosporine: Half-Life and Time to Steady State

The half-life of cyclosporine ranges from 8 to 27 hr with an average of approximately 12 hr. The half-life varies widely due to enterohepatic recycling of the drug, drug interactions, and age. Pediatric patients have a shorter half-life, often requiring every 8-hr dosing rather than the usual 12-hr interval. Patients receiving potent CYP450-3A4 inhibitors may require extended interval (e.g., 24-hr) dosing while patients receiving potent CYP450-3A4 inducers may require reduced interval (e.g., 8-hr) dosing.

Cyclosporine: Therapeutic Range

Due to the difficulty of correlating cyclosporine concentration with the immediate clinical outcome of immunosuppression, many transplant centers have established their own specific guidelines. Cyclosporine blood concentrations are no substitute for organ biopsy or organ function tests.

Patients with autoimmune diseases are often maintained at the lower end of the therapeutic range; however, no true therapeutic range has been established.

There are several different assays available; however, the consensus is that assays specific for the parent compound correlate best with clinical events. Such assays include high-performance liquid chromatography (HPLC), fluorescence polarization immunoassay, and monoclonal radioimmunoassays.[12,13]

The following are approximate values for monitoring cyclosporine concentrations. In solid organ transplantation, patients are maintained at the higher end of the therapeutic range initially, and then the desired concentration is often lowered over time to minimize nephrotoxicity and overimmunosuppression.

General: 100–500 µg/L

Transplantation
   Kidney: 100–350 μg/L
   Liver: 200–500 μg/L
   Bone marrow: 250–500 μg/L

Cyclosporine: Suggested Sampling Times[1-3]

Therapeutic efficacy and toxicity have been established according to trough serum concentrations.

Sampling times should be consistent and are usually obtained at hour 12 after a dose (trough). Although controversial and expensive, many transplant centers initially determine cyclosporine concentrations daily. After the first week posttransplantation, the need for daily concentration determinations declines.

To document acceptable steady-state values, cyclosporine serum concentrations should be assessed 3–5 days after a dosage adjustment, initiation of therapy, or discontinuation or initiation of known CYP450-3A4 inducers or inhibitors. Concentration sampling should be done immediately in any patient experiencing seizure activity. Transplant patients should be monitored more frequently in the early transplant period (3 or 4 times per week) and less frequently (every 6 months) once stable.

Some centers monitor area under the curve with limited sampling strategies at time 0, 2, and 4 hr past the dose to establish therapeutic efficacy and toxicity.

Cyclosporine: Pharmacodynamic Monitoring

Concentration-related efficacy

There are no immediate therapeutic outcome measures to use in determining relative efficacy of cyclosporine concentrations. Long-term therapeutic goals include prevention of graft rejection, graft survival, and patient survival. Many transplant centers use retrospective analyses to determine appropriate concentration-related efficacy parameters at their individual centers.[14-18]

Concentration-related toxicity

Cyclosporine possesses many concentration-related toxicities. The most common are nephrotoxicity and neurotoxicity, and these usually respond to dosage reductions. Other toxicities include dermatologic, hepatic, gastrointestinal, and hematological effects. Most of these effects resolve with dose reduction or discontinuation. The intravenous formulation is associated with sensitivity reactions in some patients due to the solubilizing agent Cremephor. Common cyclosporine toxicities and monitoring parameters are:[3,17]

Adverse Effect	Monitoring Parameter
Nephrotoxicity	S_{Cr} and urine output
Hypertension	Blood pressure
Electrolyte abnormalities	Potassium, magnesium, and bicarbonate concentrations
Neuropathy	Tremors and seizures
Hepatotoxicity	Bilirubin and liver function tests
Infections	White blood cell count and temperature
Hyperlipidemia	Triglycerides and cholesterol
Gingival hyperplasia	
Hirsutism	
Posttransplant lymphoproliferative disorder	

Cyclosporine: Drug–Drug Interactions[1-3]

Due to its extensive metabolism, other agents metabolized through the CYP450 isoenzyme pathway (particularly CYP450-3A4) may influence cyclosporine concentrations. Many interactions have been reported with cyclosporine. The following are abbreviated interaction lists.

Some drugs that may potentiate renal dysfunction:

Aminoglycosides
Amphotericin B
Cotrimoxazole (SMX–TMP)
Melphalan
Non-steroidal anti-inflammatory drugs (NSAIDs)
Tacrolimus

Some drugs that increase cyclosporine concentrations (enzyme inhibitors that decrease cyclosporine metabolism):

Antibiotics: clarithromycin, erythromycin, and quinupristin and dalfopristin
Antifungals: fluconazole, itraconazole, and ketoconazole
Ca^{++} antagonists: diltiazem, nicardipine, and verapamil
Glucocorticoids: methylprednisolone
Other drugs: allopurinol, bromocriptine, danazole, and metoclopramide

Some drugs that decrease cyclosporine concentrations (enzyme inducers that increase cyclosporine metabolism):

Antibiotics: rifampin
Anticonvulsants: carbamazepine, phenobarbital, and phenytoin
Other drugs: octreotide and ticlopidine

In addition, myositis has occurred with concomitant administration of lovastatin or simvastatin with cyclosporine.

Gingival hyperplasia has occurred frequently with concomitant use of nifedipine and cyclosporine; seizures and convulsions have occurred with high-dose methylprednisolone administered concomitantly with cyclosporine.

Cyclosporine: Drug–Disease State or Condition Interactions[1-3]

The effects of certain disease states on cyclosporine pharmacokinetics are:

Condition	Effect on Clearance	Effect on Half-Life
Renal failure	No change	No change
Hemodialysis	No change	No change
Peritoneal dialysis	No change	No change
Hepatic dysfunction	Decreased	Extended
Smoking	Increased	Shortened

Tacrolimus: Usual Dosage Range in Absence of Clearance-Altering Factors

Tacrolimus (Prograf) is a macrolide antibiotic with potent immunosuppressant properties. It is FDA approved for the prevention of rejection following kidney and liver transplantation in adults and liver transplantation in children.[18] It is also used for the treatment and prevention of rejection following heart, lung, pancreas, and small bowel transplantation in both children and adults.[19] Tacrolimus can also be used to treat graft versus host disease after bone marrow transplantation[19] and to treat severe forms of several autoimmune conditions including psoriasis,[20] refractory uveitis,[21] and atopic dermatitis.[22]

The following dosing recommendations are based on average pharmacokinetic parameters. Because there is significant interpatient variability in bioavailability, dose individualization through therapeutic monitoring is necessary.

Dosage Form[18,23]	Initial Dosage
Intravenous	For all indications: 0.03–0.05 mg/kg/day as continuous IV infusion. Adult patients should

88 CLINICAL PHARMACOKINETICS POCKET REFERENCE

receive doses at the lower end of the dosing range.[18] The concentrate must be diluted with NS or D5W to 0.004–0.02 mg/ml prior to administration.[23]

Oral Capsule — For liver (adult): 0.1–0.15 mg/kg/day (divided q12 hr); For liver (children): 0.15–0.2 mg/kg/day (divided q12 hr); For kidney (adult): 0.2 mg/kg/day (divided q12 hr)

Initial doses for other uses of tacrolimus are similar to those for the FDA-approved indications. Dosage requirements generally decline with continued therapy, and long-term administration is necessary to prevent rejection. In general, children require and tolerate higher tacrolimus maintenance doses than adults. Doses may be started lower and increased based upon concentrations in patients with renal impairment.

Tacrolimus: Dosage Form Availability[18,23]

Dosage Form	Product
Intravenous concentrate: 5 mg/ml (1-ml ampul)	Prograf
Oral capsule: 0.5, 1, and 5 mg	Prograf

As with many intravenous products containing castor oil derivatives, there is an increased risk of anaphylaxis with intravenous tacrolimus; therefore, the intravenous formulation should be used only when oral therapy is not possible.[23,24]

Tacrolimus: Bioavailability (F) of Dosage Forms

Dosage Form	Bioavailability Comments
Intravenous	100%
Oral capsules	Variable (mean 25%, range 9–43%)[24]

Oral doses are usually 3 or 4 times larger than intravenous doses due to limited bioavailability. Absorption of oral tacrolimus is variable, making therapeutic drug monitoring essential.[19]

Tacrolimus: General Pharmacokinetic Information[18,19,24–27]

Absorption

The oral absorption of tacrolimus is erratic. Oral bioavailability ranges from 9 to 43%. Intestinal CYP450-3A4 metabolism, gastric motility, and P-glycoprotein activity all affect tacrolimus absorption.

Food also reduces the absorption of tacrolimus, although the manufacturer makes no recommendation that it be taken on an empty stomach.[18] Unlike cyclosporine, the bioavailability of tacrolimus is not affected by the presence of bile salts. There is no need to adjust doses after closing the biliary diversion in liver transplant patients.

Distribution

Tacrolimus is widely distributed with a steady-state volume of distribution of >50 L when determined based on whole blood concentrations and >1000 L when determined from plasma concentrations. It is extensively bound to erythrocytes. The partitioning of tacrolimus between erythrocytes and plasma is dependent on the concentration of tacrolimus, temperature of the sample, hemoglobin count, and concentration of plasma proteins. In the plasma, it is highly bound (72–99%) to albumin and alpha-1-acid glycoprotein (AAG).

Tacrolimus crosses the placenta and is detected in breast milk.

Metabolism

Tacrolimus is extensively metabolized via the CYP450-3A4 pathway in both the gut and the liver. More than 15 active and inactive metabolites have been identified.

Excretion

Less than 1% of an intravenous dose is excreted as unchanged tacrolimus in the urine. Most of the metabolites are excreted in the bile.

Tacrolimus: Clearance (CL)

The mean clearance of tacrolimus from whole blood in adults is 0.06 L/hr/kg (range of 0.03–0.09 L/hr/kg). Children require higher doses on a milligram-per-kilogram basis than do adults. This appears to be the result of higher clearance.

Tacrolimus: Volume of Distribution (V)

The volume of distribution in whole blood is 0.85–1.0 L/kg (range of 0.5–1.4 L/kg). In plasma, the mean V is approximately 30 L/kg (range of 5.0–65 L/kg).

Tacrolimus: Half-Life and Time to Steady State

The elimination half-life of tacrolimus is variable with a mean of 12 hr (range of 4–41 hr).[19] Because tacrolimus has a long half-life with extensive distribution, dosage changes may take several days to reach steady state.

Tacrolimus: Suggested Sampling Times

For tacrolimus, a trough concentration measurement correlates well with the area under the concentration versus time curve (AUC).[19]

Tacrolimus trough concentrations should be assessed 3–5 days after initiation of therapy, after a dosage adjustment, or after discontinuation or initiation of known

CYP450-3A4 inducers or inhibitors. Therapeutic monitoring should be done more frequently in the early transplant period (3 or 4 times per week) and less frequently (every 6 months) in stable transplant recipients.[19]

Tacrolimus: Therapeutic Range

The therapeutic range for tacrolimus is 5–20 µg/L. This value represents a trough measurement in whole blood.[28] Most transplant centers strive to maintain concentrations at the higher end of this range during the initial period after transplantation (<3 months). After that time, most patients have successful outcomes and avoid toxicity with trough concentrations at the lower end of this range.[29]

Tacrolimus concentrations can be measured in plasma (processed at 37°C) or whole blood. Whole blood concentrations are generally 10–30 times higher than the corresponding plasma concentrations.[26] A consensus conference recommended whole blood use as the preferred method of tacrolimus monitoring, because it requires less lab time and a less sensitive assay due to higher concentrations.[28]

Tacrolimus: Pharmacodynamic Monitoring

Concentration-related efficacy[25,29,30]

The establishment of a concentration–efficacy (rejection) relationship for all immunosuppressants is difficult for many reasons. There is a lack of direct evidence of a correlation between a specific tacrolimus trough concentration and efficacy; however, it has been shown that higher tacrolimus concentrations are associated with lower acute rejection rates.

Concentration-related toxicity[18,23,24]

Most tacrolimus toxicities are dose and concentration dependent.

Adverse Effect	Monitoring Parameter
Nephrotoxicity	S_{Cr} and urine output
CNS toxicity	Headache, seizure, altered mental status, tremors, and altered motor function
Hyperglycemia	Blood glucose
Hypertension	Blood pressure
Hepatoxicity	Bilirubin and liver function tests
Infections	White blood cell count and temperature
Hyperlipidemia	Triglycerides and cholesterol
Electrolyte abnormalities	Potassium, magnesium, and bicarbonate concentrations
Anemia	Hemoglobin and hematocrit
Gastrointestinal	Diarrhea and nausea
Dermatologic	Pruritus and alopecia

Tacrolimus: Drug–Drug Interactions[18,19,24]

Due to its extensive metabolism, other agents metabolized through the CYP450-3A4 pathway may influence tacrolimus concentrations.

Drugs that increase tacrolimus concentrations (enzyme inhibitors that decrease tacrolimus metabolism):

>Antibiotics: clarithromycin, erythromycin, josamycin, and troleandomycin
>Antifungals: fluconazole, itraconazole, and ketoconazole
>Ca^{++} antagonists: diltiazem, nicardipine, nifedipine, and verapamil
>Corticosteroids: methylprednisolone and prednisone
>Other Drugs: bromocriptine, cimetidine, cisapride, danazole, metoclopramide, nefazodone, protease inhibitors

Drugs that decrease tacrolimus concentrations (enzyme inducers that increase tacrolimus metabolism):
>Antibiotics: nafcillin, rifabutin, and rifampin

Anticonvulsants: carbamazepine, phenobarbital, and phenytoin

In addition, rhabdomyolysis has occurred in patients receiving tacrolimus with an HMG Co-A reductase inhibitor.[23]

Like many drugs, tacrolimus absorption may be reduced from concomitant administration of aluminum hydroxide containing antacids.[19]

Like cyclosporine, tacrolimus is both an inhibitor and a substrate for P-glycoprotein. P-glycoprotein is a membrane-bound protein that acts as an active transport drug efflux pump. It is found in many tissues including intestinal luminal tissues. Drugs that affect or are affected by P-glycoprotein have the potential to interact with tacrolimus. Grapefruit juice is a known P-glycoprotein inhibitor.[31]

Tacrolimus has been shown to significantly increase mycophenolic acid concentrations in patients who are taking mycophenolate mofetil with tacrolimus. The clinical relevence of this interaction is not known, because the relationship between mycophenolic acid concentrations and efficacy or toxicity is yet to be determined.[32,33]

Drugs that may potentiate renal toxicity with tacrolimus include: ACE inhibitors, aminoglycosides, amphotericin B, cisplatin, cyclosporine, ganciclovir, and NSAIDs.

Tacrolimus: Drug–Disease State or Condition Interactions[19]

The effects of certain disease states on tacrolimus pharmacokinetics are:

Condition	Effect on Clearance	Effect on Half-Life	Effect of Absorption
Hepatic dysfunction	Decreased	Extended	No change
Gastroparesis	No change	No change	Decreased

Neither renal failure nor dialysis (hemo or peritoneal) affects the pharmacokinetics of tacrolimus.

The drug and disease state interactions with tacrolimus are complex and further support the necessity of drug concentration monitoring.

References

1. McEvoy GK, ed. AHFS drug information 99, Bethesda, MD: American Society of Health-System Pharmacists, 1999.
2. Noble S, Markham A. Cyclosporine. A review of the pharmacokinetic properties, clinical efficacy, and tolerability of a microemulsion-based formulation (Neoral). *Drugs.* 1995; 50(5):924–41.
3. Fahr A. Cyclosporine clinical pharmacokinetics. *Clin Pharmacokinet.* 1993; 24(6):472–95.
4. Mochon M, Cooney G, Lum B, et al. Pharmacokinetics of cyclosporine after renal transplant in children. *J Clin Pharmacol.* 1996; 36(7):580–6.
5. Wahlberg J, Wilczek HE, Fauchald P, et al. Consistent absorption of cyclosporine from a microemulsion formulation assessed in stable renal transplant recipients over a one-year period. *Transplantation.* 1995; 60(7):648–52.
6. Kaplan B, Lown K, Craig R, et al. Low bioavailability of cyclosporine microemulsion and tacrolimus in a small bowel transplant recipient: possible relationship to intestinal P-glycoprotein activity. *Transplantation.* 1999; 67(2):333–5.
7. Gupta SK, Manfro RC, Tomlanovich SJ, et al. Effect of food on the pharmacokinetics of cyclosporine in healthy subjects following oral and intravenous administration. *J Clin Pharmacol.* 1990; 30(7):643–53.
8. Ducharme MP, Warbasse LH, Edwards DJ. Disposition of intravenous and oral cyclosporine after administration with grapefruit juice. *Clin Pharmacol Ther.* 1995; 57(5):485–91.
9. Brunner LJ, Munar MY, Vallian J, et al. Interaction between cyclosporine and grapefruit juice requires long-term ingestion in stable renal transplant recipients. *Pharmacotherapy.* 1998; 18(1):23–9.
10. Lown KS, Mayo RR, Leichtman AB, et al. Role of intestinal P-glycoprotein (mdr1) in interpatient variation in the oral bioavailability of cyclosporine. *Clin Pharmacol Ther.* 1997; 62(3):248–60.
11. Shibata N, Minouchi T, Yamaji A, et al. Relationship between apparent total body clearance of cyclosporin A and its erythrocyte-to-plasma distribution ratio in renal transplant patients. *Biol Pharm Bull.* 1995; 18(1):115–21.
12. Shaw LM, Kaplan B, Brayman KL. Prospective investigations of concentration-clinical response for immunosuppressive drugs provide the scientific basis for therapeutic drug monitoring. *Clin Chem.* 1998; 44(2):381–7.

13. Kahan BD, Welsh M, Schoenberg L, et al. Variable oral absorption of cyclosporine. A biopharmaceutical risk factor for chronic renal allograft rejection. *Transplantation.* 1996; 62(5):599–606.
14. Kahan BD. Pharmacokinetic considerations in the therapeutic application of cyclosporine in renal transplantation. *Transplant Proc.* 1996; 28(4):2143–6.
15. Awni W, Heim-Duthoy K, Kasiske BL. Monitoring of cyclosporine by serial posttransplant pharmacokinetic studies in renal transplant patients. *Transplant Proc.* 1990; 22(3):1343–4.
16. Dunn J, Grevel J, Mapoli K, et al. The impact of steady-state cyclosporine concentrations on renal allograft outcome. *Transplantation.* 1990; 49(1):30–4.
17. Lindholm A, Welsh M, Rutzky L, et al. The adverse impact of high cyclosporine clearance rates on the incidences of acute rejection and graft loss. *Transplantation.* 1993; 55(5):985–93.
18. Prograf (tacrolimus) package insert. Deerfield, IL: Fujisawa Healthcare, Inc. 2000.
19. Venkataramanan R, Swaminathan A, Prasad T, et al. Clinical pharmacokinetics of tacrolimus. *Clin Pharmacokinet.* 1995; 29(6):404–30.
20. The European FK 506 Multicentre Psoriasis Study Group. Systemic tacrolimus (FK 506) is effective for the treatment of psoriasis in a double-blind, placebo-controlled study. *Arch Dermatol.* 1996; 132:419–23.
21. Mochizuki M, Masuda K, Sakane T, et al. A clinical trial of FK506 in refractory uveitis. *Am J Ophthalmol.* 1993; 115:763–9.
22. Ruzicka T, Bieber T, Schopf E, et al. A short-term trial of tacrolimus ointment for atopic dermatitis. *N Engl J Med.* 1997; 337:816–21.
23. Tacrolimus. In McEvoy GK, ed. AHFS drug information 2000. Bethesda, MD: American Society of Health-System Pharmacists; 2000:3441–5.
24. Spencer CM, Goa KL, Gillis JC. Tacrolimus: an update of its pharmacology and clinical efficacy in the management of organ transplantation. *Drugs.* 1997; 54(6):925–75.
25. Undre NA, Stevenson P, Schafer A. Pharmacokinetics of tacrolimus: clinically relevant aspects. *Transplant Proc.* 1999; 31(suppl 7A):21S–24S.
26. Kelly PA, Burkhart GJ, Venkataramanan R. Tacrolimus: a new immunosuppressive agent. *Am J Health-System Pharm.* 1995; 52:1521–35.
27. Winkler M, Christians U. A risk-benefit assessment of tacrolimus in transplantation. *Drug Safety.* 1995; 12(5):348–57.
28. Jusko WJ, Thompson AW, Fung J, et al. Consensus document: therapeutic monitoring of tacrolimus (FK-506). *Ther Drug Monit.* 1995; 17:606–14.
29. Oellerich M, Armstrong VW, Schultz E, et al. Therapeutic drug monitoring of cyclosporine and tacrolimus. *Clin Biochem.* 1998; 31(5):309–16.
30. Ringe B, Braun F, Lorf T, et al. FK and MMF in clinical liver transplantation: experience with a steroid sparing concept. *Transplant Proc.* 1998; 30(4):1415–6.
31. Lo A, Burkhart GJ. P-glycoprotein and drug therapy in organ transplantation. *J Clin Pharmacol.* 1999; 39:995–1005.

32. Zucker K, Rosen A, Tsaroucha A, et al. Unexpected augmentation of mycophenolic acid pharmacokinetics in renal transplant patients receiving tacrolimus and mycophenolate mofetil in combination therapy, and analogous in vitro findings. *Transplant Immunol.* 1997; 5(3):225–32.

33. Hubner GI, Eismann R, Sziegoleit W. Drug interaction between mycophenolate mofetil and tacrolimus detectable within therapeutic mycophenolic acid monitoring in renal transplant patients. *Ther Drug Monit.* 1999; 21(5):536–9.

Chapter 6
William R. Garnett

Carbamazepine
(AHFS 28:12.92)

Usual Dosage Range in Absence of Clearance-Altering Factors

Carbamazepine is the drug of choice for controlling simple, complex, and secondarily generalized partial seizures. It also may be used for some types of generalized seizures such as tonic-clonic convulsive seizures.[1] It is ineffective in absence seizures. Carbamazepine was originally marketed for the treatment of trigeminal neuralgia but was found to be effective for the treatment of seizures. Although it does not have an FDA indication for bipolar depression or peripheral pain, carbamazepine has been shown to be useful in treating these conditions. The target concentration was established for the treatment of seizures. Target concentrations have not been developed for conditions other than the treatment of seizures, so that range is employed for other uses. The therapeutic range is 4–12 mg/L. Doses are generally started at one-fourth to one-third of the expected maintenance dose to allow for completion of the autoinduction of metabolism that is unique to carbamazepine and for tolerance to the CNS effects that accompany most antiepileptic drugs.[2] The dose is titrated to a balance between the occurrence of side effects and the cessation of seizures.[3] Methods for rapid loading in critically ill patients using carbamazepine suspension[4] and tablets[5] have been described. A rapid switch-over technique using the pharmacokinetics derived from a single 10-mg/kg dose has been used to convert patients from other antiepileptic drugs to carbamazepine. The conversion to carbamazepine with the removal of other antiepileptic drugs was achieved in 6 days with no adverse effects.[6]

Dosage Form	Initial Dosage
Intravenous	None
Oral (tablets and suspension): slow titration (generally indicated)	
Week 1	One-fourth to one-third of maintenance dose
Week 2	One-third to one-half of maintenance dose
Week 3	Entire maintenance dose
Oral (suspension) or tablet: rapid loading (for critically ill patients)	
Children (≤12 years)	10 mg/kg
Adults (>12 years)	8 mg/kg

This rapid loading procedure should result in peak concentrations of around 10 mg/L. A routine maintenance dose should be started 6–8 hr after the loading dose.

Dosage Form	Maintenance Dosage
Oral (tablets and suspension)	
Children (≤15 years)	11–40 mg/kg/day
Adults (>15 years)	7–15 mg/kg/day

Since the metabolism of carbamazepine is subject to enzyme induction and inhibition, the maintenance dosage will depend on the presence or absence of concurrent antiepileptic and other drugs.

There is significant intersubject variability in the pharmacokinetics of carbamazepine that impacts on the frequency of daily dosing. Some patients may be dosed twice a day; others may require dosing as often as four times a day with immediate-release tablets. The dosage form will also affect the frequency of daily dosing. Controlled- and sustained-release dosage forms are designed for twice-a-day dosing. The suspension form will need to be given more often.

Dosage Form Availability

Dosage Form	Product
Intravenous	None available
Oral tablets 100 mg chewable	Tegretol
200 mg	Tegretol Epitol
Oral suspension: 100 mg/5 ml	Tegretol
Controlled-release tablets 100, 200, and 400 mg	Tegretol-XR
Sustained-release capsules (may be used as a sprinkle) 200 and 300 mg	Carbatrol
Rectal enema	Suspension diluted 1:1 with water

Bioavailability (*F*) of Dosage Forms

Since no intravenous form of carbamazepine is available for human trials, the absolute bioavailability is not known. A 2% oral solution was reported to be 100% bioavailable.[7]

Dosage Form	Bioavailability Comments
Intravenous	Not available
Immediate-release tablets	85–90%[8,9]
Chewable tablets	85–90%[10,11]
Oral suspension	85–90% but at a faster rate compared to immediate-release tablets[12]

Sustained-release capsules Controlled-release tablets	85–90% but may provide less variation in the concentration curve[13,14] Sustained-release and controlled-release carbamazepine given every 12 hours have been compared to immediate-release carbamazepine given every 6 hours and found to be bioequivalent
Rectal enema (must be extemporaneously compounded)	80–100% as compared to immediate-release tablets in total amount absorbed but with slower time to peak[15]

There are several generic manufacturers of immediate-release carbamazepine tablets. While there are numerous case reports of patients experiencing breakthrough seizures or side effects after a switch from one formulation to another, controlled trials have demonstrated bioequivalency of the generic formulations compared to the innovator. Although the generic formulations have been tested against the innovator, the various generic formulations have not been compared to each other. Because the standard for bioequivalency is ±20%, there is a potential that clinically important variations might occur with frequent switches of immediate-release dosage forms; however, no clinical trials indicate this problem. Also, individual patients have a narrow therapeutic range for seizure control and incidence of side effects. Therefore, it is prudent to initiate patients on one formulation and maintain them on that formulation unless they are converted to a sustained- or controlled-release dosage form.

The FDA reported that moisture may decrease the potency of carbamazepine immediate-release tablets by up to 30%; therefore, these tablets must be stored in a cool, dry place.[16]

Carbamazepine is available as a sustained-release dosage form (Carbatrol) and a controlled-release dosage form (Tegretol-XR). Carbatrol is a capsule formulation that contains immediate-release, intermediate-release, and extended-release beads of carbamazepine. Tegretol-XR utilizes the OROS system, which is a matrix system with a semipermeable membrane, for drug delivery. These formulations can be given twice a day, preferably at 12-hr intervals. When immediate-release carbamazepine administered every 6 hours was compared with either controlled- or sustained-release carbamazepine given every 12 hours, they were bioequivalent.[13,14] Results from a 5-day study of normal volunteers indicate Carbatrol is bioequivalent to Tegretol-XR but there was variability in the rate of absorption in Carbatrol.[17] Similar results were found in another study.[17] Variability in GI transient time may affect the absorption of Tegretol-XR.[18] It should not be crushed or chewed. Patients taking Tegretol-XR should be warned that the casing will be excreted in the feces and will increase in size. Carbatrol capsules may be opened and the contents used as a sprinkle. Both formulations have less peak to trough fluctuations and may be associated with fewer of the side effects related to higher peak concentrations. The twice-a-day dosing of both formulations may improve patient adherence.

General Pharmacokinetic Information

Absorption

The GI absorption of immediate-release carbamazepine is slow, erratic, and unpredictable, probably because of carbamazepine's slow rate of dissolution or anticholinergic properties.[8] There is significant inter- and intraindividual variability in the absorption rate. A circadian variation in the rate of absorption may be observed, with an evening dose being absorbed more slowly than a morning dose.[19] Absorption is prolonged and occurs throughout the upper and lower parts of the intestine, resulting in secondary peaks.[8]

There is no first-pass metabolism, and the effect of food on absorption is variable and of little clinical significance. Food may effect the rate of carbamazepine absorption. Carbamazepine may exhibit saturable absorption; doses higher than 20 mg/kg of the immediate-release tablet may be less well absorbed. A linear relationship between dose and concentration has been shown at doses between 600 and 1400 mg/day. At higher doses, the increases in the steady-state concentration tend to be less than proportional. Carbamazepine undergoes a simultaneous first-order and zero-order absorption with about 35% of the available dose being absorbed at a zero-order rate.[20] Absorption in the upper and lower part of the intestine is constant and prolonged. The rate of absorption in the colon slows significantly.[18] Absorption may be decreased in a patient with malnutrition.[21]

Distribution

Animal studies indicate that carbamazepine distributes rapidly and uniformly to various organs and tissues, achieving higher concentrations in organs of high blood flow (e.g., liver, kidney, and brain).[8]

Protein binding

Carbamazepine binds to albumin and to alpha-1-acid glycoprotein (AAG).[2] The concentration of AAG and the free fraction of carbamazepine may vary with the presence of inflammation, trauma, concurrent antiepileptic drug therapy, and age.[22] The free fraction of carbamazepine is estimated at 25%, but reports in epileptic patients have ranged from 10 to 50%.[2] The protein binding of carbamazepine in neonates is slightly less, resulting in a free fraction of 30–35%, but binding in all other age groups is comparable.[8] Monitoring of the free (unbound) concentration may be indicated when the patient's clinical presentation (e.g., the presence of side effects or the lack of response) does not coincide with the plasma concentration.[23] There is no defined target concentration range for unbound carbamazepine. Free concentrations are not routinely measured. Poorly controlled diabetic patients may have an increased free (unbound) fraction of carbamazepine because of a decrease in nonglycosylated albumin concentrations. This change may make measurement of free concentrations preferable in diabetic patients.[24]

Maternal/breast feeding/saliva
Carbamazepine rapidly crosses the placenta, achieving a concentration in the fetus equal to the concentration of the mother. The placenta does not participate in the metabolism of carbamazepine.[25] The carbamazepine concentration in breast milk is about 25–60% of the concentration in the mother's plasma.[8] Strong and highly significant correlations between saliva and plasma concentrations were found over a wide range of carbamazepine concentrations following citric acid stimulation of saliva.[26] Salivary sampling's usefulness is limited, however, and should be restricted to those occasions when a blood sample cannot be obtained.

Elimination
Carbamazepine is about 99% metabolized by oxidation, hydroxylation, direct conjugation with glucuronic acid, and sulfur conjugation pathways. Oxidation and hydroxylation pathways account for about 65% of its metabolism.[27] The most important carbamazepine metabolite is 10,11-epoxide, which appears to be active and may contribute to the efficacy and toxicity of carbamazepine.[28,29] The isoenzymes responsible for catalyzing 10,11-oxidation of carbamazepine in the human liver are CYP2C8 and CYP3A4. CYP3A4 seems to be the more important of the two.[30] While there is some polymorphic distribution of CYP2C8, it does not seem to have a major effect on the pharmacokinetics of carbamazepine. CYP1A2 and uridine diphospho-glucuronosyltransferase (UGT) are involved in forming the inactive metabolites of carbamazepine. The 10,11-epoxide metabolite is further metabolized to a diol metabolite

by a xenobiotic epoxide hydrolase. Clearance of the 10,11-epoxide metabolite is higher than that of the parent drug.[31] Drug interactions may alter the formation of the 10,11-epoxide metabolite without altering the carbamazepine concentration.[32]

The metabolism of carbamazepine may be altered by other drugs and by itself (autoinduction). Its clearance increases with continued dosing.[33] Autoinduction begins 3–5 days after the initiation of therapy and takes 2–4 weeks to complete.[33,34] The 10,11-epoxide diol pathway is induced primarily.

Additional autoinduction occurs with each dosage increase.[34] An increase in autoinduction with an increase in dose has been shown in children as well as adults.[35] Because of autoinduction, concentrations achieved initially can be expected to fall. Therefore, a drop in carbamazepine concentration may reflect autoinduction rather than patient nonadherence. Autoinduction must be considered during dosage titration. The potential for other drugs to enhance or inhibit the metabolism of carbamazepine makes drug–drug interactions likely and significant.[1] (See drug–drug interactions section.)

The variability in the pharmacokinetics of carbamazepine makes dosage prediction difficult. Statistical models and population methods are not generally useful clinically.[36,37] A Bayesian nonlinear method is clinically acceptable but needs three or four data points.[38]

Clearance (CL)

Since there is no intravenous form of carbamazepine, clearance is relative to bioavailability.

Age	Clearance
Children	
Initial dose	
0–3 years	0.320 L/hr/kg
4–9 years	0.189 L/hr/kg
10–15 years	0.123 L/hr/kg

Chronic dosing (≤15 years)　　　0.050–0.400 L/hr/kg

Adults (>15 years)
　Initial dose　　　　　　　　　0.011–0.026 L/hr/kg
　Chronic dosing　　　　　　　　0.050–0.100 L/hr/kg

The clearance of carbamazepine increases with continued dosing and is altered by enzyme-inducing or inhibiting drugs.[39] The clearance of carbamazepine decreases with increasing age and weight in children 2.3–16.3 years old.[40] In children 1–14 years old, clearance was shown to increase linearly with total body weight and nonlinearly with age; thus, older children have a lower clearance with respect to total body weight than do younger ones.[35] No effect has been shown for older patients.[41] However, older patients may have altered pharmacokinetics for carbamazepine.[42,43] Carbamazepine is metabolized by oxidative metabolism which does decrease with age.[44] A population pharmacokinetic analysis demonstrated an age-related decrease in CL/F.[45] Clearance relative to mass has been shown to decrease with an increase in body mass. Carbamazepine concentrations were significantly higher in lean subjects than those in normal weight subjects; the degree of obesity may affect serum carbamazepine concentrations.[46] Weight reduction in one patient did not affect carbamazepine clearance.[47] The relationship of clearance to dose is controversial.[48]

Volume of Distribution (V)

The volume of distribution is 0.8–2 L/kg based on total body weight. No age-related effect has been demonstrated.

Protein Binding

The free fraction of carbamazepine is normally 25% (range 10–50%). However, changes in AAG concentration result in changes in the free fraction. Protein binding of carbamazepine may be altered in poorly controlled diabetic patients.[24]

Half-Life and Time to Steady State

The half-life ($t½$) of carbamazepine changes with continued dosing and is affected by other drugs. A true half-life is difficult to measure because of the variability of absorption; absorption may continue throughout the dosing interval. The time to steady state depends on the completion of autoinduction.[39]

Dosage	Half-Life
Single dose	35 hr
Chronic dose	11–27 hr
Concurrent antiepileptic drug	5–14 hr

Therapeutic Range

The reported therapeutic range of carbamazepine is 4–12 mg/L for the treatment of seizures.[3] The exact therapeutic concentration for a given patient must be individually determined. The final target concentration is a balance between seizure control and intolerable side effects. The correlation between carbamazepine dose and concentration is poor.[49] The therapeutic range for psychiatric disorders and trigeminal neuralgia is assumed to be the same as for seizure disorders.

The 10,11-epoxide metabolite of carbamazepine is active and may contribute to efficacy as well as toxicity. Drug interactions may increase the concentration of the metabolite without changing the carbamazepine concentration. Ideally the clinician should measure both the parent drug and the metabolite, but an assay for 10,11-epoxide is not commercially available. Nevertheless, the contribution of this metabolite should be considered when the response to carbamazepine is evaluated.

Suggested Sampling Times and Effect on Therapeutic Range

The sampling time for carbamazepine depends on the duration of treatment and whether the clinician is evaluating efficacy or side effects. A blood sample is not needed for carbamazepine concentration determination after the first dose unless a rapid loading dose was given in an emergency situation. While concentrations should be determined during dosage titration to evaluate end-points, they may be expected to fall following the full effect of autoinduction. Furthermore, autoinduction must be considered when doses are changed during chronic therapy. A trough concentration measurement (i.e., one drawn just before the morning dose) is most appropriate for the evaluation of efficacy.

The dose of carbamazepine should be started low and titrated to patient response. The rate of titration will determine sample collection. If the dose is being increased weekly or every two weeks, autoinduction will occur and the concentration will change, even with good adherence. Samples may be obtained during this period to correlate dose with side effects or with seizure control, but sampling will be more meaningful after autoinduction is complete.

Numerous side effects associated with carbamazepine are concentration related.[50] Each patient apparently has a threshold for the occurrence of side effects. Therefore, for some patients the sample may be appropriately obtained when side effects are occurring. Given the variability of absorption from immediate-release tablets, it is difficult to predict when the peak carbamazepine concentration will occur. There is less peak to trough fluctuation with the sustained-release or controlled-release dosage forms. This decreased fluctuation may result in fewer peak-related side effects.

The sudden occurrence of side effects or a change in seizure frequency is an indication to monitor carbamazepine concentrations. The concentrations of carbamazepine should be monitored closely during the third trimester and postpartum in pregnant patients. Concentrations should be monitored every 6–12 months in stable adults and every 4–6 months in stable children.

Pharmacodynamic Monitoring—Concentration-Related Efficacy

The effectiveness of carbamazepine as an antiepileptic drug is associated with a concentration of 4–12 mg/L.[3] This range is intended as a guide—not as an absolute—because of the variable amount of free drug, the contribution of the 10,11-epoxide metabolite, and the intersubject variability in pharmacokinetics. The target concentration for a given patient should be achieved by titration to response and tolerance.

Pharmacodynamic Monitoring—Concentration-Related Toxicity

Concentration-related side effects include lethargy, dizziness, drowsiness, headache, blurred vision, diplopia, ataxia, and incoordination.[50] These side effects are more common at concentrations greater than 8–12 mg/L. Since each patient apparently has a threshold for the occurrence of side effects, they may be eliminated or reduced by dosage manipulation.

A slow dosage titration allows a patient time to develop some tolerance. The use of sustained-release or controlled-release dosage forms reduces the peak to trough fluctuations and may reduce side effects associated with peak concentrations. A dose reduction decreases side effects in some patients without a loss in seizure control.

Other possible concentration-related side effects include nausea, vomiting, syndrome of inappropriate secretion of antidiuretic hormone, cardiac disturbances, and osteomalacia.[2]

An exact dose and concentration effect for these side effects has not been established. However, they occur more frequently at higher doses or after prolonged exposure to carbamazepine.

Idiosyncratic reactions include bone marrow suppression (very rare), aplastic anemia, and agranulocytosis. Carbamazepine has been associated with atrioventricular block, especially in older women.[51] It is suggested that careful monitoring of the ECG and drug concentration be done in elderly patients.[52] Carbamazepine is associated with skin rash and rarely with a Stevens-Johnson reaction. The mechanism may involve reactive metabolites in the epidermis.[53] One case of skin rash was associated with an increased concentration of nicotinamide and vitamin B_6.[54] Other case reports of adverse reactions associated with carbamazepine include hypogammaglobulinaemia,[55] hearing loss,[56] tubulointerstitial nephritis (TIN),[57] alopecia,[58] and an auditory disturbance (flat A tone).[59]

Although a baseline CBC is useful, frequent CBC monitoring is not indicated for chronic carbamazepine monitoring.[60] Carbamazepine can cause a leukopenia that is not considered dangerous or a harbinger of agranulocytosis or aplastic anemia. A decrease in the WBC count is not an automatic requirement for stopping carbamazepine. Many patients taking carbamazepine routinely have low WBCs without being immunosuppressed. Carbamazepine affects the distribution of neutrophils without affecting their ability to mobilize at the time of infection.

Patients on monotherapy have fewer side effects and tolerate higher concentrations of carbamazepine than do patients on polytherapy.[49]

Drug–Drug Interactions[61–63]

Carbamazepine is an enzyme inducer and may enhance the metabolism of many drugs undergoing metabolism by CYP3A4. Because carbamazepine is extensively metabolized by CYP3A4, CYP2C8, and CYP1A2, its metabolism may be affected by drugs that induce or inhibit liver microsomal enzymes.[64–66]

Carbamazepine effects (increased clearance) on other drugs are indicated below.

Significant Effect	Moderate Effect
Alprazolam[67]	Bupropion
Bromperidol[68]	Cyclosporine
Clobazam[69]	Dicumarol
Clonazepam	Fluphenazine
Dexamethasone	Oxiracetam
Doxycycline	Thiothixene
Ethosuximide	
Felbamate[70]	
Fentanyl	
Haloperidol	
Hormonal contraceptives	
Imipramine	
Lamotrigine[71,72,73]	
Methadone	
Methylphenidate[74]	
Methylprednisolone	
Midazolam[75]	
Olanzapine[76]	
Pancuronium bromide	
Phenytoin	
Prednisolone	
Primidone	
Theophylline	
Topiramate[77]	
Valproate sodium	
Vecuronium[78]	
Warfarin sodium	

An increase in dose of the concurrent drug should be considered if carbamazepine is administered with it.

A possible synergistic effect is seen with *lithium* when carbamazepine is used in patients with bipolar depression.

The effects of other drugs on carbamazepine are listed below.

Significant Increased Clearance	Significant Decreased Clearance
Caffeine[79]	Acetazolamide
Felbamate (parent carbamazepine)[80]	Cimetidine
Phenobarbital	Clarithromycin[81]
Phenytoin	Danazol
Primidone	Dextropropoxyphene hydrochloride
	Diltiazem hydrochloride
	Erythromycin[81]
	Felbamate (10,11-diepoxide carbamazepine)[80]
Moderate Decreased Clearance	Fluvoxamine[82]
	Grapefruit juice[83] (large amounts)
	Isoniazid
Baclofen	Propoxyphene
Fluoxetine hydrochloride	Valproate sodium
Flurithromycin	Valproic acid[84]
Gemfibrozil	Verapamil hydrochloride
Niacinamide	Viloxazine

Significant amounts of carbamazepine are lost through adsorption if undiluted carbamazepine suspension is administered through polyvinyl chloride nasogastric feeding tubes. Dilution with an equal volume of diluent and flushing minimize the adsorption.[85] Enteral feedings do not appear to alter the absorption of carbamazepine suspension significantly.[86] There is a pharmacodynamic interaction with lamotrigine.

Drug–Disease State or Condition Interactions

Little information has been published concerning the interaction between carbamazepine and disease states other than epilepsy. Because carbamazepine is extensively metabolized by the liver, its clearance would be expected to decrease in patients with significant liver disease. Because almost no unchanged drug is excreted in the urine, significant renal impairment should not alter carbamazepine clearance. *Hemodialysis* does not affect the clearance of carbamazepine.[87]

Congestive heart failure that causes gut edema may contribute to the variable absorption of carbamazepine. Carbamazepine may cause sodium and water retention, aggravating congestive heart failure. *Fever* (increased metabolism) and *pulmonary disease* (decreased metabolism) have been associated with alterations of antiepileptic drug clearance. Protein binding may be altered *postoperatively*.[8] The change in protein binding and altered metabolism were believed to be responsible for carbamazepine toxicity in patients following cardiothoracic surgery and myocardial infarction.[88]

The clearance of antiepileptic drugs increases during the third trimester of *pregnancy*, so the carbamazepine concentration should be closely monitored. A dose increase should be expected. Following delivery, the clearance returns to normal and the dose should be reduced.[89]

References

1. Graves NM, Garnett WR. Epilepsy. In: DiPiro JT, Talbert RL, Yee GC, et al. eds. Pharmacotherapy: a pathophysiologic approach. 4th ed. Stamford, Ct: Appleton and Lange; 1999: 952–75.
2. MacKichan JJ. Carbamazepine. In: Taylor WJ, Caviness MHD, eds. A textbook for the clinical application of therapeutic monitoring. Irving, TX: Abbott Laboratories; 1986:211–24.
3. Loiseau P, Bernard D. Carbamazepine: clinical use. In: Levy RH, Mattson RH, Meldrum BS. Antiepileptic drugs, 4th ed. New York: Raven Press; 1995:555–66.
4. Miles MV, Lawless ST, Tennison MB, et al. Rapid loading of critically ill patients with carbamazepine suspension. *Pediatrics*. 1990; 86:263–6.
5. Cohen H, Howland MA, Luciano DJ, et al. Feasibility and pharmacokinetics of carbamazepine oral loading doses. *Am J Health-Syst Pharm*. 1998; 55:1134–40.
6. Kanner AM, Bourgeois BF, Hasegawa H, et al. Rapid switch over to carbamazepine using pharmacokinetic parameters. *Epilepsia*. 1998; 39(2):194–200.
7. Gerardin A, Dobois JP, Moppert J, et al. Absolute bioavailability of carbamazepine after oral administration of a 2% syrup. *Epilepsia*. 1990; 31:334–8.
8. Morselli PL. Carbamazepine: absorption, distribution, and excretion. In: Levy RH, Mattson RH, Meldrum BS. Antiepileptic drugs, 4th ed. New York: Raven Press; 1995:515–28.

9. Sanchez A, Duran JA, Serrano JS. Steady-state carbamazepine plasma concentration–dose ratios in epileptic patients. *Clin Pharmacokinet.* 1986; 11:411–4.
10. Maas B, Garnett WR, Pellock JM, et al. A comparative bioavailability study of carbamazepine tablets and a chewable tablet formulation. *Ther Drug Monit.* 1987; 9:28–33.
11. Patsalos PN. A comparative pharmacokinetic study of conventional and chewable carbamazepine in epileptic patients. *Br J Clin Pharmacol.* 1990; 29:574–7.
12. Garnett WR, Carson SP, Pellock JM, et al. Comparison of carbamazepine and 10,11-diepoxide levels in children following chronic dosing with Tegretol suspension and Tegretol tablets. *Neurology.* 1987; 37 (Suppl 1): 93–4. Abstract.
13. Thakker KM, Mangat S, Garnett WR, et al. Comparative bioavailability and steady state fluctuations of Tegretol commercial and carbamazepine OROS tablets in adult and pediatric epileptic patients. *Biopharm Drug Disposition.* 1992; 13:559–69.
14. Garnett WR, Levy B, McLean AM, et al. Pharmacokinetic evaluation of twice-daily extended release carbamazepine (CBZ) and four times daily immediate release CBZ in patients with epilepsy. *Epilepsia.* 1998; 39(3):274–9.
15. Neuvonen PJ, Tokola O. Bioavailability of rectally administered carbamazepine mixture. *Br J Clin Pharmacol.* 1987; 24:839–41.
16. Carbamazepine and moisture. *Medicom.* 1990; 8:442.
17. Stevens RE, Lim Sakun T, Evans G, et al. Controlled, multidose, pharmacokinetic evaluation of two extended-release carbamazepine formulations (Carbatrol and Tegretol-XR). *J Pharm Sci.* 1998; 87:1531–4.
18. Wilding IR, Davis SS, Hardy JG, et al. Relationship between systemic drug absorption and gastrointestinal transit after the simultaneous oral administration of carbamazepine as a controlled-release system and as a suspension of 15N-labelled drug to healthy volunteers. *Br J Clin Pharmacol.* 1991; 32(5):573–9.
19. Hartley R, Forsythe WJ, McLain B, et al. Daily variations in steady-state plasma concentrations of carbamazepine and its metabolites in epileptic children. *Clin Pharmacokinet.* 1991; 20:237–44.
20. Riad LE, Chan KKH, Wagner WE, et al. Simultaneous first- and zero-order absorption of carbamazepine tablets in humans. *J Pharm Sci.* 1986; 75:897–900.
21. Bano G, Raina RK, Sharma DB. Pharmacokinetics of carbamazepine in protein energy malnutrition. *Pharmacology.* 1986; 32:232–6.
22. Baruzzi A, Contin M, Perucca E, et al. Altered serum protein binding of carbamazepine in disease states associated with an increased alpha$_1$ acid glycoprotein concentration. *Eur J Clin Pharmacol.* 1986; 31:85–9.
23. Gianelli M, Gentile S, Verze L, et al. Free drug levels monitoring as a detector of false metabolic refractory epilepsy. *Eur Neurol.* 1988; 28:349–53.
24. Koyama H, Sugioka N, Uno A, et al. Effect of glycosylation on carbamazepine-serum protein binding in humans. *J Clin Pharmacol.* 1997; 37(11):1048–55.

25. Pienimaki P, Lampela E, Hakkula J, et al. Pharmacokinetics of oxcarbazepine and carbamazepine in human placenta. *Epilepsia*. 1997; 38(3):309–16.
26. Gorodischer R, Burtin P, Verjee Z, et al. Is saliva suitable for therapeutic monitoring of anticonvulsants in children: an evaluation in the routine clinical setting. *Ther Drug Monit*. 1997; 19(6):637–42.
27. Faigle JW, Feldmann KF. Carbamazepine: Chemistry and Biotransformation. In: Levy RH, Mattson RH, Meldrum BS. Antiepileptic drugs, 4th ed. New York: Raven Press; 1995:499–513.
28. Sumi M, Watari N, Umezawa O, et al. Pharmacokinetic study of carbamazepine and its epoxide metabolite in humans. *J Pharmacobiodyn*. 1987; 10:652–61.
29. Tomson T, Almkvist O, Nilsson BY, et al. Carbamazepine-10,11-epoxide in epilepsy: a pilot study. *Arch Neurol*. 1990; 47:888–92.
30. Kerr BM, Thummel KE, Wurden CJ, et al. Human liver carbamazepine metabolism. Role of CYP3A4 and CYP2C8 in 10,11 epoxide formation. *Biochem Pharmacol*. 1994; 47(11):1969–79.
31. Kerr BM, Levy RH. Carbamazepine: carbamazepine epoxide. In: Levy RH, Mattson RH, Meldrum BS. Antiepileptic drugs, 4th ed. New York: Raven Press; 1995:529–41.
32. Robbins DK, Wedlund PJ, Baumann RJ, et al. Inhibition of epoxide hydrolase by valproic acid in epileptic patients receiving carbamazepine. *Br J Clin Pharmacol*. 1990; 29:759–62.
33. Mikati MA, Browne TR, Collins JG, et al. Time course of carbamazepine autoinduction. *Neurology*. 1989; 39:592–4.
34. Bertilsson L, Tomson T, Tybring G. Pharmacokinetics: time-dependent changes—autoinduction of carbamazepine epoxidation. *J Clin Pharmacol*. 1986; 26:459–62.
35. Delgado-Iribarnegaray MF, Santo Bueldga D, Garcia Sanchez MJ, et al. Carbamazepine population pharmacokinetics in children: mixed-effect models. *Ther Drug Monit*. 1997; 19(2):132–9.
36. Racine-Poon A, Dubois JP. Predicting the range of plasma carbamazepine concentrations in patients with epilepsy. *Stat Med*. 1989; 8:1327–37.
37. Gonzalez ACA, Sanchez MJG, Hurle AD-G. Contribution of serum level monitoring in the individualization of carbamazepine dosage regimens. *Int J Clin Pharmacol Ther Toxicol*. 1988; 26:409–12.
38. Garcia MJ, Alonso AC, Maza A, et al. Comparison of methods of carbamazepine dosage, individualization in epileptic patients. *J Clin Pharm Ther*. 1988; 13:375–80.
39. Levy RH, Kerr BM. Clinical pharmacokinetics of carbamazepine. *J Clin Psychiatry*. 1988; 49(Suppl):58–61.
40. Gray AL, Botha JH, Miller R, et al. A model for the determination of carbamazepine clearance in children on mono- and polytherapy. *Eur J Clin Pharmacol*. 1998; 54(4):359–62.
41. Hockings N, Pall A, Moody J, et al. The effects of age on carbamazepine pharmacokinetics and adverse effects. *Br J Clin Pharmacol*. 1986; 22:725–8.
42. Rowan AJ. Reflections on the treatment of seizures in elderly popu-

lation. *Neurology.* 1998; 51(5)(*Suppl 4*):S28–33.
43. Thomas RJ. Seizures and epilepsy in the elderly. *Arch Intern Med.* 1997; 157(6):605–17.
44. Bernus I, Dickinson RG, Hooper WD, et al. Anticonvulsant therapy in aged patients; clinical pharmacokinetic considerations. *Drugs Aging.* 1997; 10(4):278–89.
45. Graves NM, Brundage RG, Wen Y, et al. Population pharmacokinetics of carbamazepine in adults with epilepsy. *Pharmacotherapy.* 1998; 18(2):273–81.
46. Suemaru K, Kawasaki H, Yasuhara K, et al. Steady-state serum concentrations of carbamazepine and valproic acid in obese and lean patients with epilepsy. *Acta Med Okayama.* 1998; 52(3):139–42.
47. Kuranari M, Chiba S, Ashikari Y, et al. Clearance of phenytoin and valproic acid is affected by a small body weight reduction in an epileptic obese patient: a case study. *J Clin Pharm Ther.* 1996; 21(2):83–7.
48. Summers B, Summers RS. Carbamazepine clearance in paediatric epilepsy patients: Influence of body mass, dose, sex and co-medication. *Clin Pharmacokinet.* 1989; 17:208–16.
49. Gilman JT. Carbamazepine dosing for pediatric seizure disorders: the highs and lows. *DICP Ann Pharmacother.* 1991; 25:1109–12.
50. Holmes GL. Carbamazepine: toxicity. In: Levy RH, Mattson RH, Meldrum BS. Antiepileptic drugs, 4th ed. New York: Raven Press; 1995:567–79.
51. Takayanagi K, Hisauchi I, Watanabe J, et al. Carbamazepine induced sinus node dysfunction and atrioventricular block in elderly women. *Jpn Heart J.* 1998; 39(4):469–79.
52. Hetzel W. Anticonvulsant treatment in old age—principles and differential indications. *Fortschr Neurol Psychiatr.* 1997; 65(6):261–77.
53. Wolkenstein P, Tan C, Le Coeur S, et al. Covalent binding of carbamazepine reactive metabolites to P450 isoforms in the skin. *Chem Biol Interact.* 1998; 113(1):39–50.
54. Heyer G, Simon M, Schell H, et al. Dose-dependent pellagroid skin reaction caused by carbamazepine. *Hautarzt.* 1998; 49(2):123–5.
55. van Ginneken EE, van der Meer JW, Netten PM, et al. A man with mysterious hypogammaglobulinaemia and skin rash. *Neth J Med.* 1999; 54(4):158–62.
56. de la Cruz M, Bance M. Carbamazepine induced sensorineural hearing loss. *Arch Otolaryngol Head Neck Surg.* 1999; 125(2):225–7.
57. Eijgenraam JW, Buurke EJ, van der Laan JS. Carbamazepine associated acute tubulointerstitial nephritis. *Neth J Med.* 1997; 50(1):25–8.
58. McKinney PA, Finkenbine RD, DeVane CL. Alopecia and mood stabilizer therapy. *Ann Clin Psychiatry.* 1996; 8(3):183–5.
59. Mabuchi K, Hayashi S, Nitta E, et al. Auditory disturbance induced by carbamazepine administration in a patient with secondary generalized seizure. *Rinsho-Shinkeigaku.* 1995; 35(5):553–5.
60. Pellock JM, Willmore LJ. A rational guide to routine blood monitoring in patients receiving antiepileptic drugs. *Neurology.* 1991; 41:961–4.
61. Spina E, Pisani F, Perucca E. Clinically significant pharmacokinetic drug interactions with carbamazepine: an update. *Clin Pharmacokinet.*

1996; 31(3):198–214.
62. Emilien G, Maloteaux JM. Pharmacological management of epilepsy: mechanism of action, pharmacokinetic drug interactions, and new drug discovery possibilities. *Int J Clin Pharmacol Ther*. 1998; 36(4):181–94.
63. Riva R, Albani F, Contin M, et al. Pharmacokinetic interactions between antiepileptic drugs: clinical considerations. *Clin Pharmacokinet*. 1996; 31(6):470–93.
64. Ketter TA, Post RM, Worthington K. Principles of clinically important drug interactions with carbamazepine. Part I. *J Clin Psychopharmacol*. 1991; 11:198–203.
65. Ketter TA, Post RM, Worthington K. Principles of clinically important drug interactions with carbamazepine. Part II. *J Clin Psychopharmacol*. 1991; 11:306–13.
66. Levy RH, Wurden CJ. Carbamazepine: interactions with other drugs. In: Levy RH, Mattson RH, Meldrum BS. Antiepileptic drugs, 4th ed. New York: Raven Press; 1995:543–54.
67. Furukori H, Otani K, Yasuri N, et al. Effect of carbamazepine on the single oral dose pharmacokinetics of alprazolam. *Neuropsychopharmacology*. 1998; 18(5):364–9.
68. Otani K, Ishida M, Yasuri W, et al. Interaction between carbamazepine and bromperidol. *Eur J Clin Pharmacol*. 1997; 52(3):219–22.
69. Theis JG, Koren G, Daneman R, et al. Interactions of clobazam with conventional antiepileptics in children. *J Child Neurol*. 1997; 12(3):208–13.
70. Kelley MT, Walson PD, Cox S, et al. Population pharmacokinetics of felbamate in children. *Ther Drug Monit*. 1997; 19(1):29–36.
71. Bartoli A, Guerrini R, Belmonte A, et al. The influence of dosage, age, and comedication on steady state plasma lamotrigine concentrations in epileptic children: a prospective study with preliminary assessment of correlations with clinical response. *Ther Drug Monit*. 1997; 19(3):252–60.
72. Eriksson AS, Hoppu K, Nergardh A, et al. Pharmacokinetic interactions between lamotrigine and other antiepileptic drugs in children with intractable epilepsy. *Epilepsia*. 1996; 37(8):769–73.
73. Besag FM, Berry DJ, Newberry JE, et al. Carbamazepine toxicity and lamotrigine: pharmacokinetic or pharmacodynamic interaction? *Epilepsia*. 1998; 39(2):183–7.
74. Behar D, Schaller J, Spreat S, et al. Extreme reduction of methylphenidate levels by carbamazepine (letter). *J Am Acad Child Adolesc Psychiatry*. 1998; 37(11):1128–9.
75. Backman JT, Olkkola KT, Ojala M, et al. Concentrations and effects of midazolam are greatly reduced in patients treated with carbamazepine or phenytoin. *Epilepsia*. 1996; 37(3):253–7.
76. Lucas RA, Gilfiallan DJ, Berrstrom RF. A pharmacokinetic interaction between carbamazepine and olanzapine: observations on possible mechanism. *Eur J Clin Pharmacol*. 1998; 54(8):639–43.
77. Sachdeo RC, Sachdeo SK, Walker SA, et al. Steady state pharmacokinetics of topiramate and carbamazepine in patients with epilepsy

during monotherapy and concomitant therapy. *Epilepsia*. 1996; 37(8):774–80.
78. Alloul K, Whalley DG, Shutway F, et al. Pharmacokinetic origin of carbamazepine-induced resistance to vecuronium neuromuscular blockage in anesthetized patients. *Anesthesiology*. 1996; 84(2):330–9.
79. Vaz J, Kulkami C, David J, et al. Influence of caffeine on pharmacokinetic profile of sodium valproate and carbamazepine in normal human volunteers. *Indian J Exp Biol*. 1998; 36(1):112–4.
80. Glue P, Banfield CR, Perhach JL, et al. Pharmacokinetic interactions with felbamate: in vitro-in vivo correlation. *Clin Pharmacokinet*. 1997; 33(3):214–24.
81. Amsden GW. Erythromycin, clarithromycin, and azithromycin—are the differences real? *Clin Ther*. 1996; 18(1):56–72.
82. Cottencin O, Regnaut N, Thevenon-Gignac C, et al. Carbamazepine-fluvoxamine interaction. Consequences for the carbamazepine plasma level. *Encephale*. 1995; 21(2):141–5.
83. Garg SK, Kumar N, Bhargava VK, et al. Effect of grapefruit juice on carbamazepine bioavailability in patients with epilepsy. *Clin Pharm Ther*. 1998; 64(3):286–8.
84. Bernus I, Dickinson RG, Hooper WD, et al. The mechanism of carbamazepine-valproate interaction in humans. *Br J Clin Pharmacol*. 1997; 44(1):21–7.
85. Clark-Schmidt AL, Garnett WR, Lowe DR, et al. Loss of carbamazepine suspension through nasogastric feeding tubes. *Am J Hosp Pharm*. 1990; 47:2034–7.
86. Bass J, Miles MV, Tennison MB, et al. Effects of enteral tube feeding on the absorption and pharmacokinetic profile of carbamazepine suspension. *Epilepsia*. 1989; 30:364–9.
87. Kandrotas RJ, Oles KS, Gal P, et al. Carbamazepine clearance in hemodialysis and hemoperfusion. *DICP Ann Pharmacother*. 1989; 23:137–40.
88. Wright PS, Seifert CF, Hampton EM. Toxic carbamazepine concentrations following cardiothoracic surgery and myocardial infarction. *DICP Ann Pharmacother*. 1990; 24:822–6.
89. Dam M, Christiansen J, Munck O, et al. Antiepileptic drugs: metabolism in pregnancy. *Clin Pharmacokinet*. 1979; 4:53–62.

Chapter 7
C. Lindsay Devane

Cyclic Antidepressants
(AHFS 28:16.04)

The cyclic antidepressants have multiple uses for both mental and physical disorders. The specific drugs listed (but not ranked) here in parenthesis are particularly useful for the indicated condition. However, this list is based in part on single-case reports and studies with only limited numbers of patients. While the tricyclic antidepressants continue to be available, their use is declining in favor of the selective serotonin reuptake inhibitors and newer drugs.[1]

For *children and adolescents* (younger than 18 years), the cyclic antidepressants are used for[2,3]

- Depression (not recommended for children under 12 years).
- Enuresis (imipramine).
- Attention-deficit disorder (bupropion).
- Separation-anxiety disorder or school phobia.
- Somnambulism and night terrors.
- Obsessive compulsive disorder [clomipramine and selective serotonin reuptake inhibitors (SSRIs)].

- Anorexia nervosa.
- Bulimia nervosa.

For *adults*, these drugs are used for[4]

- Mood disorders: recurrent major depression, bipolar depression, and dysthymia.
- Panic disorder (imipramine and SSRI).
- Agoraphobia.
- Obsessive compulsive disorder (clomipramine and SSRI).
- Social Anxiety Disorder (SSRI).
- Premenstrual Dysphoric Disorder (SSRI).
- Migraine headache.
- Obesity (fluoxetine).
- Peptic ulcer disease (doxepin).
- Premature ejaculation.
- Post-traumatic stress disorder.
- Sleep apnea (protriptyline).
- Chronic pain syndrome (amitriptyline and SSRI).

For some of these uses, data exist for only one drug. Therefore, therapeutic concentration ranges are difficult to predict when crossing lines of therapeutic use. Another problem for the pharmacokineticist working with cyclic antidepressants is the presence of active drug metabolites. Several metabolites may result from a single administered drug. Unfortunately, while some metabolites are recognized as pharmacologically active, their contributions to clinical response or toxicity have not all been investigated, nor are guidelines available for interpreting their concentrations.

This chapter outlines the adult population parameters for numerous cyclic antidepressants. Although these drugs are used in children and adolescents, these populations are not included here. If such information is required, primary literature that examines the specific drug in the pediatric population should be consulted. Monoamine oxidase inhibitors also are not discussed because their concentration measures have not generally been investigated for their utility in clinical practice.

Of course, the broad variability in pharmacokinetic parameters, especially clearance, demands individualization of antidepressant therapy. Many patients who receive adequate—even optimal—therapy may be outside the range of plasma concentration values considered as normal or therapeutic. When a patient is responding well, the dosage should not be altered to bring the concentration into some defined range unless toxicity is a concern. Reviews of these issues have been published.[5-7]

Usual Dosage Range in Absence of Clearance-Altering Factors[7-9]

The following oral (tablet, capsule, and solution) dosage ranges are suggested for the treatment of adult depression. Other indications may require dosage adjustment. For example, the use of fluoxetine for panic disorder requires small initial doses, 5–10 mg, to avoid excessive activation. The typical daily dose listed is that approved for adults by the FDA. Nevertheless, some patients may benefit from higher doses, especially if monitoring reveals relatively low concentrations because of rapid clearance.

Only one cyclic antidepressant, amitriptyline, is currently available in injectable form for intramuscular use, but this is not recommended for usual clinical use.

Drug	Initial Dosage[a]	Typical Daily Dosage Range
Amitriptyline	25 mg twice daily	50–300 mg
Amoxapine	50 mg two or three times daily	50–600 mg
Bupropion	100 mg twice daily	200–450 mg; 400 mg/day maximum for sustained release

Citalopram	20 mg daily	20–60 mg
Clomipramine[b]	25–100 mg daily	25–250 mg
Desipramine	25 mg three times daily	100–300 mg
Doxepin	25 mg three times daily	75–300 mg
Fluoxetine	10–20 mg daily	20–80 mg
Fluvoamine[b]	50 mg daily	50–300 mg
Imipramine	25 mg three times daily	75–300 mg
Maprotiline	25 mg three times daily	75–225 mg
Mirtazapine	15 mg daily	15–45 mg
Nefazodone	100 mg twice daily	600 mg
Nortriptyline	25 mg three times daily	75–200 mg
Paroxetine	20 mg daily	10–60 mg
Protriptyline	15 mg daily	15–60 mg
Reboxetine	4 mg twice daily	8–10 mg
Sertraline	50 mg daily	50–200 mg
Trazodone	50 mg three times daily	150–600 mg
Trimipramine	25 mg three times daily	50–300 mg
Venlafaxine	37.5–75 mg daily	75–375 mg; 225 mg/day maximum for sustained release

[a]*In geriatric patients the starting dose is generally less than the young adult dose.*
[b]*The dosage given is for obsessive-compulsive disorder. Labeling for treatment of depression has not been approved in the United States.*

Considerations in the selection of an initial antidepressant are beyond the scope of this chapter and were reviewed elsewhere.[8,10,11]

Loading doses are not used with these cyclic antidepressants. Many patients find their side effects distressing and cannot tolerate high initial doses. The daily dosage is usually titrated beginning with the smallest dose listed above. Since elderly patients are frequently sensitive to these standard initial doses, their starting doses are often reduced by one-third or one-half. In addition, reduced clearance in the elderly compared with younger patients often translates into smaller milligram maintenance doses.[12] However, the variability in clearance is great, and not all elderly patients have higher than usual concentrations from standard doses. All elderly patients should be dosed with caution.

After dosing is initiated, the daily dose is increased according to acceptance at several day intervals. The rate of dosage acceleration partly depends on the clinician's experience with the patient, the severity of symptomatology, and inpatient or outpatient status. When an acceptable dosage is reached, the plasma concentration may be checked. However, such checking is often unnecessary if the clinical response is adequate. As the SSRIs and other newer antidepressants have generally supplanted the traditional tricyclics as first-line agents for the treatment of depression, therapeutic drug monitoring for tricyclic antidepressants has become less useful.

Dosage Form Availability

The cyclic antidepressants are available from various manufacturers in several oral dosage forms including tablets with or without film coatings, capsules, and solutions. As previously mentioned, amitriptyline also is available in an injectable form for intramuscular administration.

Drug	Dosage Form	Product
Amitriptyline	Tablets: 10, 25, 50, 75, 100, and 150 mg	Elavil
	Parenteral injection: 10 mg/ml	Elavil
Amoxapine	Tablets: 25, 50, 100, and 150 mg	Asendin
Bupropion	Tablets: 75 and 100 mg	Wellbutrin
	Sustained release tablets: 100 and 150 mg	Wellbutrin SR, Zyban
Citalopram	Tablets: 20 and 40 mg	Celexa
	Oral solution: 10 mg/5 ml	
Clomipramine	Capsules: 25, 50, and 75 mg	Anafranil
Desipramine	Tablets: 10, 25, 50, 75, 100, and 150 mg	Norpramin
	Capsules: 25 and 50 mg	Pertofrane
Doxepin	Capsules: 10, 25, 50, 75, 100, and 150 mg	Adapin Sinequan
	Oral concentrated solution: 10 mg/ml	Sinequan
Fluoxetine	Capsules: 10 and 20 mg	Prozac
	Oral solution: 20 mg/5 ml	Prozac
Fluvoxamine	Tablets: 25, 50, and 100 mg	Luvox
Imipramine	Tablets: 10, 25, and 50 mg	Tofranil
	Capsules: 75, 100, 125, and 150 mg	Tofranil-PM
Maprotiline	Tablets: 25, 50, and 75 mg	Ludiomil
Mirtazapine	Tablets: 15 and 30 mg	Remeron
Nefazodone	Tablets: 50, 100, 150, 200, and 250 mg	Serzone
Nortriptyline	Capsules: 10, 25, 50, and 75 mg	Aventyl, Pamelor
	Oral solution: 10 mg/5 ml	Aventyl, Pamelor
Paroxetine	Tablets: 10, 20, 30, and 40 mg	Paxil
	Oral solution: 10 mg/5 ml	Paxil
	Sustained release: 12.5 and 25 mg	Paxil CR
Protriptyline	Tablets: 5 and 10 mg	Vivactil

Reboxetine	Expected to be marketed as tablets by 2001	Vestra
Sertraline	Tablets: 25, 50, and 100 mg Oral concentrate: 20 mg/5 ml	Zoloft
Trazodone	Capsules: 50, 100, 150, and 300 mg	Desyrel
Trimipramine	Capsules: 25, 50, and 100 mg	Surmontil
Venlafaxine	Tablets: 25, 37.5, 50, 75, and 100 mg Sustained-release capsules: 37.5, 75, and 150 mg	Effexor and Effexor-XR

General Pharmacokinetic Information

The major pharmacokinetic parameters of the cyclic antidepressants for healthy adults are summarized in Table 1.[9] Reboxetine is expected to be marketed soon as a selective norepinephrine reuptake inhibitor.[13]

The cyclic antidepressants are highly lipophilic compounds, usually basic amines with pKas of 7–10. They generally are readily and completely absorbed in the small intestine but undergo extensive presystemic elimination in the liver. This characteristic makes plasma concentrations highly variable among patients receiving the identical dose. The extent of extraction by the liver classifies these drugs as moderate to high clearance, with extraction ratios of 0.5–0.8.

These drugs are highly plasma and tissue bound, with volumes of distribution greatly exceeding body weight which implies much greater tissue than plasma concentrations. As little as 3% of the total body burden of some drugs resides in the circulating plasma. Thus, extracorporeal methods of drug elimination (hemodialysis and hemoperfusion) have little benefit in the treatment of overdosage.[16] Fortunately, the newer selective serotonin reuptake inhibitors appear to be less toxic in overdose than the older tricyclic antidepressants.[9,10,14,17,18]

While drug elimination is mostly accomplished by hepatic processes, many drugs produce pharmacologically

TABLE 1. Pharmacokinetic Parameters for Cyclic Antidepressants in Healthy Adults[5,6,14,15]

Drug	Bioavailability (F)[a]	Clearance (CL)[b]	Volume of Distribution (V)	Half-Life	Active Metabolites
Amitriptyline	30–60%	19–72 L/hr	6–36 L/kg	9–46 hr	Nortriptyline hydroxy
Amoxapine	46–82%	42–73 L/hr	c	8–14 hr	7-Hydroxy amoxapine, 8-hydroxy amoxapine
Bupropion	>90%	126–140 L/hr	27–63 L/kg	9–21 hr	Hydroxy-bupropion
Citalopram	95%	23–38 L/hr	14 L/kg	23–45 hr	Desmethyl, didesmethyl
Clomipramine	36–62%	23–122 L/hr	9–25 L/kg	15–62 hr	N-Desmethyl-
Desipramine	33–51%	78–168 L/hr	24–60 L/kg	12–28 hr	Hydroxy-
Doxepin	13–45%	41–61 L/hr	9–33 L/kg	8–25 hr	Desmethyl-
Fluoxetine	>70%	5–42 L/hr	12–42 L/kg	26–220 hr	Norfluoxetine
Fluvoxamine	>90%	33–320 L/hr	>5 L/kg	9–28 hr	None
Imipramine	30–70%	32–102 L/hr	9–23 L/kg	6–28 hr	Desipramine, 2-hydroxy-
Maprotiline	70–90%	17–34 L/hr	16–32 L/kg	27–50 hr	Desmethyl-

Mirtazapine	50%	[c]	4.5 L/kg	13–34 hr	None at significant concentrations
Nefazodone	>20%	[c]	0.2–1.0 L/kg	2–8 hr	Hydroxy, m-chlorophenylpiperazine
Nortriptyline	46–70%	17–79 L/hr	15–32 L/kg	18–56 hr	10-Hydroxy-
Paroxetine	>90%	15–92 L/hr	3–28 L/kg	7–37 hr	None
Protriptyline	75–90%	8–23 L/hr	15–31 L/kg	54–198 hr	Desmethyl-
Reboxetine	>60%	1.7 L/hr	0.5 L/kg	12–16 hr	None
Serrtraline	>44%	96 L/hr	>20 L/kg	22–36 hr	Desmethyl-
Trazodone	70–90%	7–12 L/hr	1–2 L/kg	3–14 hr	m-Chlorophenylpiperazine
Trimipramine	18–63%	40–105 L/hr	17–48 L/kg	16–40 hr	Desmethyl-
Venlafaxine	92%	40–129 L/hr	2–23 L/kg	2–11 hr	o-Desmethyl

[a] Values are misleadingly low due to extensive presystemic elimination.
[b] Values approach or exceed hepatic blood flow due to an inherent artifact in calculating clearance from oral dose data.
[c] Reliable values are not available in the literature.

active metabolites.[9-11] The concentrations of these metabolites often exceed those of the parent drug. Plasma concentrations also are relatively low, nanograms per milliliter, compared to other drugs for their usually administered daily dosages (e.g., 100–300 mg/day for the tricyclic antidepressants). Thus, analytical methods must have rigorous quality control to ensure good reproducibility.

Therapeutic Range

The use of plasma concentrations to determine adequate dosages for the cyclic antidepressants is complicated by the lack of rigorously defined therapeutic ranges. Furthermore, the use of dosage ranges with the cyclic antidepressants is complicated by the variability of patient response to various concentrations. Due to the vast differences in kinetic parameters among patient populations, clinical response may be the best predictor of adequate dosage.

The cyclic antidepressants with the most established therapeutic ranges are nortriptyline, imipramine, desipramine, and amitriptyline.[19] The SSRI and other newer antidepressants, including mirtazapine, nefazodone, reboxetine, and venlafaxine have not been reported to have a plasma concentration range correlated with clinical response or adverse events that can be used in therapeutic drug monitoring. Average steady-state concentrations from usual doses have been reported which may be useful in following compliance or assessing the presence of drug–drug interactions.

Tricyclic antidepressants

Several studies[5,20,21] confirmed that a curvilinear therapeutic window exists for nortriptyline; the best antidepressant response in frequently obtained with a concentration of 50–150 µg/L. The combined plasma concentration of imipramine and its demethylated metabolite, desipramine, is frequently 180–350 µg/L when optimal antidepressant response is observed.[19] However, the dose–response curve is thought to be more linear compared to that of nortriptyline and the upper limit of the range is less distinct. Children may respond at the same or at a lower concentration as adults.[22]

It is rarely justified for imipramine plus desipramine concentrations to exceed 350 µg/L. However, an occasional patient will have excessive concentrations from usual doses, probably due to a genetically determined poor hepatic hydroxylation ability. A concentration >500 µg/L should prompt great concern. A concentration of 1000 µg/L for any tricyclic antidepressant may herald extreme toxicity (seizures, arrhythmias, coma) and is sometimes used to define an overdose.

Desipramine concentrations of 115–250 µg/L are frequently therapeutic. Unfortunately, side effects of all TCAs can occur at any concentration and cannot be used to reflect the drug concentration.[23] Evidence for amitriptyline's therapeutic range is generally lacking.[24] At a minimum, concentrations of amitriptyline plus nortriptyline much below the 120–250 µg/L range will not be therapeutic except in a small number of patients. Concentrations much above this range, and frequently when above 450 µg/L, suggest that anticholinergic delirium is present or impending.[25]

Other antidepressants

For the remaining cyclic antidepressants, the therapeutic ranges listed reflect the concentrations obtained during chronic therapy and do not necessarily correlate strongly to clinical response. Responders will exist outside of the ranges listed, and nonresponders will have steady-state concentrations within the desired ranges. Nonetheless, drug concentration measures may be useful in monitoring adherence, documenting drug interactions, and monitoring safety in special populations such as the elderly, children, or others at high risk.

The popularity of the newer antidepressants, particularly the SSRIs, can be partly explained by their improved side effect profile and lower overdose toxicity compared with the older tricyclics. Although these drugs are extensively used, guidelines for drug concentration monitoring have not caught up with their potential clinical utility.

Three reports examined the value of monitoring bupropion concentrations.[26-28] Such monitoring is at an early stage of development, but preliminary data suggest that high hydroxymetabolite concentrations, greater than 1200 µg/L, may undermine response. Unfortunately, the assay capability for measuring bupropion's metabolites is not widely available. For bupropion alone, concentrations associated with clinical response appear to be in the 20–50 µg/L range and are usually <100 µg/L.

Seven studies examined whether a therapeutic range exists for fluoxetine.[29,30] Two reports found no relationship between drug concentrations and clinical effects. However, the other data suggest the existence of a possible therapeutic window where high concentrations of the metabolite, norfluoxetine, are associated with nonresponse. Overall, the best response appears when the combined fluoxetine plus norfluoxetine concentration is less than 500 µg/L; however plasma concentrations measured are still considered experimental and not yet justified for clinical use.[66]

With most cyclic antidepressants, the presence of active drug metabolites may be important. The hydroxylated metabolites of tricyclic antidepressants are pharmacologically active and can accumulate to concentrations higher than the parent drugs.[31-33] Their presence in cerebrospinal fluid is further evidence of their potential contribution to clinical and/or adverse effects.

When antidepressant therapy is monitored, the effects of physiological status on pharmacokinetics should be remembered. Drug interactions also can alter the expected dose–response relationships; more complete references of drug interactions should be consulted.[34]

When clinical response is adequate, dosage adjustment is unnecessary. For imipramine and nortriptyline, the dosage should be altered to bring concentrations into the therapeutic range before deciding that a patient is a true nonresponder. For the remaining drugs, the ranges listed here provide guidelines for therapy.

Drug	Average Steady-state Concentration Range[a]
Amitriptyline[35,36]	120–250 µg/L[b,c]
Amoxapine[37]	200–600 µg/L[d]
Bupropion[26,38]	20–50 µg/L, <100 µg/L[e]
Citalopram[8]	40–300 µg/L
Clomipramine[39–41]	100–250 µg/L[b,f]
Desipramine[42]	>115–250 µg/L
Doxepin[43]	>110–250 µg/L[b,d]
Fluoxetine[29]	75–450 µg/L[g]
Fluvoxamine[8]	20–500 µg/L
Imipramine[44,45]	180–350 µg/L[b,c]
Maprotiline[46]	200–600 µg/L[b,d]
Mirtazapine[8]	20–40 µg/L
Nefazodone[8]	150–1000 µg/L
Nortriptyline[19,47]	50–150 µg/L[h]
Paroxetine	10–600 µg/L
Protriptyline[48,49]	75–250 µg/L[d]
Reboxetine[8]	50–160 µg/L
Sertraline	20–200 µg/L
Trazodone[50,51]	500–1500 µg/L
Trimipramine[52]	100–300 µg/L[d]
Venlafaxine[8]	50–150 µg/L

[a]Applies to treatment of major depression. Concentration monitoring may be particularly helpful in situations of overdosage, inadequate response, diagnosis of noncompliance, and investigation of drug interactions.
[b]Parent drug plus desmethyl metabolite.
[c]Therapeutic range is less established than for nortriptyline. Concentrations greater than 450 µg/L frequently correlate with delirium and anticholinergic toxicity. Some responders occur below this range.
[d]No established therapeutic range; responders are frequently in this range.
[e]Limited data are available but suggest that high parent drug concentrations (greater than 100 µg/L) may be disadvantageous; one small study suggested that high hydroxylated metabolite concentrations correlated with the lack of antidepressant response.
[f]Parent drug concentrations. Metabolite concentrations may be somewhat higher. Therapeutic range is not well established.
[g]Sparce data are available. Metabolite concentrations may fall in the same range as for the parent drug but persist longer after discontinuance of dosing due to a prolonged half-life.
[h]Clear therapeutic window with curvilinear response. Many patients with concentrations greater than 150 µg/L show a poor response; a better response occurs if the dose is decreased to produce concentrations within the range.

Suggested Sampling Times

Any interpretation of drug concentrations should consider the average time to reach steady state. For most of the drugs listed in Table 1, the minimum time is 4–7 days. Exceptions are protriptyline and fluoxetine; because of the long half-life of the drug or metabolite, at least 2 weeks of constant dosing with protriptyline may be required before steady-state conditions occur and up to 4 weeks for fluoxetine. For antidepressants with relatively short half-lives, nefazodone and venlafaxine, steady-state concentrations of the parent drugs may be reached in 3–4 days.

For many patients, the empirically selected dosage will be adequate. However, if patient response is poor, application of the purported therapeutic ranges may be useful. For most of these drugs, the ranges listed represent the usual concentrations during treatment with usual daily doses. They are not rigorously defined ranges within which patients always show the best response.

Several methods use a concentration determined shortly after the initial dose to select a constant dosage for reaching a targeted concentration at steady state. These methods have acceptable accuracy and probably have been underutilized. They were thoroughly reviewed elsewhere.[53] They require use of a previously established mathematical relationship between the drug concentration determined one or more times after a single dose and the concentration produced at steady state following constant dosing.[22] The use of this type of predictive approach with a new patient assumes that the patient's drug disposition pattern will be similar to that of the previously tested population.

Nomograms are available, or several concentrations determined after the first dose can be used to estimate clearance and to predict a dosage for a targeted steady state with simple mathematical relationships. Any drug can be dosed according to this approach if it follows linear disposition—if a change in the daily dose, either an increase or decrease, results in a proportional change in the drug concentration. The most applicable drug for prospective dosing methods is nortriptyline with its widely accepted therapeutic concentration range.[53]

For most patients, linearity can be assumed in drug disposition with the tricyclic antidepressants, and dosage can be adjusted according to the principles outlined elsewhere in this book. Dosage changes made to achieve a new concentration should always be guided by feedback from acute and chronic pharmacological effects (presence or lack of side effects and therapeutic effects). Nonlinearity may be encountered occasionally[54] and can be manifested by an exaggerated clinical response to a dosage increase or a disproportional increase (for a given dose) in the concentration of a drug and/or metabolites. Nonlinearity has been documented for the newer antidepressants paroxetine and fluoxetine but this characteristic does not appear to be clinically significant.[9] This possibility is one reason why increasingly smaller doses should be used for dose increments.

Each patient's response to a drug follows dose–response relationships that may be steep or shallow, depending on the specific pharmacological effect observed and clinical circumstances. Clinical response always should be followed closely, including target symptoms, when a dosage change is considered. With this group of drugs, additional time often is all that is needed for improved response; pharmacodynamic effects frequently lag behind the achievement of steady-state drug conditions. Clinical experience indicates that an inadequate response with therapeutic concentrations may improve after additional treatment at the same dose and concentration.

Further Considerations for Sampling

Proper interpretation of drug concentration values requires knowledge of certain variables in the dosage regimen design. Knowledge of the length of time a constant dosage has been used is necessary to evaluate whether steady-state conditions exist. The mean estimates for half-life given in Table 1 can be used to predict the time (equal to four to five half-lives of constant dosing) necessary to elapse to approach pseudo steady state. The term "pseudo" indicates that a constant concentration is never achieved with oral dosing because the concentration is either rising or falling during a dosage interval. Thus, an accepted standardized time for drawing blood is approximately 12 hr after the previous dose, usually early in the morning.

Analytical methods used to quantify cyclic antidepressant concentrations in plasma vary in their expense, sensitivity, reliability, and ease of operations. Currently employed methods include radioimmunoassay, high performance liquid chromatography, gas chromatography, and enzyme and fluorescence immunoassay methods (EMIT and TDX). All are sensitive enough to provide reliable data for routine monitoring purposes, but the laboratory must maintain an internal and external quality control program.

Drug–Drug Interactions

Pharmacodynamic and pharmacokinetic interactions of antidepressants are summarized in Table 2. The capacity for some newer drugs to inhibit isoforms of the cytochrome (CYP) P450 system in recent years has stimulated much research in this field. More in-depth discussions have been published.[55–60]

Among the SSRIs, fluoxetine and paroxetine strongly inhibit CYP2D6. Fluoxetine also has been shown to be a mild inhibitor of CYP2C9; its metabolite in high concentrations is a potential CYP3A4 inhibitor, but there is little documentation that fluoxetine interacts with CYP3A4. Sertraline is only a mild inhibitor of

TABLE 2. Selected Drug Interactions of Cyclic Antidepressants

Drug	Combined Therapy	Interaction	Suggested Action
Bupropion	Carbamazepine, phenobarbital, phenytoin	Reduce antidepressant concentration	Monitor effects closely
	Monoamine oxidase inhibitors[b]	Potential toxicity	Contraindicated
	Drugs with seizure activity	Combined increased risk	Use with caution
Mirtazapine	Benzodiazepines	Increased sedation, other side effects	Avoid or lower doses and monitor
	Monoamine oxidase inhibitors[b]	Potential serotonin syndrome	Contraindicated
Nefazodone	Alprazolam, triazolam	Increased anxiolytic concentration	Use reduced benzodiazepine doses
	Monoamine oxidase inhibitors[b]	Toxicity	Contraindicated
SSRIs[a]	Alprazolam	Increased anxiolytic concentration with fluvoxamine and nefazodone	Monitor effects, may require reduced dosage
	Antiarrhythmics (Type IC), beta-blockers	Some combinations result in enhanced concentration	Consider non-interacting SSRI, or monitor and adjust doses
	Carbamazepine	Increased concentration in some patients	Monitor carbamazepine concentration
	Cimetidine	Increased SSRI concentration	Usually no action required
	Clozapine	Increased concentration from fluvoxamine and fluoxetine	Monitor clozapine concentration
	Codeine	Inhibited metabolism to morphine by CYP2D6 inhibitors	Use non-interacting SSRI or other antidepressant
	Monoamine oxidase inhibitors[b]	Possible serotonin syndrome	Contraindicated combination
	Phenytoin	Increased concentration with fluoxetine, possible with fluvoxamine and sertraline	Monitor anticonvulsant concentration

TABLE 2. (*continued*)

Drug	Combined Therapy	Interaction	Suggested Action
	Theophylline	Increased concentration with fluvoxamine	Monitor theophylline concentration, use lower doses as needed
	Tricyclic antidepressants	Reciprocal inhibition	Monitor, use lower doses as needed
	Warfarin	Increased warfarin effects	Monitor prothrombin time
Tricyclic antidepressants	Anticholinergics	Increased adverse effects	Use lower initial doses
	Antipsychotics	Mutual inhibition with some concentration	Use lower initial doses
	Carbamazepine, barbiturates	Decreased tricyclic antidepressant concentration	Monitor effects and concentrations as needed
	Cimetidine, disulfiram, methadone, quinidine, SSRIs[a]	Increased concentration of some drugs or metabolites	Monitor concentrations when appropriate
	Monoamine oxidase inhibitors[b]	Fatal reaction possible	Contraindicated combination
	Valproate	Tricyclic antidepressants can increase	Monitor concentration and effects
Venlafaxine	Cimetidine	Increased venlafaxine concentration	No action usually required, monitor
	Haloperidol	Increased haloperidol concentration	Monitor and adjust doses as needed
	Monoamine oxidase inhibitors	Toxicity	Contraindicated

[a]SSRIs = selective serotonin reuptake inhibitors.
[b]Severe reactions, including death, have occurred when monoamine oxidase inhibitors have been combined with antidepressants. Symptoms that suggest a serotonin syndrome include tremore, myoclonus, diaphoresis, nausea, vomiting, dizziness, and hyperthermia.

CYP2D6 while fluvoxamine is unique among the SSRIs in its potent inhibition of CYP1A2. It also inhibits CYP2C9 and CYP3A4. Citalopram appears to have the least potential to participate in cytochrome P450 mediated drug interactions among the SSRIs. Nefazodone is a potent CYP3A4 inhibitor while the other newer antidepressants, venlafaxine, mirtazapine, and reboxetine appear to have the least liability for pharmacokinetic interactions. The labeling for buproprion notes the possibility of CYP2D6 inhibition but patient reports are lacking.

Drug–Disease State or Condition Interactions

Adolescence

Milligram per kilogram requirements may be higher compared with adult doses due to more efficient hepatic elimination. Chronic therapy may require increased doses to maintain the same concentration.[61]

Advanced age

Geriatric patients have decreased ability to metabolize cyclic antidepressants. Drug concentrations are higher due to decreased clearance and prolonged half-life. The elderly (older than 65 years) should receive smaller initial doses (one-third to one-half reduction); however, some elderly will show no apparent impairment in clearance compared to younger patients.[12,62] This is because CYP450 enzymes do not decrease in activity uniformly with age. CYP2D6 is still preserved in the elderly while total P450 content decreases markedly after age 70 years.[62]

Alcoholism, alcoholic liver disease

The usual result is impairment of drug metabolism accompanied by a longer half-life and higher concentrations. Worse adverse drug reactions are possible.[63]

Cardiac disease

Little data exist on alterations of pharmacokinetic parameters. Orthostatic hypotension may become worse, especially with tricyclic antidepressants and trazodone. Caution is required due to tachycardia and anticholinergic effects of tricyclics. Tricyclic antidepressants may be relatively contraindicated in severe conduction defects. The safest drugs are bupropion and the SSRIs in comparison to the tricyclic antidepressants.[64]

Inflammatory disease states

Protein binding may be altered due to increases in alpha-1-acid glycoprotein, but the importance of protein binding changes is not supported by extensive literature documentation.

Nutritional status

Severe malnutrition may alter protein binding. Although literature documentation is limited, caution is warranted.

Renal failure

Parent drug concentrations of most cyclic antidepressants are not greatly affected, but conjugated metabolites can show excessive accumulation. In severe renal failure, more adverse consequences occur from normal doses. Dosages should be reduced.[65]

Smoking status

Smoking has an inductive effect on hepatic microsomal enzymes responsible for metabolizing cyclic antidepressants. A decreased steady-state concentration and more rapid drug elimination may result. Initial doses do not need to be higher in smokers compared to nonsmokers.[63]

Thyroid disease

Documentation of effects on pharmacokinetics is lacking. Hypothyroidism may mimic depression and result in a lack of antidepressant response until the underlying problem is treated. L-Triiodothyronine (T_3) is sometimes used as an adjunct to antidepressant therapy in relatively nonresponders.[66]

References

1. Hirschfeld RMA. Efficacy of SSRI's and newer antidepressants in severe depresssion: Comparison with TCAs. *J Clin Psychiatry.* 1999; 60:326–35.
2. DeVane CL, Sallee FR. Serotonin selective reuptake inhibitors in child and adolescent psychopharmacology: a review of published experience. *J Clin Psychiatry.* 1996; 57:55–66.
3. Green WH. Child and adolescent clinical psychopharmacology. Baltimore, MD: Williams & Wilkins; 1991.
4. United States pharmacopeia dispensing information: drug information for the health care professional, 17th ed. Rockville, MD: United States Pharmacopeial Convention; 1997.
5. DeVane CL, Jarecke R. Cyclic antidepressants. In: Evans WE, Schentag JJ, Jusko WJ, eds. Applied pharmacokinetics, principles of therapeutic drug monitoring, 3rd ed. Vancouver, WA: Applied Therapeutics; 1992.
6. Preskorn SH, Dorey RC, Jerkovich GS. Therapeutic drug monitoring of tricyclic antidepressants. *Clin Chem.* 1988; 34:822–8.
7. DeVane CL. Fundamentals of monitoring psychoactive drug therapy. Baltimore, MD: Williams & Wilkins; 1990.
8. Frazer A. Pharmacology of antidepressants. *J Clin Psychopharmacol.* 1997; 17(*Suppl 1*):2–18.
9. DeVane CL. Differential pharmacology of newer antidepressants. *J Clin Psychiatry.* 1998; 59 (*Suppl 20*):85–93.
10. Potter WZ, Manji HK, Rudorfer MV. Tricyclics and Tetracyclics. In: Schatzberg AF, Nemeroff CB, eds. American psychiatric press textbook of psychopharmacology, 2nd ed. Washington, DC: APA Press; 1998: 199–218.
11. Tollefson GD, Rosenbaum JF. Selective serotonin reuptake inhibitors. In: Schatzberg AF, Nemeroff CB, eds. American psychiatric press textbook of psychopharmacology, 2nd ed. Washington DC: APA Press; 1998:219–37.
12. DeVane CL, Pollock BG. Pharmacokinetic considerations of antidepressant use in the elderly. *J Clin Psychiatry.* (in press, 1999).
13. Riva M, Brunello N, Rovescalli AC, et al. Effect of reboxetine, a new antidepressant drug, on the central noradrenergic system: behavioural and biochemical studies. *J Drug Develop.* 1989; 1:243–53.

14. DeVane CL. Metabolism and pharmacokinetics of selective serotonin reuptake inhibitors. *Cell Mol Neurobiol.* 1999; 19:443–66.
15. Rudorfer MV, Potter WZ. Metabolism of tricyclic antidepressants. *Cell Mol Neurobiol.* 1999; 19:373–409.
16. Pentel PR, Bullock ML, DeVane CL. Hemoperfusion for imipramine overdose: elimination of active metabolites. *J Toxicol Clin Toxicol.* 1982; 19:239–48.
17. Borys DJ, Setzer SC, Ling LJ, et al. The effect of fluoxetine in the overdose patient. *J Toxicol Clin Toxicol.* 1990; 28:331–40.
18. Barbey JT, Roose SP. SSRI safety in overdose. *J Clin Psychiatry.* 1998; 59:42–8.
19. Glassman AH, Schildkraut JJ, Orsulak PJ, et al. Tricyclic antidepressant blood level measurements and clinical outcome. *Am J Psychiatry.* 1985; 142:155–63.
20. Kragh-Sorensen P, Hansen CE, Baastrup PC, et al. Self-inhibiting action of nortriptyline's antidepressant effect at high plasma levels. *Psychopharmacology:* 1976; 45:305–14.
21. Perry PJ, Browne JL, Alexander B, et al. Two prospective dosing methods for nortriptyline. *Clin Pharmacokinet.* 1984; 9:555–63.
22. Preskorn SH, Weller EB. Depression in children: relationship between plasma imipramine levels and response. *J Clin Psychiatry.* 1982; 43:450–3.
23. Nelson JC, Jatlow PI, Bock J, et al. Major adverse reactions during desipramine treatment. *Arch Gen Psychiatry.* 1982a; 39:1055–61.
24. Breyer-Pfaff U, Giedke H, Gaertner HJ, et al. Validation of a therapeutic plasma level range in amitriptyline treatment of depression. *J Clin Psychopharmacol.* 1989; 9:116–21.
25. Preskorn SH, Irwin HA. Toxicity of tricyclic antidepressants— kinetics, mechanism, intervention: a review. *J Clin Psychiatry.* 1982; 43:151–6.
26. Golden RN, DeVane CL, Laizure SC, et al. Bupropion in depression. II. The role of metabolites in clinical outcome. *Arch Gen Psychiatry.* 1988; 45:145–9.
27. Goodnick PJ. Blood levels and acute response to bupropion. *Am J Psychiatry.* 1992; 149:399–400.
28. Preskorn SH. Antidepressant response and plasma concentrations of bupropion. *J Clin Psychiatry.* 1983; 44(*Suppl 5*): 137–9.
29. Goodnick PJ. Pharmacokinetics of second generation antidepressants: fluoxetine. *Psychopharmacol Bull.* 1991; 27:503–12.
30. Amsterdam JD, Fawcett J, Quitkin FM, et. al. Fluoxetine and norfluoxetine plasma concentrations in major depression: a multicenter study. *Am J Psychiatry.* 1997; 154:963–9.
31. DeVane CL, Jusko WJ. Plasma concentration monitoring of hydroxylated metabolites of imipramine and desipramine. *Drug Intell Clin Pharm.* 1981; 15:263–6.
32. Young RC. Hydroxylated metabolites of antidepressants. *Psychopharmacol Bull.* 1991; 27:521–32.
33. Nelson JC, Bock J, Jatlow PI. Clinical implications of 2-hydroxydesipramine plasma concentrations. *Clin Pharmacol Ther.* 1983; 33:183–9.

34. DeVane CL, Nemeroff CB. Psychotropic drug interactions. *Primary Psychiatry.* 1998; 5:36–70.
35. Ziegler VE, Co BT, Taylor JR, et al. Amitriptyline plasma levels and therapeutic response. *Clin Pharmacol Ther.* 1976; 19:795–801.
36. Kupfer DJ, Hanin I, Spiker DG, et al. Amitriptyline plasma levels and clinical response in primary depression. *Clin Pharmacol Ther.* 1977; 22:904–11.
37. Boutelle WE. Clinical response and blood levels in the treatment of depression with a new antidepressant drug, amoxapine. *Neuropharmacology.* 1980; 19:1229–31.
38. Preskorn SH. Should bupropion dosage be adjusted based upon therapeutic drug monitoring? *Psychopharmacol Bull.* 1991; 27:637–43.
39. Reisby N, Gram LF, Beck P, et al. Clomipramine: plasma levels and clinical effects. *Common Psychopharmacol.* 1979; 5:341–51.
40. Traskman L, Asberg M, Bertilsson L, et al. Plasma levels of clomipramine and its desmethyl metabolite during treatment of depression. Differential biochemical and clinical effects of the two compounds. *Clin Pharmacol Ther.* 1979; 26:600–10.
41. Stern RS, Marks IM, Mawson D, et al. Clomipramine and exposure for compulsive rituals II: plasma levels, side effects and outcome. *Br J Psychiatry.* 1980; 136:161–6.
42. Nelson JC, Jatlow P, Quinlan DM, et al. Desipramine plasma concentration and antidepressant response. *Arch Gen Psychiatry.* 1982b; 39:1419–22.
43. Linnoila M, Seppala T, Mattila MJ, et al. Clomipramine and doxepin in depressive neurosis: plasma levels and therapeutic response. *Arch Gen Psychiatry.* 1980; 37:1295–9.
44. Reisby N, Gram LF, Beck P, et al. Imipramine: clinical effects and pharmacokinetic variability. *Psychopharmacology.* 1977; 54:263–72.
45. Glassman AH, Perel JM, Shostak M, et al. Clinical implications of imipramine plasma levels for depressive illness. *Arch Gen Psychiatry.* 1977; 34:197–204.
46. Gwirtsman HE, Ahles S, Halaris A, et al. Therapeutic superiority of maprotiline versus doxepin in geriatric depression. *J Clin Psychiatry.* 1983; 44:449–53.
47. Montgomery S, Braithwaite R, Dawling, et al. High plasma nortriptyline levels in the treatment of depression. *Clin Pharmacol Ther.* 1978; 23:309–14.
48. Biggs JT, Holland WH, Sherman WR. Steady-state protriptyline levels in an outpatient population. *Am J Psychiatry.* 1975; 132:960–2.
49. Moody JP, Whyte SF, MacDonald AJ, et al. Pharmacokinetic aspects of protriptyline plasma levels. *Eur J Clin Pharmacol.* 1977; 11:51–6.
50. Putzolu S, Pecknold JC, Baiocchi L. Trazodone: clinical and biochemical studies II. Blood levels and therapeutic responsiveness. *Psychopharmacol Bull.* 1976; 12:40–1.
51. Mann JJ, Georgotas A, Newton R, et al. A controlled study of trazodone, imipramine, and placebo in outpatients with endogenous depression. *J Clin Psychopharmacol.* 1981; 1:75–80.
52. Suckow RF, Cooper TB. Determination of trimipramine and metabolites

in plasma by liquid chromatography with electrochemical detection. *J Pharm Sci.* 1984; 73:1745–8.
53. DeVane CL, Rudorfer MV, Potter WZ. Dosage regimen design for cyclic antidepressants: a review of pharmacokinetic methods. *Psychopharmacol Bull.* 1991; 27:619–31.
54. Nelson JC, Jatlow PI. Nonlinear desipramine kinetics: prevalence and importance. *Clin Pharmacol Ther.* 1987; 41:666–70.
55. Nemeroff CB, DeVane CL, Pollock BG. Antidepressants and the cytochrome P450 system. *Am J Psychiatry.* 1996; 153:311–20.
56. Ereshefsky L, Riesenman C, Lam YW. Antidepressant drug interactions and the cytochrome P450 system: the role of cytochrome P450 2D6. *Clin Pharmacokinet.* 1995; 29(Suppl 1):10–9.
57. Brosen K. Are pharmacokinetic drug interactions with the SSRIs an issue? *Int Clin Psychopharmacol.* 1996; 11(Suppl 1):23–7.
58. Mitchell PB. Drug interactions of clinical significance with selective serotonin reuptake inhibitors. *Drug Safety.* 1997; 17:390–406.
59. Wong SL, Cavanaugh J, Shi H. Effects of divalproex sodium on amitriptyline and nortriptyline phramacokinetics. *Clin Pharmacol Therap.* 1996; 60:48–53.
60. Ereshefsky L, Riesenman C, Lam YW. Antidepressant drug interactions and the cytochrome P450 system. The role of cytochrome P450 2D6. *Clin Pharmacokinet.* 1995; 29(Suppl 1):10–8, 18–9.
61. Geller B. Psychopharmacology of children and adolescents: pharmacokinetics and relationships of plasma/serum levels to response. *Psychopharmacol Bull.* 1991; 27:401–10.
62. DeVane CL, Pollock BG. Pharmacokinetic considerations of antidepressant use in the elderly. *J Clin Psychiatry.* 1999; 60(Suppl 20):38–44.
63. Shoaf SE, Linnoila M. Interaction of ethanol and smoking on the pharmacokinetics and pharmacodynamics of psychotropic medications. *Psychopharmacol Bull.* 1991; 27:577–94.
64. Roose SR, Glassman AH. Cardiovascular effects of tricyclic antidepressants in depressed patients with and without heart disease. *J Clin Psychiatry Monograph.* 1989; 7:1–18.
65. Lane EA. Renal function and the disposition of antidepressants and their metabolites. *Psychopharmacol Bull.* 1991; 27:533–40.
66. Goodwin FK, Prange A, Post R, et al. Potentiation of antidepressant effects by L-triiodothyronine in tricyclic nonresponders. *Am J Psychiatry.* 1982; 139:34–8.

Chapter 8
Martin L. Job

Digoxin (AHFS 24:04)

Usual Dosage Range in Absence of Clearance-Altering Factors

Digoxin, the most commonly used cardiac glycoside, is primarily used in the treatment of congestive heart failure (CHF), and controlling the ventricular response in atrial fibrillation and flutter. Digoxin has a narrow therapeutic index and requires reasonably cautious dosage determination.[1] The following dosage ranges are based on lean or ideal body weight and may need substantial modification. These dosages are based on administration of the tablet or elixir form of digoxin; when the intravenous or capsule formulation is used, differences in bioavailability must be considered. Dosage adjustment should be determined by individual response to digoxin.

Dosage Form	Loading Dose[a]	Maintenance Dosage[a]
Intravenous		
Premature neonates (<4 weeks)[2]	15–30 µ/kg	5–10 µ/kg[b]
Full-term neonates[3]	10–30 µ/kg	8–10 µ/kg[b]
Oral (elixir)[c]		
Infants (≤2 years)[3]	38–63 µ/kg	13–15 µ/kg[b]
Children (2–10 years)[3]	25–44 µ/kg	10–13 µ/kg[b]
Children (≥10 years)[3]	10–15 µ/kg	4–13 µ/kg[b]

Oral (tablets)
    Adults[4]   10–15 μ/kg[d]   0.25 mg/day[e]

[a]Based on ideal body weight (IBW).
[b]Divided q 12 hr for children <10 yr.
[c]Doses adjusted according to bioavailability.
[d]Three divided doses.
[e]Administered qd.

For adults with normal renal function, the usual approach is administration of a total loading dose of 1–1.5 mg orally (e.g., 0.5 mg followed by 0.25 mg 6 and 12 hr later) followed by 0.25 mg/day. For patients with impaired renal function (CrCl <20 ml/min), a 0.5-mg loading dose (two 0.25-mg doses 6 hr apart) is followed by 0.125 mg/day.[4–6] Larger loading doses may be required to control the ventricular rate in atrial fibrillation and flutter. Maintenance doses should be based on CrCl, digoxin, serum concentrations, and patient response. The following maintenance dosages and interval adjustments, based on CrCl, have been proposed.[5]

CrCl	Percentage of Normal Recommended Maintenance Dose	Interval
>50 ml/min	100%	24 hr
10–50 ml/min	25–75%	24–36[a] hr
<10 ml/min	10–25%	48 hr

[a]The 36-hr interval is not recommended by author due to complicated dosing schedules.

Dosage Form Availability[7]

Dosage Form	Product
Intravenous	
0.25 mg/ml	Digoxin Injection
	Lanoxin
0.1 mg/ml	Lanoxin Injection Pediatric
Oral capsules	
0.05, 0.1, and 0.2 mg	Lanoxicaps
Oral tablets	
0.125, 0.25, and 0.5 mg	Lanoxin

Oral elixir
    0.05 mg/ml   Digoxin Elixir

                                    Lanoxin Elixir Pediatric

Bioavailability (F) of Dosage Forms[6]

Dosage Form	Bioavailability
Intravenous	100%
Intramuscular	Not recommended
Oral capsules[a]	95 ± 13%
Oral tablets[a]	75 ± 14%
Oral elixir[a]	80 ± 16%

[a]*Several agents may decrease absorption and erythromycin and tetracycline can increase it.[8] (See section on drug–drug interactions.) Food may reduce peak level without affecting total absorption.*

When patients are changed from one route to another, differences in bioavailability should be considered.

General Pharmacokinetic Information[6,9]

Parameter	Outcome	Comments
Protein binding	25%	Reduced during hypoalbuminemia but not clinically significant
Distribution	Highly distributed to lean organ tissues (e.g., heart, muscle, kidneys, and liver)	Serum to cardiac tissue approximately 1:100; distribution decreased by coadministration of quinidine and in patients with renal impairment
Excretion (renal unchanged)	70%	Primarily glomerular filtration with some tubular secretion
Elimination (nonrenal)	30%	Primarily through biliary and intestinal tracts with some gut flora elimination; small amount through metabolism

Clearance (CL)

Age	Clearance
Neonates[10] (<4 weeks)[a]	1.8 L/hr/m^2
Infants[10] (4 weeks–1 year)[a]	11.2 L/hr/m^2
Children[10] (1–12 years)[a]	8 L/hr/m^2

[a]*In patients with normal renal function for age.*

For adults (>12 years of age), several methods based on population pharmacokinetic parameters have been proposed.

Method 1:[11]

CL = [1.303 × CrCl (ml/min)] + 41 ml/min
(CHF absent)

CL = [1.303 × CrCl (ml/min)] + 20 ml/min
(CHF present)

Method 2:[12]

CL = 1.94 L/hr/m^2 + [CrCl (L/hr/m^2) × 1.02]
(CHF absent)

CL = 0.78 L/hr/m^2 + [CrCl (L/hr/m^2) × 0.88]
(CHF present)

Method 3:[13]

CL = 3.0 ml/min + [0.0546 × CrCl (ml/min)]
(if concomitant quinidine, multiply by 0.559)

Oral bioavailability was assumed to be 0.6 for Methods 1 and 2 and 0.82 for Method 3. Methods 1 and 2 were developed prior to the identification of the digoxin–quinidine interaction and may underpredict serum digoxin concentrations (SDCs).[14] Method 3 may be a better predictor of SDCs across all populations.[15]

Volume of Distribution (V)

Age	Volume (mean ± SD)
Neonates[15] (<4 weeks)	10.0 ± 1.0 L/kg
Infants[10] (4 weeks–1 year)	16.3 ± 2.1 L/kg
Children[10] (1–12 years)	16.1 ± 0.8 L/kg
Adults[7] (>12 years)	6.7 ± 1.4 L/kg

*a*When patient weight is used in V calculations, IBW is used for patients whose actual weight >IBW.

The volume of distribution is decreased in patients with renal impairment, so a reduced total loading dose is required.[16] The following equations correspond to the calculated V from the above clearance methods.

Method 1:[17]

$$V(/_{1.73\,m^2}) = V_{min} + \frac{V_n(CrCl)}{K_d + CrCl}$$

where

$V_{min} = 226$ L/1.73 m^2
$V_n = 298$ L/1.73 m^2
$K_d = 29.1$ ml/min/1.73 m^2
CrCl in ml/min/1.73 m^2

Method 2:[13]

$$V(L) = (153\ L/m^2 + 29.5\ L/m^2 \times CrCl) \times BSA$$

where BSA = body surface area in m^2

Method 3:[14]

$$V(L) = (5.05 + 0.0882 \times CrCl) \times IBW$$

where CrCl = ml/min, IBW = kg

Half-Life and Time to Steady State

Age	Half-Life (mean ± SD)	Time to Steady State
Premature neonates[18] (<4 weeks)	61 ± 16.1 hr	225–385 hr

Full-term neonates[15] (<4 weeks)	44 ± 13 hr	157–283 hr
Infants[10] (4 weeks–1 year)	18 ± 9 hr	45–135 hr
Children		
>1–<1.5 years	Not available	Not available
1.5–2.5 years[10]	36 ± 11 hr	124–232 hr
2.5–<7 years[19]	37 ± 16 hr	104–267 hr
7–12 years	Not available	Not available
Adults[7] (>12 years)	36 ± 8 hr	140–220 hr

Although not verified, the half-life ($t\frac{1}{2}$) and time to steady state for children 7–12 years old are probably similar to the values found in adults. SDCs may decrease during pregnancy because of increased renal clearance.[20] Reductions in renal function below the average for age and size lead to lengthening of the half-life.

Therapeutic Range[21, 22]

Disease or Condition	Therapeutic Range	Comment
CHF	0.8–2 µg/L	Significant overlap between therapeutic and toxic ranges[21, 22]
		A recent analysis suggests that a lower therapeutic range (0.5–1.0 µg/L) may be as effective as higher concentrations and is associated with a lower risk of toxicity[23]
Atrial fibrillation	0.8–2 µg/L	Patients may require concentrations as high as 2.6 µg/L to control ventricular response;[21] neonates and infants can tolerate higher concentrations than adults, though this may be due in part to endogenous digoxin-like substances[24]

Suggested Sampling Times

Because of digoxin's long half-life, concentrations vary only slightly over a few hours, except during the first 4–6 hr after a dose when initial distribution is slow. Concentrations shortly after an intravenous dose can be greater than 10 µg/L. Therefore, to ensure that drug distribution is complete, no sampling should occur during the first 6 hr after a dose.[25]

The variation from the peak after distribution to the trough before the next dose is usually 30% or less. However, evaluation of a patient's digoxin clearance will be improved if all concentrations are taken at approximately the same time after doses. A variation in the collection time of only 2–3 hr will generally be inconsequential.

For outpatients, an annual SDC measurement is sufficient for those on a stable dose of digoxin.[26] Appointments should be scheduled to ensure that the daily dose has not been taken before sampling; if necessary, outpatients can hold the dose for a few hours. For hospitalized patients, trough concentrations should usually be scheduled 1–4 hr before the usual morning daily dose.

Pharmacodynamic Monitoring—Concentration-Related Efficacy

Patients with CHF should be monitored for heart and lung sounds, changes in urine output, edema, and neck vein distention. Patients with hyperthyroidism may have reduced myocardial responsiveness to digoxin therapy. Digoxin response may be improved by treating the hyperthyroidism. The opposite applies when treating hypothyroidism.[9,26]

Patients with atrial fibrillation should be monitored for decreased ventricular rate and ECG changes.[24]

Patients receiving digoxin should have serum creatinine, potassium, SDCs, and general fluid and electrolyte status monitored periodically to avoid toxicity. Changes in status can indicate need to increase or reduce doses or to monitor SDCs.

Pharmacodynamic Monitoring—Concentration-Related Toxicity

Toxicity in all patients taking digoxin can be noted as a decrease in heart rate, other ECG changes, and arrhythmias; anorexia, nausea, vomiting, and diarrhea; and visual disturbances. Toxicity can occur within the normal therapeutic range, especially in patients with metabolic derangement (e.g., hypokalemia) or severe underlying disease.[9,26] Because the volume of distribution is decreased in hypothyroidism, patients should be monitored to avoid increased digoxin concentrations and toxicity.[9] Digoxin Immune Fab (ovine) may be used to treat life-threatening digoxin toxicity due to iatrogenic or purposeful overdosing.[1]

Falsely elevated SDCs can be caused by endogenous, digoxin-like substances (EDLS) in patients with renal[27] or liver[28] impairment, pregnant women,[29] and neonates.[30] SDC measurements taken during the distribution phase after digoxin dosing can be quite high and may not be indicative of toxicity.[31] SDC elevations due to drawing during the distribution phase must not be incorrectly diagnosed and treated with Digoxin Immune Fab. Signs and symptoms of digoxin toxicity should be present before such treatment.

Drug–Drug Interactions[8,22]

Some important digoxin–drug interactions are listed here.

Drug	Effect on Digoxin	Comments
Amiodarone	Reduced renal and non-renal clearances	Interaction is dose dependent; digoxin concentrations may increase >70%

Antacids	Absorption reduced by 25%	Doses should be separated by ≥2 hr
Cholestyramine	Absorption reduced (most when given concomitantly)	Reduction may be minimized by twice-daily dosing of cholestyramine 8 hr before and after digoxin
Diltiazem	Reduced renal and nonrenal clearances	Interaction is dose dependent; increased digoxin concentrations
Macrolides[32] Erythromycin and Clarithromycin	Reduced intestinal metabolism; increased serum concentrations	Effects may be minimized by use of encapsulated liquid concentrate (Lanoxicap)[32]
Kaolin-pectin	Time-dependent decrease in absorption (62% when given concomitantly; 20% when given 2 hr apart)	Doses should be separated by ≥2 hr
NSAIDs	Decreased renal clearance	Increased concentrations
Propafenone[33]	Reduced renal and nonrenal clearances; decreased V	Interaction is dose dependent; digoxin concentrations may increase >80%; obtain SDC within 48-96 hrs of adding or removing propafenone
Quinidine	Reduced renal clearance and tissue binding	Concentrations should be monitored carefully; digoxin dose may need to be decreased by 50%
Spironolactone	Decreased renal clearance; reduced tissue binding; increased serum concentrations	Also falsely elevated concentrations due to interference with some immunoassay tests
Tetracycline	Increased absorption; reduced intestinal metabolism; increased serum concentrations	Eradication of gut flora (e.g., *Eggerthella lenta*)

Verapamil	Reduced renal and extrarenal clearances	Interaction is dose dependent; digoxin concentrations may increase 70%; increased concentrations may decline over a period of weeks with concomitant therapy
St. John's Wort[34]	Reduced absorption	May be mediated by inducing P-glycoprotein; monitor clinical response and SDC in patients titrated to effective dose who suddently discontinue St. John's Wort

References

1. Hauptman PJ, Kelly RA. Digitalis. *Circulation.* 1999; 99:1265–70.
2. Pinsky WW, Jacobsen JR, Gillette PC. Dosage of digoxin in premature infants. *J Pediatr.* 1979; 96:639–42.
3. Digoxin. In: Phelps SJ, Hak EB. Guidelines for administration of intravenous medications to pediatric patients, 5th ed. Bethesda, MD: American Society of Health-System Pharmacists; 1996:46.
4. Jellife RW. Therapeutic Guideline. Administration of digoxin. *Dis Chest.* 1969;56:56–60.
5. Aronoff GR, Berns JS, Brier ME. Antihypertensive and cardiovascular agents. In: Drug prescribing in renal failure, 4th ed. Philadelphia, PA: American College of Physicians 1999:34.
6. Reuning RH, Geraets DR. Digoxin. In: Evans WE, Schentag JJ, Jusko WJ, eds. Applied pharmacokinetics: principles of therapeutic drug monitoring, 2nd ed. Spokane, WA: Applied Therapeutics; 1986: 570–623.
7. Digoxin. In: McEvoy GK, ed. American hospital formulary service drug information 99. Bethesda, MD: American Society of Health-System Pharmacists; 1999:1363.
8. Rodin SM, Johnson BF. Pharmacokinetic interactions with digoxin. *Clin Pharmacokinet.* 1988; 15:227–44.
9. Mooradian AD. Digitalis. An update of clinical pharmacokinetics, therapeutic monitoring techniques and treatment recommendation. *Clin Pharmacokinet.* 1988; 15:165–79.
10. Morselli PL, Asbael BM, Gomeni R, et al. Digoxin pharmacokinetics during human development. In: Morselli A, Garibatini S, Serini F, eds. Basic and therapeutic aspects of perinatal pharmacology. New York: Raven Press; 1975:377–92.
11. Koup J, Greenblatt D, Jusko W, et al. Pharmacokinetics of digoxin in normal subjects after intravenous bolus and infusion doses. *J Pharmacokinet Biopharm.* 1975; 3:181–92.

12. Sheiner LB, Rosenburg B, Marathe V. Estimation of population characteristics of pharmacokinetic parameters from routine clinical data. *J Pharmacokinet Biopharm.* 1977; 5:445–79.
13. Williams PJ, Lane J, Murray W, et al. Pharmacokinetics of the digoxin-quinidine interaction via mixed-effects modeling. *Clin Pharmacokinet.* 1992; 22:66–74.
14. Williams PJ, Lane JR, Capparelli EV, et al. Direct comparison of three methods for predicting digoxin concentrations. *Pharmacotherapy.* 1996; 16:1085–92.
15. Wettrell G. Distribution and elimination of digoxin in infants. *Eur J Clin Pharmacol.* 1977; 11:329–35.
16. Cheng JWM, Charland SL, Shaw LM, et al. Is the volume of distribution of digoxin reduced in patients with renal dysfunction? Determining digoxin pharmacokinetics by fluorescence polarization immunoassay. *Pharmacotherapy.* 1997;17:584–90.
17. Jusko WJ, Szefler SJ, Goldfarb AL. Pharmacokinetic design of digoxin dosage regimens in relation to renal function. *J Clin Pharmacol.* 1974; 14: 525–35.
18. Lang D, Bernuth G. Serum concentrations and serum half-life of digoxin in premature and mature newborns. *Pediatrics.* 1977; 59:902–6.
19. Dungan WT, Doherty JE, Harvey C. Triitated digoxin XVIII. Studies in infants and children. *Circulation.* 1972; 46:983–9.
20. Chow T, Galvin J, McGovern B. Antiarrhythmic drug therapy in pregnancy and lactation. *Am J Cardiol.* 1998; 82:581–621.
21. Dobbs JR, O'Neill CSA, Deshmukh AA, et al. Serum concentration monitoring of cardiac glycosides. How helpful is it for adjusting dosage regimens? *Clin Pharmacokinet.* 1991; 20:175–93.
22. Caufield JS, Gums PG, Grauer K. The serum digoxin concentration. Ten questions to ask. *Am Fam Physician.* 1997; 56:495–503.
23. Terra SG, Washam JB, Dunham GD, et al. Therapeutic range of digoxin's efficacy in heart failure: What is the evidence? *Pharmacotherapy.* 1999; 19(10):1123–26.
24. Halkin H, Radomsky M, Blieden L, et al. Steady-state serum digoxin concentration in relation to digitalis toxicity in neonates and infants. *Arch Dis Child.* 1973; 48:55–7.
25. Williamson KM, Thrasher KA, Fulton KB, et al. Digoxin toxicity—an evaluation in current clinical practice. *Arch Intern Med.* 1998; 158:2444–9.
26. Cañas F, Tanasijevic MJ, Ma'luf N, et al. Evaluating the appropriateness of digoxin level monitoring. *Arch Intern Med.* 1999; 159:363–8.
27. Graves SW, Brown B, Valdes R. An endogenous digoxin-like substance in patients with renal impairment. *Ann Intern Med.* 1983; 99:604–8.
28. Nikou GC, Yyssoulis GP, Venetikou MS, et al. Digoxin-like substance(s) interfere(s) with serum estimations for the drug in cirrhotic patients. *J Clin Gastroenterol.* 1989; 114:430–3.
29. Graves SW, Valdes R, Brown BA, et al. Endogenous digoxin immunoreactive substance in human pregnancy. *J Clin Endocrinol Metab.* 1984; 58:148–50.

30. Valdes R, Graves SW, Brown B, et al. Endogneous substance in newborn infants causing false-positive digoxin measurements. *J Pediatr.* 1983; 102:947–50.

31. Longley JM, Murphy JE. Falsely elevated digoxin levels: another look. *Ther Drug Monitoring.* 1989; 11:572–3.

32. Bizjak ED, Mauro VF. Digoxin-macrolide drug interaction. *Ann Pharmacother.* 1997; 31:1077–9.

33. Belz GG, Matthews J, Dosing W, et al. Digoxin–antiarrhythmic: pharmacodynamic and pharmacokinetic studies with guanidine, propafenone, and verapamil. *Clin Pharmacol Ther.* 1982; 31:202–3.

34. Johne A, Brockmöller J, Bauer S, et al. Pharmacokinetic interaction with an herbal extract from St. John's Wort (Hypericum perforatum). *Clin Pharmacol Ther.* 1999; 66:338–45.

Chapter 9
William R. Garnett

Ethosuximide
(AHFS 28:12.20)

Usual Dosage Range in Absence of Clearance-Altering Factors

Ethosuximide is the drug of choice for controlling absence seizures, and its therapeutic range is 40–100 mg/L. A loading dose is not needed for absence seizures. The starting dose should be low so that the patient can accommodate to the initial CNS depression seen with most antiepileptic drugs. The dose should be titrated to the individual patient's response.[1,2]

Based on the half-life of ethosuximide, a once-daily dosage regimen can be used successfully. However, GI side effects increase with the dose in some patients. Therefore, ethosuximide may need to be given twice a day.[3]

Dosage Form	Initial Maintenance Dosage
Intravenous	None
Oral (capsules and solution)	
Children (≤11 years)	20–40 mg/kg/day
Adolescents and adults (>11 years)	15–30 mg/kg/day

The actual dose may depend on the dosage form available. A rough guideline is to initiate therapy with 250 mg/day in children 3–6 years old and with 500 mg/day in patients older than age 6. While a maximum dose of 1.5 g/day has been suggested,[4] a better guide to the maximum dose is the achieved ethosuximide concentration, control of seizures, and occurrence of side effects. The 1.5-g/day dose may be exceeded to achieve the desired concentration for seizure control if the patient does not have side effects.

Dosage Form Availability

Dosage Form	Product
Intravenous	None available
Oral capsules: 250 mg	Zarontin
Oral solution: 250 mg/5 ml	Zarontin

Bioavailability (*F*) of Dosage Forms[5]

Dosage Form	Bioavailability Comments
Intravenous	Not available
Oral capsules and solution	Assumed complete (100%)

General Pharmacokinetic Information

The pharmacokinetics of ethosuximide are poorly understood, even though it is an old antiepileptic drug and there is a sensitive and specific assay for it. Ethosuximide has been described as following a one-compartment model with first-order elimination.[2,5]

Absorption

In humans, ethosuximide is rapidly absorbed; peak concentrations are achieved in 3–7 hr.[2] The time to peak concentration is somewhat faster with a single dose than after repeated dosing. Absorption from the syrup is faster than from the capsule, but the extent of absorption is the same.

Distribution

Ethosuximide does not bind to plasma proteins. A cerebrospinal fluid to plasma to saliva ratio of 1 indicates that most of the drug in the plasma is in the unbound form. Except for body fat, ethosuximide is uniformly distributed throughout the body. Ethosuximide does not distribute into body fat.

The apparent volume of distribution (V) of ethosuximide is approximately 70% of ideal body weight, which is equivalent to total body water. The apparent V is 0.69 L/kg in children younger than 10 years of age and 0.62–0.67 L/kg in adults older than 18 years of age.[2]

Ethosuximide crosses the placenta and passes into breast milk, achieving a concentration similar to that in the mother's plasma.[5] Spinal fluid, saliva, and tears have concentrations similar to that in plasma.

Metabolism

Ethosuximide is poorly extracted by the liver and, therefore, does not undergo first-pass metabolism. The apparent clearance of ethosuximide in normal adults has been estimated at 0.010 ± 0.004 L/hr/kg, which is less than hepatic blood flow and demonstrates that the elimination is not flow dependent. Ethosuximide is first hydroxylated and then conjugated to inactive metabolites before being excreted into the urine.[6] CYP3A and CYP2E are primarily involved in ethosuximide metabolism with CYP2B and CYP2C playing a minor role.[6]

The half-life in children was reported to be 30 hr versus 60 hr in adults. Data for neonates are derived from case reports and indicate that the half-life is between 32 and 41 hr. The total body clearance of ethosuximide was reported to be 0.016 L/hr/kg in children and 0.010–0.013 L/hr/kg in adults. The half-life of ethosuximide was reported to be unaffected by dose size and to be constant with repeated dosing. However, a 15% decrease in total body clearance also was described and attributed to a decrease in the non-renal clearance.[2]

Two studies suggested that ethosuximide may display nonlinear clearance at the upper end of the therapeutic range. Smith et al. reported that, in individual patients, successive dose increments of equal size produced disproportionately greater increases in steady-state concentrations.[7] Bauer et al. found that seven of 10 patients demonstrated evidence of nonlinearity.[8] Therefore, the dose and steady-state concentration relationship of ethosuximide may vary significantly, especially at the upper end of the therapeutic range.

The asymmetric center in ethosuximide is quaternary, making racemization unlikely.[9] The metabolism of ethosuximide does not appear to be stereoselective. Therefore, the measurement of total ethosuximide is adequate for therapeutic monitoring.

Attempts to predict dosing in epileptic patients have not been successful.

Clearance (CL)

Age	Clearance
Children (<10 years)	0.016 L/hr/kg
Adults (>18 years)	0.010–0.013 L/hr/kg

Volume of Distribution (V)

Age	Volume
Children (<10 years)	0.69 L/kg (IBW)
Adults (>18 years)	0.62–0.67 L/kg (IBW)

Protein Binding

Protein binding of ethosuximide is negligible (0%) in both children and adults.

Half-Life and Time to Steady State

Age	Half-Life	Time to Steady State
Children (<10 years)	30 hr	6 days
Adults (>18 years)	60 hr	12 days

Therapeutic Range

The therapeutic range of ethosuximide is 40–100 mg/L for the treatment of absence seizures.[1,2] Within this range, 80% of patients will achieve partial control and 60% will become seizure free. However, concentrations up to 150 mg/L or higher may be needed for complete seizure control in some cases. These concentrations have been used without signs of toxicity, but patients with high concentrations should be monitored closely. Factors that predict therapeutic success are (1) absence seizures as the only seizure type, (2) normal EEG background activity, and (3) normal intelligence.[1,2]

The exact concentration where a given patient will respond is not predictable, so the dose must be titrated to individual response. While ethosuximide may be assumed to follow a first-order pharmacokinetic model, dosage adjustments should be made gradually to allow for patient tolerance. Steady state should be achieved, and the patient's response (both efficacy and toxicity) should be assessed. Dosage increases may be made until the patient achieves seizure control or develops intolerable side effects. If side effects occur, the dose of ethosuximide should be reduced. After the patient has been free of absence seizures for 2–4 years, ethosuximide may be discontinued. Dosage reduction should occur gradually.

Suggested Sampling Times and Effect on Therapeutic Range[2]

The indications for monitoring ethosuximide concentrations include

- A poor response to therapy.
- Questionable compliance.
- Low doses.
- Maintenance of optimal concentrations.

Ethosuximide has a long half-life. This half-life should be considered in determining when to collect blood samples after therapy is initiated or the dosage is changed. The initial sample or the sample after a dosage change should not be drawn for at least 6 days in children or 12 days in adults so that the patient can reach steady state. Samples may be drawn earlier if the patient experiences unexpected side effects.

The long half-life of ethosuximide would suggest minimal changes in the peak to trough ratio. However, trough concentrations are recommended for monitoring, particularly if the patient is on a once-a-day regimen.

There is no indication that serum ethosuximide concentrations differ from plasma concentrations.

Because of the negligible protein binding of ethosuximide, there is no indication for determining unbound ethosuximide. The concentration of ethosuximide in saliva or tears equals its serum concentration and may be used in some patients if blood sampling is not possible.

Once the desired therapeutic response has been achieved, concentrations should be monitored every 4–6 months. A change in response or the onset of unusual side effects indicates a need to monitor concentrations.

Pharmacodynamic Monitoring— Concentration-Related Efficacy[1,2]

The desired therapeutic end-point for ethosuximide is the abolition of absence seizures. In some cases, EEG monitoring may be required. Ethosuximide is indicated only for the treatment of absence seizures; it may exacerbate other seizure types. Ethosuximide is very effective as monotherapy for absence seizures. In refractory patients, however, the combination of ethosuximide and valproate may be more effective than either drug alone.

Pharmacodynamic Monitoring— Concentration-Related Toxicity[10]

Patients should be monitored for ethosuximide side effects. The most frequent side effects, nausea and vomiting, may be related to the dosage size. Other side effects that may be dose or concentration related are abdominal discomfort, anorexia, drowsiness, fatigue, lethargy, dizziness, hiccups, and headache. Headaches may persist after a dosage reduction.

Behavioral and cognitive side effects of ethosuximide are not well documented.

Rare side effects include skin rashes, systemic lupus erythematosus, blood dyscrasias, and changes in liver function tests.

Drug–Drug Interactions

Animal studies indicate that the metabolism of ethosuximide may be induced or inhibited. However, clinical reports of drug interactions with ethosuximide are rare and often poorly documented. The ratio of ethosuximide concentrations to dose was significantly higher when ethosuximide was given alone than when it was administered with *carbamazepine, primidone,* or *valproic acid*.[11] Other studies found increased ethosuximide concentrations when ethosuximide was given with valproic acid. The interaction with valproic acid may be complex and may require the presence of other concurrent antiepileptic drugs or high concentrations of valproic acid.[12-14]

Isoniazid increased ethosuximide concentrations[15] and ethosuximide increased *phenytoin* concentrations[16] in single-case studies.

Drug–Disease State or Condition Interactions

Patients on *hemodialysis* lose about 50% of their ethosuximide stores during a 6-hr dialysis.[17] Therefore, they require increased monitoring both pre- and postdialysis as well as supplemental dosing. The study was done in 4 patients who were on dialysis. They were each given a single test dose of 500 mg. The efficacy of removal of ethosuximide was 61% in one patient, 78% in one patient, and close to 100% in two patients. The authors state that 50% was removed during a 6 hour dialysis period. A replacement of one dose may be warranted after hemodialysis.

Pregnancy is reported to increase the clearance of all antiepileptics. Based on two case reports,[18,19] this effect appears to be true for ethosuximide.

Ethosuximide is 80% metabolized by the liver and 20% excreted unchanged. Therefore, although unconfirmed by clinical studies, patients with *impaired liver* or *renal* function may require altered dosing.[2]

References

1. Sherwin AL. Ethosuximide—clinical use. In: Levy R, Mattson R, Meldrum B, et al., eds. Antiepileptic drugs, 4th ed. New York: Raven Press; 1995:667–73.
2. Garnett WR. Ethosuximide. In: Taylor WJ, Caviness MHD, eds. A textbook for the clinical application of therapeutic drug monitoring. Irving, TX: Abbott Laboratories; 1986:225–35.
3. Dooley JM, Camfield PR, Camfield CS, et al. Once-daily ethosuximide in the treatment of absence epilepsy. *Pediatr Neurol*. 1990; 6:38–9.
4. McEvoy GK, ed. American hospital formulary service drug information 93. Bethesda, MD: American Society of Hospital Pharmacists; 1993:1285.
5. Bialer M, Xiaodona S, Perucca E. Ethosuximide—absorption, distribution, and excretion. In: Levy R, Mattson R, Meldrum B, et al., eds. Antiepileptic drugs, 4th ed. New York: Raven Press; 1995:659–65.
6. Pisani F, Bialer M. Ethosuximide: Chemistry and Biotransformation. In: Levy R, Mattson R, Meldrum B, et al., eds. Antiepileptic drugs, 4th ed. New York: Raven Press; 1995:655–8.
7. Smith GA, McKauge L, Dubetz D, et al. Factors influencing plasma concentrations of ethosuximide. *Clin Pharmacokinet*. 1979; 4:38–52.
8. Bauer LA, Harris C, Wilensky AJ, et al. Ethosuximide kinetics: possible interaction with valproic acid. *Clin Pharmacol Ther*. 1982; 31: 741–5.

9. Villen T, Bertilsson L, Sjoqvist F. Nonstereoselective disposition of ethosuximide in humans. *Ther Drug Monit.* 1990; 12:514–6.
10. Dreifuss FE. Ethosuximide—toxicity. In: Levy R, Mattson R, Meldrum B, et al., eds. Antiepileptic drugs, 4th ed. New York: Raven Press; 1995:675–9.
11. Battino D, Cusi C, Franceschetti S, et al. Ethosuximide plasma concentrations: Influence of age and associated concomitant therapy. *Clin Pharmacokinet.* 1982; 7:176–80.
12. Mattson RH, Cramer JA. Valproic acid and ethosuximide interaction. *Ann Neurol.* 1980; 7:583–4.
13. Bourgeois BFD. Combination of valproate and ethosuximide: antiepileptic and neurotoxic interaction. *J Pharmacol Exp Ther.* 1988; 247:1128–32.
14. Pisani F, Narbone MC, Trunfio C, et al. Valproic acid–ethosuximide interaction: a pharmacokinetic study. *Epilepsia.* 1984; 25:229–33.
15. Van Wieringen A, Vriglandt CM. Ethosuximide intoxication caused by interaction with isoniazid. *Neurology.* 1983; 33:1227–8.
16. Dawson GW, Brown HW, Clark BG. Serum phenytoin after ethosuximide. *Ann Neurol.* 1978; 4:583–4.
17. Marbury TC, Lee CC, Perchalski RJ, et al. Hemodialysis clearance of ethosuximide in patients with chronic renal failure. *Am J Hosp Pharm.* 1981; 38:1757–60.
18. Koup JR, Rose JQ, Cohen ME. Ethosuximide pharmacokinetics in a pregnant patient and her newborn. *Epilepsia.* 1978; 19:535–9.
19. Rane A, Tulnell R. Ethosuximide in human milk and in plasma of a mother and her nursed infant. *Br J Clin Pharmacol.* 1981; 12:855–8.

Chapter 10
James B. Groce III

Heparin and Low Molecular Weight Heparin (AHFS 20:12.04)

Heparin: Usual Dosage Range in Absence of Clearance-Altering Factors

Heparin is used primarily as an anticoagulant to treat active thrombosis and to prevent clot formation in patients at high risk (e.g., due to surgery, prolonged bed rest, or pregnancy) or during extracorporeal circulation [e.g., hemodialysis, cardiopulmonary bypass procedures in adults, and extracorporeal membrane oxygenation (ECMO) in neonates]. Additionally, heparin may help to prolong the patency of arterial and venous catheters.

When heparin therapy is initiated for active thrombosis, a loading dose of 70–100 units/kg should be given. Current guidelines of the American College of Chest Physicians (ACCP) Fifth ACCP Consensus Conference on Antithrombotic Therapy recommend an 80-unit/kg– loading dose for treatment of venous embolic disease. In some instances (e.g., cardiology) loading doses are as low as 70 units/kg, especially in situations

The contributions made by Peter Gal and Robert J. Kandrotas to this chapter are gratefully acknowledged.

for which concomitant Glycoprotein IIb/IIIa inhibitor drug therapy or thrombolytic drug therapy may be coadministered.[1]

Though the current ACCP guidelines do not address the issue of ideal body weight (IBW) versus total body weight (TBW), some have suggested using an adjusted *dosing weight* to account for obesity (e.g., 30–40% of the difference between the TBW and IBW is added to the IBW to result in the dosing weight).

For maintenance heparin therapy, dosage requirements are dictated by the specific treatment indication (Table 1).

TABLE 1. Usual Maintenance Dosage Range in the Absence of Clearance-Altering Factors

Age	Indication	Usual Maintenance Dosage Range
Neonates and infants (<2 months)	Thrombosis and ECMO Catheter patency[b]	28 units/kg/hr[a] 0.5–1 unit/ml
Children and adolescents (≥2 months–<18 years)	Thrombosis Catheter patency[b] Hemodialysis	20 units/kg/hr[a] Adult values initially Adult values initially
Adults (≥18–≤65 years)	Deep vein thrombosis (DVT) Pulmonary embolism (PE) Thrombosis prevention Cardiopulmonary bypass Hemodialysis Catheter patency[b]	10–25 units/kg/hr 15–30 units/kg/hr 5000 units/8–12 hr 100–400 units/kg as single bolus dose 50–100 units/kg as single bolus dose 1–10 units/ml
Geriatrics (>65 years)	DVT and PE	May require 25–33% smaller doses than younger adults

[a] *TBW.*
[b] *E.g., arterial and venous line patency.*

The use of heparin in each individual patient must be understood since target end-points differ for its various therapeutic uses and assays. Furthermore, the laboratory test preferred for monitoring heparin's effect depends on the drug's use [e.g., activated coagulation time (ACT) is more commonly used for cardiopulmonary bypass surgery or hemodialysis, while activated partial thromboplastin time (aPTT) is more commonly used for treating active thrombosis].

aPTT responsiveness to heparin's effect may be impacted by several technical variables that include: the type of clot detection system used within the instrumentation on which the aPTT is being performed, the contact activator for the reagent being used, and the phospholipid composition of the reagent being used. The response of the aPTT to heparin can be reduced by elevated concentrations of factor VIII that can occur in a number of clinical states, including pregnancy, malignancy, acute thrombosis, and major surgery.[2] Clot burden or size, duration of therapy, and concomitant disease states may also affect aPTT responsiveness.

Treating thromboembolic disease

For treatment of venous thromboembolic disease (VTED), concomitant heparin and warfarin therapy is used except during pregnancy or when warfarin is contraindicated. Patients with proven VTED should receive anticoagulant therapy with heparin and warfarin as follows.[25]

Disease Suspected:
- Obtain baseline aPTT, PT/INR, CBC; check for contraindications to heparin therapy.
- Give heparin 5000 units intravenous bolus; order imaging study.

Disease Confirmed:
- Rebolus with heparin, 80 units/kg intravenous, and start maintenance infusion at 18 units/kg/hr.

- Check aPTT at 6 hr and maintain a range corresponding to a therapeutic heparin level.
- Check platelet count daily.
- Start warfarin therapy on day 1; adjust subsequent daily dosing based on INR, and stop heparin after 4 or 5 days overlap, when INR is >2.0 on 2 consecutive days.
- Anticoagulate with warfarin for 3–6 months (patient/disease-state specific).

Heparin: Dosage Form Availability

Heparin is available only as a solution for injection. It usually is administered intravenously or subcutaneously, but it also has been administered by the intrapulmonary route.[3] Heparin should not be given intramuscularly (IM). Giving heparin IM will potentiate the likelihood of hematoma formation and can cause pain and irritation. Heparin sodium and heparin calcium for injection are supplied by several manufacturers in concentrations ranging from 1000 to 40,000 units/ml. Preparations are then diluted to the desired concentration in a dextrose or saline solution.

Heparin is also marketed as a heparin sodium flush solution in concentrations of 10–100 units/ml. This flush solution, diluted to 1 unit/ml or less, can be used to maintain the patency of intravenous catheters.

Heparin preparations are available from different sources including beef lung and pork intestine. Some reports note important differences between these preparations (e.g., the incidence of thrombocytopenia is greater with heparin from beef lung).[3] The molecular weight of heparin ranges from 5,000 to 30,000 daltons with a mean molecular weight of 15,000 daltons (approximately 50 monosaccharide chains).[2]

Heparin also is available as low molecular weight preparations (≈4500 daltons). Four low molecular weight heparins (LMWHs) are currently commercially available (ardeparin, dalteparin, enoxaparin, and tinzaparin). The molecular weights for the currently available products vary between 4,200 and 6,500 daltons. Further discussion of LMWHs may be found in the section "Low Molecular Weight Heparins."

Heparin: Bioavailability (F) of Routes of Administration

Dosage Form	Bioavailability Comments
Intravenous	100%
Subcutaneous	30%

Heparin: General Pharmacokinetic Information

The pharmacokinetic parameters of heparin have been determined using methods that (1) measure a coagulation test parameter such as aPTT, (2) directly measure heparin by activation of a single clotting factor such as factor X, or (3) directly measure neutralization of heparin by protamine titration. Tables 2 and 3 illustrate the differences in pharmacokinetic parameters that may be found depending on direct (Table 2)[4-7] or indirect (Table 3)[4-12] measurement of the heparin concentration. These tables illustrate the inter- and intra-patient variability possible with heparin therapy.

Heparin is cleared by both zero-order and first-order elimination processes. In the zero-order process, heparin is metabolized and depolymerized by endothelial cells and macrophages. In the first-order process heparin is cleared renally. The plasma half-life of heparin varies from 30 to 150 minutes as the administered dose increases from 25 to 400 U/kg.[13-15] In addition, patient-specific variables (e.g., age, thromboembolic disease state, hepatic or renal impairment, and obesity) may significantly alter heparin pharmacokinetic parameters of clearance, volume of distribution, and half-life. Heparin binding proteins are acute

TABLE 2. Heparin Pharmacokinetics in Different Patient Populations Assuming a Linear One-Compartment Model and Directly Measured Heparin Concentration[a]

Patient Population	N[b]	Clearance (mean ± SD)	Volume of Distribution (mean ± SD)	Half-Life (mean ± SD)	Assay Used
Neonates[4]					
33–36 weeks	8	0.082 ± 0.028 L/hr/kg	0.058 ± 0.032 L/kg	0.59 ± 0.15 hr	X_a[c]
29–32 weeks	7	0.086 ± 0.023 L/hr/kg	0.073 ± 0.025 L/kg	0.60 ± 0.11 hr	X_a
25–28 weeks	10	0.089 ± 0.052 L/hr/kg	0.081 ± 0.041 L/kg	0.69 ± 0.24 hr	X_a
Adults					
Healthy[4]	8	0.026 ± 0.005 L/hr/kg	0.037 ± 0.007 L/kg	1.06 ± 0.26 hr	X_a
Healthy[5]	12	0.038 ± 0.007 L/hr/kg	0.070 ± 0.007 L/kg	1.78 ± 0.28 hr	X_a
PE[5]	11	0.048 ± 0.014 L/hr/kg	0.068 ± 0.015 L/kg	1.33 ± 0.32 hr	X_a
PE[6]	4	0.158 ± 0.059 L/hr/kg	0.141 ± 0.047 L/kg	0.63 ± 0.03 hr	Protamine titration
DVT[5]	14	0.033 ± 0.011 L/hr/kg	0.062 ± 0.011 L/kg	1.77 ± 0.47 hr	X_a
DVT[6]	15	0.078 ± 0.034 L/hr/kg	0.124 ± 0.068 L/kg	1.16 ± 0.28 hr	Protamine titration
Healthy[1,d]	11	0.023 L/hr/kg	0.050 L/kg	1.51 ± 0.57 hr	X_a
Hemodialysis[7]	21	0.028 ± 0.013 L/hr/kg	0.066 ± 0.023 L/kg	1.81 ± 0.98 hr	X_a
Liver disease[5]	7	0.052 ± 0.002 L/hr/kg	0.078 ± 0.012 L/kg	1.33 ± 0.35 hr	X_a
Obese females[1]	10	0.015 L/hr/kg	0.046 L/kg	2.13 ± 0.56 hr	X_a
Renal disease[5]	12	0.036 ± 0.008 L/hr/kg	0.071 ± 0.012 L/kg	1.83 ± 0.30 hr	X_a

[a]This assumption is acceptable within the therapeutic range.[5]
[b]The number of patients treated in the referenced study.
[c]This assay measures heparin concentration by measuring inactivation of factor X_a by the heparin-antithrombin III (ATIII) complex from a previously known amount of factor X_a.[2]
[d]Pharmacokinetic estimates are extrapolated based on area under the curve data from 0 to 7 hr.
[e]The prolonged half-life in obese patients may reflect the higher heparin concentrations achieved and nonlinear elimination.

TABLE 3. Heparin Pharmacokinetics in Different Patient Populations Using a Linear One-Compartment Model and Coagulation Tests as Indirect Measures of Heparin Concentration

Patient Population	N^a	Clearance (mean ± SD)	Volume of Distribution (mean ± SD)	Half-Life (mean ± SD)	Assay Used
Neonates					
33–36 weeks[4]	8	0.059 ± 0.020 L/hr/kg	0.056 ± 0.007 L/kg	0.71 ± 0.36 hr	One-stage clotting time
29–32 weeks[4]	7	0.067 ± 0.030 L/hr/kg	0.067 ± 0.019 L/kg	0.81 ± 0.31 hr	One-stage clotting time
25–28 weeks[4]	10	0.060 ± 0.025 L/hr/kg	0.068 ± 0.013 L/kg	0.85 ± 0.25 hr	One-stage clotting time
On ECMO[8]	5	0.228 ± 0.114 L/hr/kg	N/A^b	N/A	ACT
Off ECMO[8]	5	0.096 ± 0.030 L/hr/kg	N/A	N/A	ACT
Adults					
Healthy[4]	8	0.024 ± 0.004 L/hr/kg	0.036 ± 0.004 L/kg	1.03 ± 0.15 hr	One-stage clotting time
Healthy[9]	18	N/A	N/A	1.61 ± 0.07 hr	Whole blood clot time
		N/A	N/A	1.71 ± 0.10 hr	Whole blood clot time
		N/A	N/A	1.34 ± 0.10 hr	Plasma aPTT
		N/A	N/A	1.32 ± 0.07 hr	Plasma aPTT
PE[10]	13	0.042 ± 0.020 L/hr/kg	0.048 ± 0.024 L/kg	0.86 ± 0.34 hr	aPTT
PE[6]	4	N/A	N/A	0.88 ± 0.51 hr	aPTT
DVT[10]	7	0.041 ± 0.009 L/hr/kg	0.055 ± 0.016 L/kg	0.93 ± 0.19 hr	aPTT
DVT[6]	15	N/A	N/A	1.55 ± 1.29 hr	aPTT
Male[10]	12	0.047 ± 0.019 L/hr/kg	0.052 ± 0.025 L/kg	0.78 ± 0.23 hr	aPTT
Female[10]	8	0.034 ± 0.010 L/hr/kg	0.048 ± 0.016 L/kg	1.04 ± 0.33 hr	aPTT
Smoker[10]	5	0.052 ± 0.014 L/hr/kg	0.047 ± 0.017 L/kg	0.62 ± 0.16 hr	aPTT
Nonsmoker[10]	15	0.038 ± 0.017 L/hr/kg	0.052 ± 0.023 L/kg	0.97 ± 0.28 hr	aPTT
Healthy[11]	10	N/A	N/A	0.61 ± 0.08 hr	ACT
Renal failure[11]	13	N/A	N/A	0.79 ± 0.28 hr	ACT
Extracorporeal circulation[12]	50	N/A	N/A	2.1 ± 0.08 hr	ACT

^{a}The number of patients treated in the referenced study.
^{b}N/A = not available.

phase reactants and may be elevated in acutely ill patients.[16] While hepatic or renal impairment may influence the pharmacokinetic parameters delineated above, no significant dosage modification is necessary for unfractionated heparin.

Since heparin products are mixtures of a wide range of molecular weights, pharmacokinetic parameters may vary with the particular preparation used. The variability of pharmacokinetic parameters brought about by heparin is caused by its nonspecific binding to proteins and cells. Heparin-binding proteins are quite variable in their concentration during acute illness. This accounts for the unpredictable anticoagulant response and the potential for heparin resistance that may be seen in some patients. The impact of LMWH to address these concerns will be discussed in the section "Low Molecular Weight Heparins."

The volume of distribution (V) of heparin closely approximates blood volume.[7] Estimation of blood volume provides a reasonable estimation of V when pharmacokinetic calculations are performed.

Heparin: Therapeutic Range

In general, the targeted pharmacologic effect for heparin is a prolongation of the selected clotting test to 1.5–2.5 times the patient's normal baseline value.[2-4] However, the target effect varies with the specific indication for its use (Table 5).[17-24] Current recommendations of the American College of Chest Physicians and the College of American Pathologists indicate that patients should be treated with unfractionated IV heparin to prolong the aPTT to a range that corresponds to a whole-blood heparin concentration of 0.2–0.4 U/ml or 0.3–0.7 U/ml by chromogenic/amidolytic anti-X_a heparin assay. These recommendations are based on well-controlled, randomized trials in patients with both pulmonary embolism and deep venous thrombosis.[2,25]

TABLE 5. Therapeutic End-Points for Specific Treatment Indications

Disease or Condition	Therapeutic Range	Comments
Prevention of catheter clotting	Nonspecific low doses	No studies on survival of catheters related to degree of anticoagulation
ECMO in neonates	ACT 180–240 sec[17]	Range apparently based on anecdotal experience
Cardiopulmonary bypass in adults or pediatrics	ACT 400–600 sec[18,19]	Range based on animal studies and anecdotal experience
Hemodialysis	ACT 180–240 sec	
Treatment of DVT and PE	Prolong the aPTT to a range that corresponds to a whole blood heparin concentration of 0.2–0.4 U/ml by protamine titration or a plasma X_a concentration of 0.3–0.7 U/ml by amidolytic assay	Recommendation based on studies in patients with DVT and PE and on the relationship between the aPTT and effectiveness.[25]
Treatment of MI	CIUFH sufficient to prolong the aPTT 1.5–2 times control.	'With or without thrombolytic therapy having been administered.[35]

Several coagulation tests are used for monitoring heparin's effect, and each has different limitations (Table 6).[3,23,26–30] Heparin concentration measurements may be used to reach a target therapeutic range (e.g., 0.3–0.7 unit/ml), especially in unusual coagulation situations such as pregnancy[24] where the reliability of clotting studies is questionable. For DVT or PE, it may be

TABLE 6. Coagulation Tests Used to Regulate Heparin Dosing[2, 23, 25-29]

Test	Range	Advantages	Disadvantages
aPTT	28–42 sec Patient's own baseline should be used[a,b]	DVT and PE studies done using this test; recognized standards available; laboratory control equipment and quality control better; extensive clinical experience	Lacks reproducibility with different reagents, instruments, and laboratories; nonlinear relationship to increasing heparin concentration; loss of accuracy of value above 150 sec
ACT	80–130 sec Patient's own baseline should be used[b]	Rapid bedside test; linear increase with heparin concentration in usual therapeutic range; extensive experience in hemodialysis, cardiopulmonary bypass, and ECMO patients	Lacks reproducibility with ACT of >600 sec and with different reagents and instruments; limited clinical trials in DVT or PE patients.
Whole blood heparin concentration	0.2–0.4 U/ml	Overcomes inadequacies of aPTTs Useful in heparin resistance Useful in setting of pregnancy	Labor intensive
Plasma heparin concentration	0.3–06 U/ml	Overcomes inadequacies of aPTTs Useful in heparin resistance Useful in setting of pregnancy Useful in setting of lupus antibodies/Antiphospholipid Antibody Syndrome	Labor intensive

TABLE 6. (*continued*)

Test	Range	Advantages	Disadvantages
		Less labor intensive than whole blood test	

ᵃIf unavailable or elevated, laboratory control values may be used.
ᵇCIUFH = continuous infusion unfractionated heparin.

preferable to correlate heparin concentrations with a target aPTT;[3,31–33] pharmacokinetic information derived from heparin concentrations may help to achieve therapeutic aPTT values more rapidly.[34]

Heparin: Suggested Sampling Times and Monitoring

Specific sampling times for patients receiving heparin therapy vary according to the treatment indication. The times suggested for PE, DVT, extracorporeal circulation, and prophylaxis of venous thrombosis are listed in Table 7.[34]

TABLE 7. Suggested Sampling Times for Patients Receiving Heparin for Various Indications

Indication	Sampling Time
PE or DVT	Continuous infusion heparin: coagulation test obtained 6 hr after start of infusion or after change in infusion rateᵃ (refer to dosing method 2) Intermittent subcutaneous heparin: coagulation test obtained 6 hr after any dose
Extracorporeal circulation	Neonatal ECMO or cardiopulmonary bypass: ACT obtained every 30–60 min during dialysis Hemodialysis: ACT obtained at least every 60 min during dialysis

TABLE 7. (*continued*)

Prophylaxis of venous thrombosis	Coagulation test obtained 6 hr after subcutaneous heparin dose

If heparin is being dosed by a combined pharmacokinetic and pharmacodynamic approach (see pharmacokinetic dosing approaches section), samples for heparin concentrations and clotting studies should be obtained 1, 4, and 12 hr after initiation of a continuous infusion. Doses should be adjusted after 1- and 4-hr samples, and precision should be checked with 12-hr samples.[33]

Monitoring

The anticoagulant effects of heparin are most frequently monitored by aPTT. Adjustments are predicated upon the results of aPTT values. When heparin is administered in fixed doses, the anticoagulant response to heparin varies among patients and within the same patient (inter- and intrapatient variability). This variability is caused by differences in heparin concentrations, neutralizing proteins, and rates of heparin clearance.

For many aPTT reagents, a therapeutic effect is achieved with an aPTT ratio of 1.5–2.5 (measured by dividing the patient's observed aPTT by the mean of the normal laboratory control aPTT). With very sensitive aPTT reagents, the therapeutic range is higher, while for less sensitive reagents, the therapeutic range is lower, prompting the necessity of heparin concentration determinations.

Since aPTT reagents may vary in their sensitivity, it is inappropriate to use the same aPTT ratio (1.5–2.5) for all reagents. The therapeutic range for each aPTT reagent should be calibrated to be equivalent to a heparin concentration of 0.2–0.4 units/ml by whole blood (protamine titration) or to an anti-factor X_a level (plasma heparin concentration) of about 0.3–0.7 units/ml.[47]

Anti-X_a plasma heparin concentrations are another method of monitoring the anticoagulant effects of heparin. Consensus guidelines (American College of Chest Physicians as well as the College of American Pathologists) are increasingly calling for monitoring of both unfractionated heparin as well as low molecular weight heparin with anti-X_a plasma heparin concentrations. There are misconceptions regarding the availability and costs of anti-X_a plasma heparin concentrations. These misconceptions have been addressed in the literature and dispelled.[48]

While there is evidence relating a higher heparin dose to the likelihood of a bleeding complication, there is stronger evidence supporting the contributions of patient-related factors such as recent surgery, generalized hemostatic abnormalities, peptic ulcers, neoplastic lesions, and use of concomitant antithrombotic medications (e.g., glycoprotein IIb/IIIa inhibitors, thrombolytic agents, and antiplatelet agents) to an increase in the likelihood of a bleeding complication.[2] Given these observations, most published guidelines, especially in the setting of cardiology, advocate a lowered dose of unfractionated heparin when coadministering these agents. Specific guidelines exist and should be adhered to when treating the corresponding patient population.[49]

Heparin: Pharmacodynamic Monitoring—Concentration-Related Efficacy

Thrombus formation, extension, or embolization can be markers of inadequate heparinization or development of heparin-associated thrombocytopenia. Factors that affect heparin concentrations and the anticoagulant effect relationship include ATIII and platelet factor 4 (PF4). Technical variables that affect the aPTT response to heparin include the type of clot detection system used in the instrumentation, the contact activator, and the phospholipid composition of the reagent. Elevated concentrations of factor VIII can occur in a number of clinical states, including pregnancy, malignancy, acute thrombosis, and major surgery.[36,37] These and other factors are discussed in Table 8.[38–46]

TABLE 8. Factors to Consider when Interpreting Heparin Pharmacodynamics

Factor	Comments
ATIII (obtained with baseline coagulation studies and on day 3)[38-42]	If ATIII concentrations are low (<84%), heparin may not exert its anticoagulant effect at usual doses and concentrations (i.e., heparin resistance).[38] ATIII concentrations may fall due to heparin therapy.[39] Decreased ATIII predisposes the patient to thrombus formation[38] and PE during heparin therapy for DVT.[39] ATIII is easily replaced with administration of blood, plasma, or ATIII concentrates.
PF4 (not routinely measured)[43, 44]	PE4 neutralizes heparin effect and promotes thrombus formation. When PF4 is increased (e.g., during disseminated intravascular coagulation or immune thrombocytopenia), patient may be relatively heparin resistant.[43, 44] Elevated PF4 in plasma also may inactivate heparin concentrations in vitro, giving falsely low heparin concentration results.
Heparin cofactor II (not routinely measured)[45]	This factor plays a minor role when ATIII concentrations are adequate but can be important if ATIII deficiency occurs.
Coagulation tests	Correlation of heparin concentrations with coagulation tests shows at least a fivefold variation in clotting tests at the same concentration.[3]
Pregnancy	During the third trimester, pregnant patients display relative heparin resistance.[24]
Circadian effect	Effects of heparin on coagulation tests may be greater (up to 50–60%) at night than during the daytime.[46]

Heparin: Pharmacodynamic Monitoring—Concentration-Related Toxicity

Table 9 outlines heparin-related toxicities.

TABLE 9. Heparin-Related Toxicities

Toxicity	Monitoring and Detection	Prevention and Management
Major bleeding[50] (leading to blood transfusion, heparin discontinuation, prolonged hospital stay, or death)	Clinical signs depend on site of bleeding. Increased risk correlated with increased dose, but studies of relationship to coagulation tests are limited. Risk factors include female >60 years old, dose of >25 units/kg/hr, concomitant aspirin, heavy alcohol use, increased length of use, and intermittent intravenous bolus dosing.	• Coagulation tests kept below 2.5 times baseline • Length of use limited by early initiation of warfarin • Heparin effects reversed with protamine sulfate (see reversing heparin's effect section)
Minor bleeding[50]	Relationship to heparin dose and coagulation studies was noted in some reports. Guaiac-positive stool and bleeding from nose, gums, puncture sites, urine, sputum, etc, occur.	• Intramuscular route avoided for medications • Coagulation tests kept below 2.5 times baseline
Thrombocytopenia[51]	Direct platelet effect is not dose related, with onset 1–20 (usual 5–9) days after start of heparin. Effect is often transient. Platelet counts should be monitored at least every other day while patient receives heparin.[52]	• Pork intestine heparin used instead of beef lung heparin when possible • Heparin stopped if platelets are <100,000 or bleeding occurs[52]

TABLE 9. (continued)

Toxicity	Monitoring and Detection	Prevention and Management
Thrombosis due to immune thrombocytopenia[53,54]	Triad of decreased platelets, high heparin dose requirements, and formation of arterial thrombi is present. If platelet count decreases, platelet aggregation testing should be done if possible. A positive test confirms diagnosis.	• Initiate warfarin early to decrease risk • Heparin avoided in patients with prior history • If thrombosis is suspected, all heparin stopped immediately, including flushes and arterial catheters; danaproid or lepirudin for venous embolic disease started to aspirin and dipyridamole started to inhibit platelet aggregation; thrombolytic therapy provided for life-threatening thrombus until warfarin effect is adequate;[54] warfarin should not be used alone[2]
Osteoporosis[57]	Problem only occurs with long-term use (>6 months) of doses over 20,000 units/day. Bone films in otherwise at risk patients may be appropriate.	• Risk minimized by assuring adequate calcium intake
Hyperkalemia	Monitoring at least every 3–4 days is necessary during therapy.	• Fluids adjusted

Increased aspartate aminotransferase (AST) and alanine aminotransferase (ALT)	Monitoring of laboratory values probably is not routinely necessary.	• Warfarin introduced and heparin stopped as soon as possible (probably not due to liver disease)
Transient alopecia	No special monitoring is necessary.	• No special treatment performed
Other side effects Skin lesions Skin necrosis Hypersensitivity Priapism	Observation	• Supportive therapy

Reversing Heparin's Effect

Protamine is used to neutralize heparin following severe heparin overdosing. Overdosing of protamine must be avoided, however, because it can cause bleeding.

Each milligram of protamine sulfate neutralizes 90 units of beef lung heparin sodium, 100 units of heparin calcium, or 115 units of heparin sodium derived from porcine intestinal mucosa or roughly 1 mg (100 units) of low molecular weight heparin. For low molecular weight heparin there is approximately 60% reversal of the effect on Factor X_a.

Overdose of protamine may potentiate bleeding. Protamine must be administered slowly over 1 hr minimally to avoid anaphylaxis and not exceed a total dose of 50 mg.

Time after Heparin Dose	Protamine Sulfate Dose[a]
<30 min	1–1.5 mg for each 100 units of heparin in last dose
30–120 min	0.5–0.75 mg for each 100 units of heparin in last dose
>120 min	0.25–0.375 mg for each 100 units of heparin in last dose
Heparin intravenous infusion	25–50 mg after infusion is stopped

[a]*In the event of major bleeding, some clinicians recommend using the lower end of these ranges to avoid potential bleeding caused by excess protamine sulfate.*

Heparin: Drug–Drug Interactions

Use of the drugs listed in Table 10[56–59] in patients receiving heparin may warrant adjustments in dosing or sampling procedures.

TABLE 10. Heparin-Drug Interactions

Drug	Interaction	Prevention and Management
Nitroglycerin (intravenous)[56,57]	Resistance to anticoagulant effect of heparin.	• Infuse drugs at different sites • Adjust doses for therapeutic aPTT
Platelet function inhibitors[58] (e.g., aspirin and nonsteroidal anti-inflammatory agents)	Risk of bleeding increases	• Avoid if possible • Salsalate, an alternative anti-inflammatory agent, does not inhibit platelet aggregation
Decreased in vitro[59] binding of basic and acidic drugs (e.g., propranolol and quinidine); in vivo effect not shown	Increased lipoprotein lipase activity by heparin increases free fatty acid (FFA) formation, leading to displacement by FFAs	• Heparinized samples should be processed rapidly when analyzing for free drug • Results interpreted cautiously
Warfarin[60]	aPTT is prolonged	• Heparin doses reduced, if necessary, to prevent excessive aPTT.
Thrombolytics GPIIb/IIIa antagonists	Risk of bleeding increases	• Heparin doses reduced

Heparin: Drug–Disease State or Condition Interactions

Heparin's pharmacokinetic parameters may be influenced by a patient's condition or underlying disease state. Table 11 provides adjustment factors for several such conditions and disease states.

TABLE 11. Drug-Disease State or Condition Interactions with Comparisons Made to Average DVT Patients

Disease State or Condition	Assay	Adjustment Factors[a]		
		Clearance	Volume of Distribution[b]	Half-Life
PE	X_a	1.5	1	0.75
	ACT	1	1	1
Liver disease	X_a	1.5	1	0.75
Renal disease	X_a	1	1	1
Hemodialysis	X_a	1	1	1
	ACT	Not available	Not available	1
Neonates				
>32 weeks	X_a	2.5	1	0.33
≤32 weeks	X_a	2.6	1.3	0.33
	Clotting time	1.6	1.2	0.85
Neonates on ECMO	ACT	5.5	Not available	Not available
Adults				
Male	ACT	1.1	1	0.85
Female	ACT	0.8	1	1.1
Smoker	ACT	1.2	1	0.67
Nonsmoker	ACT	1	1	1

[a]Standard values for adjustments are CL = 0.03 L/hr/kg, V = 0.07 L/kg, and t½ = 1.6 hr. To correct pharmacokinetic parameters for underlying condition these values are multiplied by the adjustment factors.
[b]The V of heparin is similar to the patient's blood volume.

Heparin: Pharmacokinetic Dosing Approaches

Heparin dosing can be adjusted either empirically or by pharmacokinetic calculations using one of several approaches:

1. For practical dosing, heparin's therapeutic effect is hastened by a loading dose. This dose may be empiri-

cally selected (e.g., 5000 units) as an intravenous bolus, or loading doses may be individualized using the patient's weight. Such an approach has utilized 70–100 units/kg. In some instances, the weight-based approach to loading patients is based on the indication for use; 70 units/kg is used for all thrombotic indications other than suspected or proven pulmonary embolism, for which the 100-units/kg dose is utilized. Variable approaches to continuous dosing have been employed. Empiric dosing of 1000–1333[61] units/hr may be used. The lowest dose may result in outcomes (i.e., aPTT values) that are below or above the therapeutic ranges.

Other approaches to continuous dosing include the use of a weight-based dosing nomogram, which is variable between 15 and 25 units/kg/hr. The lowest doses are usually used for the majority of thrombotic indications except pulmonary embolism where the patient could receive 25 units/kg/hr due to increased clearance.

Heparin dosing adjustment nomograms assist the initial weight-based dosing efforts. All such nomograms should be developed for a specific aPTT reagent. Examples are depicted in Tables 12[61] and 13[62].

2. The necessary infusion rate (R_2) for a target ACT (ACT_2) can be calculated from the actual steady-state ACT (ACT_1) at a known heparin dosing rate (R_1) using the formula[2,13]

$$R_2 = R_1 \times \frac{(\log ACT_2 - \log ACT_0)}{(\log ACT_1 - \log ACT_0)}$$

where ACT_0 is the baseline pretreatment ACT.

3. If aPTT monitoring of heparin's effect is used, doses must be adjusted with the understanding that aPTT rises disproportionately to the heparin concentration and dose in a nonlinear manner. The changes noted in aPTT with adjustments in heparin doses are unpre-

TABLE 12. Heparin Dosage Adjustment Protocol[61, a]

Patients aPTT[b]	Repeat Bolus Dose	Hold Infusion (minutes)	Change Rate (dose) of Infusion (units/hr)	Timing of Next aPTT
<50	5000 units	0	+120	6 hr
50–59	0	0	+120	6 hr
60–85[c]	0	0	0	Next morning
86–95	0	0	−80	Next morning
96–120	0	30	−80	6 hr
>120	0	60	−160	6 hr

[a]*Starting dose of 5000 units intravenous bolus followed by 1333 units/hr (32,000 units/24 hr) as a continuous infusion. An aPTT was performed 6 hr after the bolus injection, dosage adjustments were made according to protocol, and the aPTT was repeated as indicated in the right-hand column.*
[b]*Normal range for aPTT with Dade Actin FS reagent is 27–35 seconds equivalent to 40 units/ml of heparin. Therapeutic range of 60–85 seconds is equivalent to a heparin concentration of 0.2–0.4 units/ml by whole blood protamine titration or 0.3–0.7 units/ml as a plasma anti-factor X_a concentration. The therapeutic range varies with the responsiveness of the aPTT reagent to heparin.*
[c]*The therapeutic range in seconds should correspond to a plasma heparin concentration of 0.2–0.4 IU/ml by protamine sulfate or 0.3–0.7 IU/ml by plasma-amidolytic assay. When aPTT is checked at 6 hr or longer, steady state can be assumed.*

dictable; such guidelines are only rough estimates. Therefore, the clinician may have to deviate frequently. Cruickshank et al.[63] described a protocol where 66 and 81% of the patients were above the lower limit of the therapeutic range by 24 and 48 hr, respectively. Of 350 aPTT measurements following the initial dosing adjustments using the protocol, 59.4% were within the therapeutic range, 25.2% were below the therapeutic range, and 15.4% were above the therapeutic range.

4. If heparin concentrations can be measured concomitantly with coagulation studies, a combined pharma-

TABLE 13. Body Weight-Based Dosing Scheme for Heparin[62,a]

aPTT (seconds)	Dose Change (units/kg/hr)	Additional Action	Next aPTT, (hr)
<35 (<1.2 × mean normal)	+4	Rebolus with 80 IU/kg	6
35–45 (1.2–1.5 × mean normal)	+2	Rebolus with 40 IU/kg	6
46–70 (1.5–2.3 × mean normal)	0	0	6[b]
71–90 (2.3–3.0 × mean normal)	−2	0	6
> 90 (>3 × mean normal)	−3	Hold infusion 1 hr	6

[a] *Initial dosing: loading dose is 80 IU/kg; maintenance infusion is 18 IU/kg/hr (aPTT in 6 hr).*
[b] *During the first 24 hr, repeat aPTT every 6 hr. Thereafter, monitor aPTT once every morning unless it is outside of the therapeutic range.*

cokinetic–pharmacodynamic model can be used. The target heparin concentration is determined from the relationship of heparin concentrations and coagulation studies drawn 1 and 4 hr after initiation of heparin.[34] Subsequent heparin infusion rates to achieve the targeted concentrations are then calculated using the pharmacokinetic infusion model developed by Chiou et al.:[64]

$$CL = [2R / (C_1 + C_2)] + [2V(C_1 - C_2) / (C_1 + C_2)(t_2 + t_1)]$$

where

CL = apparent heparin clearance in units per hour
R = heparin infusion rate in units per hour
V = volume of distribution equal to patient's estimated blood volume in milliliters (0.07 L/kg)
C_1 = first heparin concentration, drawn at time 1 (t_1), 1 hr after initiation of heparin
C_2 = second heparin concentration, drawn at t_2, 4 hr after initiation of heparin

The clearance may then be used to determine a dose to produce heparin concentrations in the therapeutic range.

maintenance dose = (target heparin concentration) (CL)

The validity of this method was confirmed with plasma heparin concentrations using a factor X_a assay, which is more readily adapted to routine clinical applications.[65]

5. Heparin dosing also may be estimated using blood volume calculations to estimate V and population half-life estimates (Tables 2 and 3) to calculate K. The correction factors in Table 11 can be used. Target heparin concentrations are usually 300–600 unit/L, and heparin doses can be calculated with these formulas:

loading dose = (V × target heparin concentration)
= (0.07 L/kg) (patient's weight)(600 U/L)[11]
maintenance dose = (target heparin concentration) $(V)(K)$[66]

This dosing approach may be particularly useful for morbidly obese patients[66] where underdosing may be a problem.

Summary of Heparin Dosing and Monitoring

Heparin and warfarin therapy is used except during pregnancy or when warfarin is contraindicated. Patients with proven thromboembolic disease should receive therapy with heparin and warfarin and monitored as follows:

1. Patient specific indication(s) for heparin and warfarin therapy should be addressed, and where appropriate: give weight based, nomogram driven, or pharmacokinetic modeling to achieve desired outcome of efficacy and safety.
2. Baseline coagulation studies (aPTT, PT/INR, CBC) in all patients prior to initiating therapy.

- Continue monitoring aPTT at 6-hour intervals and maintain an aPTT range corresponding to a therapeutic heparin concentration.

- Check platelet count by day 4 in heparin naïve patients, and daily in patients with prior heparin exposure.
3. Initiate warfarin within first 24–48 hours[67], adjust subsequent daily dosing based on INR response, and stop heparin after 4 or 5 days overlap, when INR is >2.0 for two consecutive days. (See Chapter 21, Warfarin.)
4. Monitor for clinical outcomes of efficacy and safety (Tables 9 and 10).

Low Molecular Weight Heparins (LMWH)

LMWHs are now widely used if not in deference then at least as an option compared to heparin for the prevention and treatment of venous and arterial embolic disease. LMWHs are obtained by fractionating or depolymerizing UFH, which is a heterogeneous mixture of heparin chains with molecular weights of 5,000–30,000 daltons. The mean molecular weight (daltons) of LMWH is approximately 4,000–5,000. LMWH indications vary by manufacturer. Each of the LMWHs has been evaluated in numerous randomized clinical trials and has been proven to be safe and efficacious for the prevention and treatment of venous thromboembolism. LMWHs are used for prevention of deep venous thrombosis after hip replacement, knee replacement, abdominal surgery, and trauma, oncology, medical, and spinal cord injury patients. In addition, LMWHs are used to treat patients who have unstable angina, non-q-wave myocardial infarction, deep venous thrombosis, and pulmonary embolism.

The LMWHs are often viewed as a homogeneous group, but their derivation from unfractionated heparin using different methods of enzymatic or hydrolytic cleavage results in different molecular weight profiles for each product. These variations may result in clinically relevant, different pharmacokinetic and pharmacodynamic effects. Compared with unfractionated heparin, which has a ratio of anti-factor X_a to anti-factor II_a activity of approximately 1:1, the various commercial LMWHs have anti-factor X_a to anti-factor II_a ratios varying between 2:1 and 4:1, depending on their molecular size distribution (Table 14).[68]

Pharmacokinetic parameters for different LMWHs are documented in the literature, but few studies have directly compared different agents in human subjects. The pharmacokinetics of heparin and LMWHs differ. LMWHs are less protein bound than heparin. Because of their long elimination half-lives, some LMWHs may be administered as single daily doses, which is an advantage over heparin.[69]

Doses of heparin and LMWHs are not interchangeable because of differences in their anticoagulant activity.[70] Routine monitoring of coagulation tests (e.g., aPTT) or heparin concentration assays during prophylactic LMWH therapy is generally considered unnecessary.[71]

Subcutaneous injection of the LMWHs produce only minimal effects on aPTT, and, as such, aPTT values

TABLE 14. LMWH Comparison of Pharmacokinetic/Pharmacodynamic Parameters[a]

LMWH	Brand Name	Avg Molecular Weight, daltons	Bioavailability (F), %	Half-Life, hr	Xa:IIa Binding Affinity Ratio
Ardeparin	Normiflo	6000	90	3	1.9:1
Dalteparin	Fragmin	6000	87	3	2.7:1
Enoxaparin	Lovenox	4500	92	4.5	3.8:1
Tinzaparin[85]	Innohep	6500	8.7	3.5	1.9:1

[a]*Adapted with permission from reference 68.*

cannot be used reliably to monitor or document efficacy and safety of LMWHs. LMWHs can be monitored by heparin concentration assay (anti-factor X_a assay by either whole blood or plasma determinations) for patients treated with LMWHs. Though routine monitoring with heparin concentration assay is not necessary, it may be warranted in patients with renal impairment (CrCl <30 ml/min) because LMWHs are renally eliminated. It may also be warranted in morbidly obese patients.

The therapeutic range for anti-factor X_a assay by whole blood protamine titration is 0.2–0.4 units/ml, whereas the therapeutic range for plasma heparin determinations by amidolytic assay is 0.3–0.7 units/ml.[72]

LMWH: Usual Dosage Range in Absence of Clearance-Altering Factors

LMWHs have a longer plasma half-life and a more predictable anticoagulant response to weight-adjusted doses than standard heparin. These characteristics allow some LMWHs to be administered once daily and without laboratory monitoring.

LMWHs are disease state and product specific, with different doses being administered based upon the specific indication and the manufacturer.

Table 15 shows manufacturers' suggested dosing for specific indications. Guidelines for treating venous thromboembolic disease (VTED) follow.

For suspected VTED

- Obtain baseline aPTT, PT/INR, and CBC.
- Check for contraindication to heparin therapy.
- Give *unfractionated heparin* (UFH), 5000 IU, intravenous push.
- Order imaging study.

TABLE 15. LMWHs Manufacturers' Dosing and Disease-State Indications[a]

	Prophylaxis against DVT in setting of:		
LMWH	General Surgery	Orthopedic Surgery	Treatment of DVT
Ardeparin	Not indicated	50 units/kg twice daily	Not indicated
Dalteparin	2500 IU subcutaneously daily	2500 IU subcutaneously twice daily	120 IU/kg subcutaneously twice daily
		-or-	-or-
		5000 IU subcutaneously daily	200 IU/kg subcutaneously daily
Enoxaparin	40 mg subcutaneously daily	30 mg subcutaneously every 12 hr	1 mg/kg subcutaneously every 12 hr
			-or-
			1.5 mg/kg subcutaneously daily
Tinzaparin[85]	Not indicated	Not indicated	175 IU/kg subcutaneously once daily

[a]*Adapted with permission from: Hirsch J. Low molecular weight heparins. St. Louis, MO: B.C. Decker; 1999:35.*

For confirmed VTED

- Give LMWH (enoxaparin)[a], 1 mg/kg subcutanously every 12 hr for outpatient treatment or 1.5 mg/kg subcutanously daily for inpatient treatment of DVT with or without PE.

[a]*Current Guidelines, Fifth American college of chest physicians consensus conference on antithrombotic therapy (1998). Adapted from* Chest. 1998; 114 *(Suppl):439S–769S.*

- Start warfarin therapy on day 1; adjust subsequent daily dosing according to INR.
- Consider checking platelet count between days 1 and 5.
- Stop LMWH after at least 5–7 days of combined therapy when INR is >2.0 on two consecutive days.
- Anticoagulate with warfarin for at least 3 months (goal INR = 2.5, range 2.0–3.0).

LMWH: Dosage Form Availability

LMWHs are available only as solutions for injection. Currently, LMWHs are administered subcutaneously, although trials examining their role via the intravenous route of administration have been conducted or are underway. LMWHs for injection are supplied at different concentrations by several manufacturers.

LMWH: Bioavailability (F) of Dosage Forms

The bioavailability of subcutaneous doses of LMWHs (87–100%) is greater than that of doses of UFH (30%) which may translate into lower LMWH dosage requirements.[73,74]

LMWH: General Pharmacokinetic Information

The plasma recoveries and pharmacokinetics of LMWHs differ from heparin because of differences in the binding properties of the two sulfated polysaccharides to plasma proteins and endothelial cells. LMWHs bind much less avidly to heparin-binding proteins than heparin, a property that contributes to the superior bioavailability of LMWHs at low doses and their more predictable anticoagulation response. LMWHs also do not bind to endothelial cells in culture, a property that could account for their longer plasma half-life and their dose-independent clearance.[68] LMWHs are cleared renally and their biologic half-life is increased in patients with

TABLE 16. Comparison of the Pharmacokinetic Profiles of Dalteparin and Enoxaparin Administered Subcutaneously in Volunteers (Doses for Prevention of Thromboembolic Disease)[a]

Pharmacokinetic Parameter	Dalteparin 2500 units	Enoxaparin 40 mg
A_{max} (units/ml)	0.22 ± 0.07	0.57 ± 0.14[b]
t_{max} (hr) (median and range)	2.5 (1.5–6.0)	3.0 (2.0–4.5)
$T_{\frac{1}{2}a}$ (hr)	0.91 ± 0.20	0.74 ± 0.44
CL/F (ml/min)	33.33 ± 11.83	13.83 ± 3.17[b]
$T_{\frac{1}{2}}$ (hr)	2.81 ± 0.84	4.37 ± 0.47[b]
V (L)	7.74 ± 2.50	5.24 ± 1.20[b]

[a] Adapted with permission from reference 78.
[b] Statistically significant.
A_{max} = maximum plasma activity; t_{max} = time to maximum activity; $T_{\frac{1}{2}a}$ = apparent absorption half-life; CL/F = apparent total body clearance; $T_{\frac{1}{2}}$ = apparent elimination half-life; and V = volume of distribution.

renal failure.[75–77] Pharmacokinetic and pharmacodynamic differences existing for the LMWHs are shown in Table 14.

Table 16 shows differences found in one study of two commercially available products. The study demonstrated that dalteparin and enoxaparin differed significantly from each other in their pharmacokinetic profiles. These differences may contribute to different safety and efficacy balances reported in clinical studies. In view of these variations, LMWHs currently must be considered as different medications, each characterized by its own safety and efficacy profile.[78]

LMWH: Therapeutic Range

Therapeutic LMWHs levels have been monitored by use of a heparin concentration assay:[78]

Whole blood anti-factor X_a assay	0.2–0.4 units/ml
Plasma anti-factor X_a assay	0.3–0.7 units/ml

LMWH: Suggested Sampling Times and Effects on Therapeutic Range

LMWHs are not monitored by aPTT determinations. Heparin concentration assays, although not necessarily based upon manufacturer's recommendations, should be obtained at midinterval of the dosing regimen if done at all. The heparin concentration should be obtained before the third dose of oral anticoagulant therapy with warfarin. This recommendation is because heparin assays measure factor X_a. By the third dose of warfarin, factor X_a activity is no longer clinically detectable by assay because it has been suppressed by warfarin.

LMWH: Pharmacodynamic Monitoring—Concentration-Related Efficacy

It is generally accepted that a minimum level of LMWH must be maintained to achieve an effective antithrombotic state and that inadequate anticoagulant therapy results in unacceptably higher rates of thromboembolic disease recurrence. Animal experiments support the concept that a plasma concentration of heparin between 0.2 and 0.4 IU/ml (measured by protamine sulfate titration) is necessary to interrupt an ongoing thrombotic process.[79]

Studies examining the efficacy of LMWHs for treatment of thromboembolic disease have used symptomatic recurrent disease as the end-point. No differences in outcomes for recurrence of thromboembolic disease have been noted for LMWHs when compared to UFH.[80,81]

For prophylaxis against thromboembolic disease, development of VTED has been the end-point for determining efficacy. Compared to traditional prophylaxis with UFH or oral anticoagulant therapy with warfarin, LMWHs have been demonstrated to be as or more efficacious in their ability to prevent occurrence of VTED.

For treatment of unstable angina, non-q wave myocardial infarction, LMWHs achieve therapeutic heparin concentrations (by anti-factor X_a assay in the therapeutic range 0.3–0.7 units/ml) as soon as 30 minutes after subcutaneous administration.[82] Currently, trials examining the role of intravenous LMWH in unstable angina, non-q wave myocardial infarction reveal an immediate antithrombotic effect after intravenous administration.

LMWH: Pharmacodynamic Monitoring—Concentration-Related Toxicity

The antithrombotic and hemorrhagic effects of heparin have been compared with LMWHs in various experimental animal models. When compared on a gravimetric basis, LMWHs are said to cause decreased potential for hemorrhagic episodes in animal models. Contemporary studies evaluating alternative regimens of continuous infusion unfractionated heparin (CIUFH) versus LMWHs reveal rates of major bleeding ranging from 0 to 7% for CIUFH and rates of fatal bleeding ranging from 0 to 2%. For LMWHs, the rates of major bleeding range from 0 to 3% and fatal bleeding from 0 to 0.8%. These data support the inference that LMWH does not result in increased risk of major bleeding compared to UHF.[83] Differences in the relative antithrombotic to hemorrhagic ratios among these polysaccharides could be explained by the observations that LMWHs have less inhibitory effects on platelet function and vascular permeability.[69] For all LMWHs there exist the potential for neuraxial hematoma if epidural, spinal anesthesia, or other spinal punctures are performed while patients are anticoagulated with LMWHs or heparinoids for prevention of thromboembolic complications. LMWHs have been found to have a lessened incidence of thrombocytopenia when compared to UFH,[69] but it is important to realize that patients having antibodies to UFH may similarly have reactions to LMWHs, producing heparin-induced thrombocytopenia (HIT).

TABLE 18. Protamine Dose for Reversal of LMWH

LMWH	<8 hr	8–12 hr	>12 hr
Ardeparin	1 mg/100 anti-factor X_a IU	0.5 mg/100 anti-factor X_a IU	Not necessary
Dalteparin	1 mg/100 anti-factor X_a IU	0.5 mg/100 anti-factor X_a IU	Not necessary
Enoxaparin	1 mg/1 mg	0.5 mg/1 mg	Not necessary
Tinzaparin	1 mg/100 anti-factor X_a IU	0.5 mg/100 anti-factor X_a IU	Not necessary

LMWH: Reversing the Effect of LMWHs

LMWHs may be reversed by protamine sulfate. Care should be taken to avoid overdosage with protamine sulfate. Administration of protamine sulfate can cause severe hypotension and anaphylactic reactions. Slow intravenous injection of protamine sulfate (1% solution) at 1 mg of protamine for every 100 anti-factor X_a IU of dalteparin or 1 mg of enoxaparin has been recommended by its manufacturer for reversal. Based on timing of the LMWH relative to the hemorrhagic complication, protamine sulfate may not be necessary. Table 18 gives guidelines for reversal of LMWHs with respect to time since the last LMWH dose.

LMWH: Drug–Drug Interactions

LMWHs do not have definitively identified drug interactions as is the case for UFH, although platelet-inhibiting drugs or GI irritant drugs could in theory potentiate any likelihood of complications.

LMWH: Drug–Disease State or Condition Interaction

LMWHs, unlike UFH, bind less avidly to acute phase reactant plasma proteins, which are often increased during illness. Endogenous plasma proteins, platelet factor 4 (released from activated platelets) and vonWillebrand's factor are circulating substances released during illness and clotting respectively. Thromboembolic disease as well as comorbid conditions account for variability of these plasma proteins which, in turn, causes variable anticoagulant responsiveness with UFH. Such variability is seen less often with LMWHs because of their decreased binding to these acute phase reactant substances and their improved bioavailability.

Smaller doses of LMWHs are used for prophylaxis than those used for documented thromboembolic disease.[84]

Summary of LMWH Dosing and Monitoring

Development of LMWHs is a breakthrough in the management of venous and arterial thromboembolic disease. These drugs have better bioavailability, a longer half-life, and a more predictable anticoagulant effect than standard UFH. LMWHs are safe and effective in preventing recurrent venous thromboembolic disease when compared to standard UFH dosed by weight-adjusted nomograms. With these findings, LMWHs administered subcutaneously, without laboratory monitoring, in a dose determined by body weight for treatment indications, will shift management strategies from standard UFH to LMWHs in both inpatient and outpatient settings.[84]

References

1. Proceedings of the American College of Chest Physicians 5th consensus on antithrombotic therapy. *Chest* 1998 Nov;114(5 Suppl): 439S–769S.
2. Hirsh J, Warkentine TE, Raschke R, et al. Heparin and low-molecular-weight-heparin: Mechanisms of action, pharmacokinetics, dosing considerations, monitoring, efficacy, and safety. *Chest* 1998; 114:489S–510S.
3. Cipolle RJ, Rodvold KA. Heparin. In: Evans WE, Schentag JJ, Jusko WJ, eds. Applied pharmacokinetics: principles of therapeutic drug monitoring, 2nd ed. Spokane, WA: Applied Therapeutics; 1986:908–43. *Blood:* 1979; 53:525–44.

4. McDonald MM, Jacobson IJ, Hay WW Jr, et al. Heparin clearance in the newborn. *Pediatr Res.* 1981; 15:1015–8.
5. Simon TL, Hyers TM, Gaston JP, et al. Heparin pharmacokinetics: increased requirements in pulmonary embolism. *Br J Haematol.* 1978; 39:111–20.
6. Hirsh J, Van Aken WG, Gallus AS, et al. Heparin kinetics in venous thrombosis and pulmonary embolism. *Circulation.* 1976; 53:681–95.
7. Kandrotas RJ, Gal P, Douglas JB, et al. Heparin pharmacokinetics during hemodialysis. *Ther Drug Monit.* 1989; 11:674–9.
8. Green TP, Isham-Schopf B, Irmiter RJ, et al. Inactivation of heparin during extracorporeal circulation in infants. *Clin Pharmacol Ther.* 1990; 48:148–54.
9. Estes JW. Kinetics of the anticoagulant effect of heparin. *JAMA.* 1970; 212:1492–5.
10. Cipolle RJ, Seifert RD, Nellan BA, et al. Heparin kinetics: variables related to disposition and dosage. *Clin Pharmacol Ther.* 1981; 29:387–93.
11. Perry PJ, Herron GR, King JC. Heparin half-life in normal and impaired renal function. *Clin Pharmacol Ther.* 1974; 16:514–9.
12. Bull BS, Korpman RA, Huse WM, et al. Heparin therapy during extracorporeal circulation. *J Thorac Cardiovasc Surg.* 1975; 69:674–84.
13. de Swart CAM, Nijmeyer B, Roelofs JMM, et al. Kinetics of intravenously administered heparin in normal humans. *Blood* 1982; 60:1251–58.
14. Olsson P, Lagergren H, Ek S. The elimination from plasma of intravenous heparin: an experimental study on dogs and humans. *Acta Med Scand* 1963; 173:619–30.
15. Bjornsson TO, Wolfram BS, Kitchell BB. Heparin kinetics determined by three assay methods. *Clin Pharmacol Ther* 1982; 31:104–13.
16. Young E, Prins MH, Levine MN, et al. Heparin binding to plasma proteins, an important mechanism for heparin resistance. *Thromb Haemost* 1992;67:639–43.
17. Green TP, Isham-Schopf B, Steinhorn RH, et al. Whole blood activated clotting time in infants during extracorporeal membrane oxygenation. *Crit Care Med.* 1990; 18:494–8.
18. Young JA, Kisker CT, Doty DB. Adequate anticoagulation during cardiopulmonary bypass determined by activated clotting time and the appearance of fibrin monomer. *Ann Thorac Surg.* 1978; 26:231–40.
19. Cohen JA. Activated coagulation time method for control of heparin is reliable during cardiopulmonary bypass. *Anesthesiology.* 1984; 60:121–4.
20. Basu D, Gallus A, Hirsh J, et al. A prospective study of the value of monitoring heparin treatment with the activated partial thromboplastin time. *N Engl J Med.* 1986; 287:324–7.
21. Hull RD, Raskob GE, Hirsh J, et al. Continuous intravenous heparin compared with intermittent subcutaneous heparin in the initial treatment of proximal-vein thrombosis. *N Engl J Med.* 1986; 315:1109–14.
22. Taberner DA, Poller L, Thomson JM, et al. Randomized study of adjusted versus fixed low dose heparin prophylaxis of deep vein thrombosis in hip surgery. *Br J Surg.* 1989; 76:933–5.

23. Leyvrez P, Jacques R, Fedor B, et al. Adjusted versus fixed-dose subcutaneous heparin in the prevention of deep-vein thrombosis after total hip replacement. *N Engl J Med.* 1983; 309:954–8.
24. Hahn CLA. Pulsatile heparin administration in pregnancy: a new approach. *Am J Obstet Gynecol.* 1986; 155:283–7.
25. Hyers TM, Agnelli G, Hull RD, et al. Antithrombotic therapy for venous thromboembolic disease. Chest. 1998; 114 (*Suppl*):561S–78S.
26. Brandt JT, Triplett DA. Laboratory monitoring of heparin effect of reagents and instruments on the activated partial thromboplastin time *Am J Clin Pathol.* 1981; 76(Suppl):530–7.
27. Banez EI, Triplett DA, Koepke J. Laboratory monitoring of heparin therapy—the effect of different salts of heparin on the activated partial thromboplastin time. *Am J Clin Pathol.* 1980; 74:569–74.
28. Bain B, Forster T, Sleigh B. Heparin and the activated partial thromboplastin time—a difference between the *in-vitro* and *in-vivo* effects and implications for the therapeutic range. *Am J Clin Pathol.* 1980; 74:668–73.
29. Hattersley PG. Progress report: the activated coagulation time of whole blood (ACT). *Am J Clin Pathol.* 1976; 66:899–904.
30. Uden DL, Payne NR, Kriesmer P, et al. Procedural variables which affect activated clotting time test results during extracorporeal membrane oxygenation therapy. *Crit Care Med.* 1989; 17:1048–51.
31. Hasegawa H, Oguma Y, Takei H, et al. Assay of heparin in plasma using a chromogenic substrate and its clinical applications. *Jpn Heart J.* 1980; 21:367–80.
32. Holm HA, Abildgaard U, Larsen ML, et al. Monitoring of heparin therapy: should heparin assays also reflect the patient's antithrombin concentration? *Thromb Res.* 1987; 46:669–75.
33. Kandrotas RJ. Heparin pharmacokinetics and pharmacodynamics *Clin Pharmacokinet.* 1992; 22:359–74.
34. Groce JB, Gal P, Douglas JB, et al. Heparin dosage adjustment in patients with deep-vein thrombosis using heparin concentrations rather than activated partial thromboplastin time. *Clin Pharm.* 1987; 6:216–22.
35. Cairns JA, Theroux P, Lewis HD, et al. Antithrombotic agents in coronary artery disease. *Chest* 1998; 114:611S–633S.
36. Young E, Wells P, Holloway S, et al. Ex vivo and in-vitro evidence that low molecular weight heparins exhibit less binding to plasma proteins than unfractionated heparin. *Thromb Haemost* 1994; 71:300–4.
37. Levine M, Hirsh J, Gent M, et al. A randomized trial comparing activated thromboplastin time with heparin assay in patients with acute venous thromboembolism requiring large daily doses of heparin. *Arch Intern Med* 1994; 154:49–56.
38. Thaler E, Lechner K. Antithrombin III deficiency and thromboembolism. *Clin Haematol.* 1981; 10:369–90.
39. Holm HA, Kalvenes S, Abildgaard U. Changes in plasma antithrombin (heparin cofactor activity) during intravenous heparin therapy: observations in 198 patients with deep venous thrombosis. *Scand J Haematol.* 1985; 35:564–9.

40. Rosenberg RD. Heparin, antithrombin, and abnormal clotting. *Ann Rev Med*. 1978; 29:367–78.
41. Rosenberg RD. Biochemistry of heparin antithrombin interactions, and the physiologic role of this natural anticoagulant mechanism. *Am J Med*. 1989; 87(3B):2S–9S.
42. Batist G, Bothe A Jr, Bern M, et al. Low antithrombin III in morbid obesity: return to normal with weight reduction. *J Parenter Enter Nutr*. 1983; 7:447–9.
43. Triplett DA. Heparin: biochemistry, therapy, and laboratory monitoring. *Ther Drug Monit*. 1979; 1:173–97.
44. Levine SP, Sorenson RR, Harris MA, et al. The effect of platelet factor 4 (PF4) on assays of plasma heparin. *Br J Haematol*. 1984; 57:585–96.
45. Andersson TR, Bangstad H, Larsen ML. Heparin cofactor II, antithrombin and protein C in plasma from term and preterm infants. *Acta Paediatr Scand*. 1988; 77:485–8.
46. Decousus HA, Croze M, Levi FA, et al. Circadian changes in anticoagulant effect of heparin infused at a constant rate. *Br Med J*. 1985; 290:341–4.
47. Brill-Edwards P, Ginsburg JS, Johnston M, et al. Establishing a therapeutic range for heparin therapy. *Ann Intern Med*. 1993; 119:104–9.
48. Rosborough TK. Monitoring unfractionated heparin therapy with antifactor X_a activity results in fewer monitoring tests and dosage changes than monitoring with the activated partial thromboplastin time. *Pharmacotherapy* 1999; 19:760–6.
49. Ryan TJ, Antman EM, Brooks NH, et al. 1999 update: ACC/AHA guidelines for the management of patients with acute myocardial infarction. A report of the American College of Cardiology/American Heart Association task force on practice guidelines (committee on management of acute myocardial infarction). *J Am Coll Cardiol*. 1999 Sep; 34(3):890–911.
50. Levine MN, Hirsh J. Hemorrhagic complications of anticoagulant therapy. *Semin Thromb Hemost*. 1986; 12:39–57.
51. Nelson JC, Lerner RG, Goldstein R, et al. Heparin-induced thrombocytopenia. *Arch Intern Med*. 1978; 138:548–52.
52. Carter BL. Therapy of acute thromboembolism with heparin and warfarin. *Clin Pharm*. 1991; 10:503–18.
53. Silver D, Kapsch DN, Tsoi EKM. Heparin-induced thrombocytopenia, thrombosis, and hemorrhage. *Ann Surg*. 1983; 198:301–6.
54. Clifton GD, Smith MD. Thrombolytic therapy in heparin-associated thrombocytopenia with thrombosis. *Clin Pharm*. 1986; 5:597–601.
55. Griffith GC, Nichols G, Asher JD, et al. Heparin osteoporosis. *JAMA*. 1965; 193:91–4.
56. Habbab MA, Haft JI. Heparin resistance induced by intravenous nitroglycerin. *Arch Intern Med*. 1987; 147:857–60.
57. Becker RC, Corrao JM, Bovill EG, et al. Intravenous nitroglycerin-induced heparin resistance: a qualitative antithrombin III abnormality. *Am Heart J*. 1990; 119:1254–61.

58. Colburn WA. Pharmacologic implications of heparin interactions with other drugs. *Drug Metab Rev.* 1976; 5:281–93.
59. Naranjo CA, Sellers EM, Khouw V, et al. Variability in heparin effect on serum drug binding. *Clin Pharmacol Ther.* 1980; 28:545–50.
60. Mungall D, Floyd R. Bayesian forecasting of APTT response to continuously infused heparin with and without warfarin administration. *J Clin Pharmacol.* 1989; 29:1043–7.
61. Hirsh J, ed. Guidelines for antithrombotic therapy. 1st ed. Hamilton, Ontario, CANADA: Decker Periodicals, Inc.; 1993:19–20.
62. Raschke RA, Reilly BM, Guidry JR, et al. The weight-based heparin nomogram compared with a "standard care" nomogram: a randomized controlled trial. *Ann Intern Med.* 1993; 119:874–81.
63. Cruickshank MK, Levine MN, Hirsh J, et al. A standard heparin nomogram for the management of heparin therapy. *Arch Intern Med.* 1991; 151:333–7.
64. Chiou WL, Gadella MAF, Peng GW. Method for the rapid estimation of the total body clearance and adjustment of dosage regiments in patients during a constant-rate intravenous infusion. *J Pharmacokinet Biopharm.* 1978; 6:135–51.
65. Kandrotas RJ, Groce JB, Douglas JB, et al. Rapid determination of maintenance heparin infusion rates with the use of non-steady-state heparin concentrations. *Pharmacotherapy.* 1991; 11:280.
66. Ellison MJ, Sawyer WT, Mills TC. Calculation of heparin dosage in a morbidly obese woman. *Clin Pharm.* 1989; 8:65–8.
67. Hull RD, Raskob GE, Rosenbloom D, et al. Heparin for 5 days as compared with 10 days in the initial treatment of proximal venous thrombosis. *N Engl J Med.* 1990; 322:1260–4.
68. Weitz JI. Low-molecular-weight-heparins. *N Engl J Med.* 1997; 337:688–98.
69. Hirsh J, Warkentin TE, Raschke R, et al. Heparin and low-molecular-weight-heparin: Mechanism of action, pharmacokinetics, dosing considerations, monitoring, efficacy, and safety. *Chest.* 1998; 114 (*Suppl*):489S–510S.
70. Nightingale SL. From the food and drug administration. *JAMA.* 1993; 270:1672.
71. McEvoy GK, ed. American Hospital Formulary Service Drug Information 99. Bethesda, MD: American Society of Health-System Pharmacists; 1999:1255–6.
72. Hyers TM, Agnelli G, Hull RD, et al. Antithrombotic therapy for venous thromboembolic disease. *Chest* 1998; 114(*Suppl*):561S–78S.
73. Cziraky MJ, Spinler SA. Low-molecular-weight-heparins for the treatment of deep vein-thrombosis. *Clin Pharm.* 1993; 12:892–9.
74. Hoppensseadt D, Walenga JM, Fareed J. Low-molecular-weight-heparins: An overview. *Drugs Aging.* 1992; 2:406–22.
75. Boneu B, Caranobe C, Cadroy Y, et al. Pharmacokinetic studies of standard unfractionated heparin and low-molecular-weight-heparin in the rabbit. *Semin Thromb Hemost.* 1998; 14:18–27.
76. Caranobe C, Barret A, Gabaig AM, et al. Disappearance of circulating anti-X_a activity after intravenous injection of unfractionated heparin

and low-molecular-weight heparin (CY216) in normal and nephrectomized rabbits. *Thromb Res.* 1985; 40:129–33.

77. Dalen M, Mattsen CH. Pharmacokinetics of heparin and low-molecular-weight-heparin fragment (Fragmin) in rabbits with impaired renal or metabolic clearance. *Thromb Haemost.* 1987; 58:932–5.

78. Collignon F, Caplain H, Ozoux ML, et al. Comparison of the pharmacokinetic profiles of two low-molecular-weight-heparins–dalteparin and enoxaparin–administered subcutaneously in healthy volunteers (doses for prevention of thromboembolism). *Thromb Haemost.* 1995; 73(4):630–40.

79. Chiu HM, Hirsh J, Yung WL, et al. Relationship between the anticoagulant and antithrombotic effects of heparin in experimental venous thrombosis. *Blood.* 1977; 49:171–84.

80. Levine M, Jent M, Hirsh J, et al. A comparison of low-molecular-weight-heparin administered primarily at home with unfractionated heparin administered in the hospital for proximal deep-vein thrombosis. *N Engl J Med.* 1996; 334:677–81.

81. Koopman MMW, Prandoni P, Piovella F, et al. Treatment of venous thrombosis with unfractionated heparin administered in the hospital as compared with subcutaneous low-molecular-weight-heparin administered at home. *N Engl J Med.* 1996; 334:682–7.

82. Cohen M, Demers C, Gurfinkel EP, et al. A comparison of low-molecular-weight-heparin with unfractionated heparin for unstable coronary artery disease. *N Engl J Med.* 1997; 337:447–52.

83. Levine MN, Raskob G, Landefeld S, et al. Hemorrhagic complications of anticoagulant treatment. *Chest* 1998; 114(*Suppl*):511S–23S.

84. Hitchens K, Merli JG, Groce JB, et al. Implementing outpatient treatment of deep vein thrombosis. *Hosp Pharm Report* 1999, 13 (*suppl*): 1S–14S.

85. Innohep [package insert]. Wilmington, Delaware: DuPont Pharma; 2000.

Chapter 11
Paul E. Nolan, Jr. & Toby C. Trujillo

Lidocaine (AHFS 24:04)

Usual Dosage Range in Absence of Clearance-Altering Factors[1]

Lidocaine, a class I (membrane-stabilizing/sodium channel blocking) antiarrhythmic agent, exhibits electrophysiologic characteristics of the class IB subgroup of antiarrhythmic agents. Lidocaine controls ventricular arrhythmias by suppressing both automaticity in the His–Purkinje system and spontaneous depolarization of ventricles during diastole.

The following dosage ranges are suggested for the treatment of ventricular arrhythmias; dosages should be adjusted according to individual requirements.

Dosage Form	Initial Dosage (lidocaine hydrochloride)
Intravenous (bolus)	
Children (≤18 years)	0.5–1 mg/kg slow intravenous push at 25–50 mg/min, with dose repeated every 3–5 min if needed; total dose should not exceed 3–5 mg/kg
Adults (>18 years)	50–100 mg (1–1.5 mg/kg) slow intravenous push at 25–50 mg/min, with dose repeated every 3–5 min if needed; total dose should not exceed 300 mg in any hour

Intravenous (maintenance)
Children (≤18 years) — Infusion of 1.2–3 mg/kg/hr, with an additional 1-mg/kg bolus if clinically indicated
Adults (>18 years) — Infusion of 1.5–3 mg/kg/hr or 60–240 mg/hr

Intramuscular
Children (≤18 years) — Not FDA approved
Adults (>18 years) — 200–300 mg (4 mg/kg) injected into deltoid muscle (or lateral thigh if autoinjector device is used), with dose repeated in 60–90 min if clinically indicated

Oral — None

Lidocaine has also been administered via an endotracheal tube during cardiac arrest.[2] Although no dosage recommendations are established for this route, it is discussed in the dosing strategies section.

Dosage Form Availability[1]

All listed preparations are intended for cardiac use. Lidocaine preparations containing epinephrine (intended for anesthesia) should never be used for cardiac purposes. All lidocaine parenteral preparations are available as the hydrochloride salt and provide 86% lidocaine base ($S = 0.86$).

Dosage Form	Product
Intramuscular: 100 mg/ml in 3 ml (contains edetate disodium and methylparaben)	LidoPen Autoinjector (Survival Technology)
Intravenous (bolus): 10 and 20 mg/ml	various manufacturers
Intravenous (for infusion preparation) 40 and 200 mg/ml (1 or 2 g) 100 mg/ml (1 g)	various manufacturers

Intravenous (premixed infusion
   solution)　　　　　　　　　　　　　various manufacturers
   2 and 4 mg/ml in dextrose
     5% (1 or 2 g)　　　　　　　　　　various manufacturers
   8 mg/ml in dextrose 5%
     (2 or 4 g)
                                  Not available
Oral

Bioavailability (*F*) of Dosage Forms

Dosage Form	Bioavailability Comments
Intravenous[3]	100%
Intramuscular	Absolute bioavailability not determined
Oral[3]	91 ± 6% for hepatically impaired patients 39 ± 5% for normal patients

     Since the intramuscular method of drug administration avoids the first-pass metabolism of the liver, bioavailability should be similar to that for intravenous lidocaine. The deltoid muscle is preferred for intramuscular administration, resulting in a superior rate and extent of absorption compared to the gluteus and vastus lateralis muscles.[4,5]

     Although the oral bioavailability of lidocaine averages 39% in patients without hepatic impairment, a large intersubject variability exists due to first-pass hepatic metabolism.[3] Therapeutic lidocaine concentrations may not be rapidly and predictably attained in many patients, thus preventing its use as an oral agent.

General Pharmacokinetic Information

Distribution

     Following intravenous administration, the disposition of lidocaine is usually described by an open, two-compartment model.[6] However, some studies best describe lidocaine disposition by a three-compartment model.[6,7] For this text, a two-compartment model is assumed.

Elimination

Determination of the total body or systemic clearance (CL_{total} or $CL_{systemic}$) of lidocaine depends on the method of administration. Compared to a single intravenous bolus dose, the CL_{total} decreases during a prolonged (longer than 24 hr) constant-rate infusion. This phenomenon is referred to as time-dependent pharmacokinetics. The magnitude of the reduction in CL_{total} with a continuous infusion may depend on its absolute duration as well as on the patient's underlying clinical condition.[7,9]

The mechanism for the time-dependent reduction in CL_{total} of lidocaine is a reduction in its intrinsic clearance mediated by either lidocaine itself[10] or monoethylglycinexylidide (MEGX), its principal metabolite.[11]

Metabolism

Lidocaine is extensively metabolized hepatically through sequential deethylation by the cytochrome P450 enzyme system.[6] The hepatic extraction ratio is high, ranging from 62 to 81% of the dose administered.[3] As with other highly extracted drugs, hepatic blood flow appears to be the primary determinant of clearance.[12,13] However, changes in lidocaine clearance also can result from hepatic enzyme induction or inhibition.[6,13] Therefore, alterations in either hepatic blood flow or intrinsic hepatic metabolic capacity can influence the elimination of lidocaine.

The hepatic metabolism of lidocaine results in the formation of two active metabolites, MEGX and glycinexylidide (GX)[14,15] (Table 1). MEGX may contribute to both the therapeutic and toxic effects of lidocaine, whereas GX may contribute to the toxicity of lidocaine and/or MEGX.

TABLE 1. Formation and Activity of Lidocaine Metabolites[11, 16-19]

Compound	Amount Excreted in Urine[a]	Antiarrhythmic Activity
Lidocaine	2%	Yes
MEGX	4%	Yes
GX	2.5%	No[b]
4-OH 2,6-xylidine	73%	No
Others	10–20%	No

[a]*Percentage of administered lidocaine dose.*
[b]*GX has only 10% of the antiarrhythmic activity of lidocaine. GX's antiarrhythmic activity is not clinically significant.*

Conditions that decrease lidocaine clearance also may potentially decrease MEGX clearance, resulting in increased adverse effects secondary to accumulation of MEGX.[11,15] On the other hand, patients with renal impairment may be at greater risk of adverse effects secondary to accumulation of GX.[15,16]

Protein binding

Protein binding of lidocaine depends on many variables, including drug concentration, type and concentration of plasma proteins, sample collection method, pH, and quantification method.[6] Lidocaine exhibits concentration-dependent binding; that is, the degree of binding decreases as the total (bound plus unbound) drug concentration increases.[20] Although lidocaine binds to albumin (approximately 25%), alpha-1-acid glycoprotein (AAG), an acute phase reactant, serves as the primary binding protein (approximately 50%).

The concentration of AAG may be significantly altered by disease, stress, or other clinical situations.[21-29] Decreased concentrations of AAG result in a higher unbound fraction of lidocaine (increased free drug concentration) and possibly increased pharmacologic and/or toxic effects at any given total lidocaine concentration. Conversely, increased AAG levels decrease the proportion of unbound (active) drug and may decrease the pharmacologic effect at any given total lidocaine concentration.

Displacement of lidocaine bound to AAG by another drug (e.g., disopyramide, quinidine, propranolol, and tricyclic antidepressants) results in a higher free fraction of lidocaine and may rarely enhance the pharmacologic or toxic effect.[22–24,30]

Clearance (CL)

The clearance values of lidocaine in different patient populations via different administration techniques are presented in Table 2.

TABLE 2. Clearance of Lidocaine

Population[a]	Clearance (mean ± SD)	Mode of Administration
Adults[8]	0.72 ± 0.15 L/hr/kg	Single dose
Adults[9]	0.51 ± 0.13 L/hr/kg	Continuous infusion
Adults (endotracheal tube)[2]	0.55 ± 0.18 L/hr/kg	Single dose
Children[31]	0.71 ± 0.2 L/hr/kg	Single dose
Neonates[32]	0.61 ± 0.38 L/hr/kg	Single dose
Morbidly obese adult males[33]	0.69 ± 0.22 L/hr/kg[b]	Single dose
Morbidly obese adult females[33]	0.68 ± 0.17 L/hr/kg[b]	Single dose
Chronic CHF[34]	0.38 L/hr/kg[c]	Single dose
Chronic CHF[35]	0.23 ± 0.08 L/hr/kg	Continuous infusion
Mild to moderate chronic CHF[35]	0.35 L/hr/kg[d]	Continuous infusion
Severe chronic CHF[35]	0.12 L/hr/kg[d]	Continuous infusion
Chronic hepatic dysfunction[34]	0.42 ± 0.19 L/hr/kg	Single dose
Chronic renal failure[34]	0.82 L/hr/kg[c]	Single dose
Acute myocardial infarction without heart failure[36]	0.54 ± 0.12 L/hr/kg[e]	Continuous infusion
Acute myocardial infarction with heart failure[36]	0.33 ± 0.09 L/hr/kg[e]	Continuous infusion

[a]*Most studies had small numbers of patients.*
[b]*Based on total body weight.*
[c]*Only mean data reported.*
[d]*Calculated from reported mean data.*
[e]*Blood to plasma conversion applied.*

Volume of Distribution (V)

Lidocaine is widely distributed into body tissue following distribution from the central compartment (i.e., heart, lungs, and kidneys). Table 3 presents the volume of distribution after administration of a single lidocaine dose to different patient populations.

TABLE 3. Volume of Distribution of Lidocaine

Population	Volume (mean ± SD)
Adults[8]	V_c = 0.50 ± 0.21 L/kg V_β = 1.66 L/kg[a] V_{ss} = 1.32 ± 0.27 L/kg
Adults (endotracheal tube)[2]	V_β = 1.06 ± 0.54 L/kg
Children[31,37]	V_c = 0.31 ± 0.07 L/kg V_β = 1.10 ± 0.11 L/kg V_{ss} = 1.18 ± 0.36 L/kg
Neonates[32]	V_β = 2.75 ± 1.61 L/kg
Elderly males[38]	V_β = 2.91 ± 0.88 L/kg
Elderly females[38]	V_β = 3.45 ± 0.79 L/kg
Morbidly obese adult males[33]	V_β = 2.67 ± 0.82 L/kg[b]
Morbidly obese adult females[33]	V_β = 2.88 ± 1.03 L/kg[b]
Chronic CHF[34]	V_c = 0.30 L/kg[c] V_{ss} = 0.88 L/kg[c]
Chronic hepatic dysfunction[34]	V_c = 0.61 L/kg[c] V_{ss} = 2.31 L/kg[c]
Chronic renal failure[34]	V_c = 0.55 L/kg[c] V_{ss} = 1.20 L/kg[c]

[a]*Calculated using* $V_\beta = (CL_{total})/k$
[b]*Based on total body weight.*
[c]*Only mean data reported.*

Half-Life and Time to Steady State

Unless otherwise stated, the half-lives and anticipated times to steady state in Table 4 are based on intravenous bolus dosing. As previously described, clearance decreases with prolonged infusions of lidocaine, thus increasing the half-life and time to steady state. When time to steady state

TABLE 4. Half-Life and Time to Steady State for Lidocaine

Population	Terminal Half-Life (mean ± SD)	Time to Steady State (3 to 5 $t\frac{1}{2}$'s)
Adults[8]	1.6 ± 0.4 hr	4.8–8 hr
Adults (endotracheal tube)[2]	1.2 ± 0.5 hr	3.6–6 hr
Children[31]	1.0 ± 0.3 hr	3.1–5.2 hr
Neonates[32]	3.2 ± 0.1 hr	9.5–15.8 hr
Elderly males[38]	2.7 ± 0.5 hr	8.1–13.5 hr
Elderly females[38]	2.3 ± 0.6 hr	6.8–11.4 hr
Morbidly obese adult males[33]	2.7 ± 0.8 hr	8.1–13.5 hr
Morbidly obese adult females[33]	3.0 ± 1.0 hr	8.9–14.8 hr
Chronic CHF[34]	1.9 hr[a]	5.8–9.6 hr
Chronic hepatic dysfunction[34]	4.9 hr[a]	14.8–24.7 hr
Chronic renal failure[34]	1.3 hr[a]	3.9–6.5 hr
Acute myocardial infarction without heart failure[b,39]	3.2 ± 0.5 hr	9.6–16 hr
Acute myocardial infarction with heart failure[b,40]	10.2 ± 5.3 hr	31–51 hr

[a]Only mean data reported.
[b]Infusion of longer than 24 hr.

is assessed, the method of drug administration must be considered along with patient population characteristics.[5,9,41]

Therapeutic Range

When a therapeutic range for lidocaine is determined, it is important to note that plasma, serum, and whole blood concentrations are not interchangeable. For conversion from blood (C_b) to serum (C_s) concentrations, a factor of 1.3 should be applied:[20]

$$C_s = (C_b)(1.3)$$

The usual therapeutic range in serum is 1.5–6 mg/L (total)[42] or 0.5–2 mg/L (free or unbound).

Suggested Sampling Times and Effect on Therapeutic Range

Lidocaine concentrations should be measured and assessed in the following situations:[6,43]

- Patient potentially at increased risk for developing lidocaine toxicity (e.g., patient with shock, CHF, or hepatic disease).
- Patient concomitantly receiving medications with potentially major or moderately significant drug interactions. (See drug–drug interactions section.)
- Prolonged infusion (longer than 24 hr) of lidocaine, especially in patients with underlying disease states or conditions that may affect lidocaine clearance.
- Patient requiring doses that exceed the maximum recommended amount.
- Assessment or confirmation of toxicity and/or efficacy.
- Research investigation.

The following sample collection time[43] recommendations are only guidelines for the clinician in assessing lidocaine efficacy and toxicity. They are not to be employed without thorough clinical evaluation of the patient and consideration of conditions that alter lidocaine pharmacokinetics.

Monitoring Goal	Suggested Sampling Time
Assessment of efficacy	1–2 hr following initiation of therapy in patients who fail to respond to lidocaine[a]
Dosage adjustment	12–24 hr following initiation of therapy to assess steady-state concentration 24–48 hr following initiation of ongoing continuous infusion to avoid drug accumulation resulting from time-dependent reduction in clearance
Confirmation of toxicity	When clinical signs and symptoms of suspected lidocaine toxicity appear

[a]*Failure to respond may result from the "therapeutic gap," high systemic lidocaine clearance, or intrinsic resistance to lidocaine therapy.*

Clinical Use

Intravenous lidocaine is currently indicated for use in the acute management of ventricular tachycardia and/or fibrillation in the setting of acute myocardial infarction (AMI).

Lidocaine is no longer recommended in the treatment of isolated ventricular premature beats, couplets, or nonsustained VT or as prophylaxis against ventricular arrhythmias in the setting of AMI.[44] The rationale for this change in practice is that, although lidocaine used prophylactically can decrease the incidence of ventricular arrhythmias in the setting of AMI, overall mortality may not be altered and may, in fact, be increased.[44-48]

Lidocaine is also listed as drug of choice for the management of hemodynamically stable VT and a variety of other ventricular arrhythmias in the *Textbook of Advanced Cardiac Life Support* (ACLS).[49] However, it is postulated that this recommendation will change when the ACLS guidelines are updated. This anticipated change is based on data that demonstrate that lidocaine is relatively ineffective compared to other antiarrhythmics in the treatment of ventricular arrhythmias in the absence of ischemia and the availability of amiodarone in an intravenous formulation.[50,51]

Pharmacodynamic Monitoring: Concentration-Related Efficacy and Toxicity

Lidocaine concentrations associated with the control of ventricular arrhythmias have generally fallen in the range of 1.5 to 6 mg/L.[42,49,52]

Adverse effects with lidocaine principally involve the CNS or cardiovascular system. CNS effects include confusion, dizziness, slurred speech, numbness of the lips and tongue, diplopia, tremor, severe nausea and vomiting, and seizures. Cardiovascular adverse effects include sinus bradycardia, sinus arrest, and atrioventricular conduction disturbances. Adverse effects have been weakly correlated to bound and unbound lidocaine concentrations.[6,53] In Table 5, possible signs of toxicity are correlated to total serum lidocaine concentrations.

TABLE 5. Lidocaine Concentration–Toxicity Correlation[1,6,53]

Total Serum Lidocaine Concentration	Underlying Toxicity
<1.5 mg/L	Idiosyncratic
1.5–4 mg/L	Mild CNS and cardiovascular effects
>4–6 mg/L	Mild CNS toxicity[a]; cardiovascular toxicity[b] common with preexisting disease present
>6–8 mg/L	Major CNS[c] and cardiovascular depressant effects
>8 mg/L	Seizures, obtundation, hypotension, respiratory depression, and decreased cardiac output

[a]*Mild CNS toxicity includes somnolence, dizziness, numbness, slurred speech, and confusion.*
[b]*Cardiovascular toxicity includes sinus bradycardia, sinus arrest, atrioventricular conduction disturbances, hypotension, and decreased cardiac output.*
[c]*Major CNS toxicity includes severe confusion, severe slurred speech, tremor, diplopia, respiratory arrest, and seizure.*

Drug–Drug Interactions

Pharmacokinetic interactions with lidocaine largely result from alterations in hepatic clearance. Hepatic clearance depends on three factors:[13]

- Free fraction of the drug.
- Hepatic blood flow.
- Intrinsic metabolic clearance.

Changes in blood flow would be expected to yield more important interactions (moderate to major), whereas changes in free fraction or intrinsic clearance due to drug interactions may be less significant (mild to moderate). Drug–drug interactions with lidocaine are listed in Table 6 along with the clinical significance of the interaction.

Although maintenance infusion rates may have to be adjusted for lidocaine when it is administered concomitantly with drugs that result in interactions of major or moderate clinical significance, no data describe a generalized dose reduction. Therefore, careful monitoring of signs

TABLE 6. Drug–drug Interactions with Lidocaine

Agent	Interaction	Significance
Amiodarone[54-56]	Clearance decreased due to inhibition of CYP3A4	Mild to moderate
Beta-adrenergic blockers[9,57-59]	Clearance decreased due to decreased hepatic blood flow	Moderate to major
Cimetidine[60-62]	Clearance decreased due to decreased hepatic blood flow	Moderate to major
Erythromycin[63]	Increased concentrations of MEGX metabolite; mechanism unknown	Clinical significance unknown
Protease inhibitors[64]	AUC of lidocaine may be increased up to threefold; mechanism unknown	Mild to moderate
Rifampin[65]	Clearance increased due to cytochrome P450 enzyme induction	Mild to moderate
Succinylcholine[66,67]	Prolongation of succinylcholine-induced neuromuscular blockade; mechanism unknown	Mild to moderate

and symptoms of toxicity and lidocaine concentrations is particularly important for these drug interactions. Furthermore, the significance of any drug interaction may increase in the presence of other clearance-altering factors, which may necessitate dose adjustments.

Drug–Disease State or Condition Interactions

Congestive heart failure (CHF)
An inverse relationship exists between cardiac index and lidocaine concentrations.[57] For example, in adult patients with CHF, the increasing severity of CHF results in an increased potential for drug accumulation and decreased dosing requirements.[35]

For adult patients with mild to moderate CHF, an initial maintenance infusion of 1.4 mg/kg/hr is suggested for these patients to achieve a steady-state lidocaine concentration of 4 mg/L.

For patients with severe CHF, the initial maintenance infusion should be 0.6 mg/kg/hr for these patients to achieve a steady-state lidocaine concentration of 4 mg/L. As always, careful individual assessment of efficacy and toxicity is prudent. Loading doses may need to be reduced due to smaller central volume in patients with CHF.

Acute myocardial infarction (AMI)
For adult patients with AMI without CHF, a constant rate infusion of 2.6 mg/kg/hr should achieve steady-state lidocaine concentrations of 4 mg/L. Patients with AMI and CHF require lower continuous infusion rates. Therefore, an initial continuous infusion rate of 1.5 mg/kg/hr is suggested for this patient population. Furthermore, in this group, loading doses of lidocaine may need to be reduced approximately 40% because of a decreased central volume of distribution.[34]

In addition, AAG concentrations increase following AMI.[23] The implications of altered binding were previously addressed. (See general pharmacokinetic information section.) Since binding alterations are unpredictable and may not be of great clinical significance, especially in patients receiving prophylactic lidocaine, empiric dosage adjustment recommendations are not needed. However, clinical and laboratory parameters must be monitored carefully, with appropriate reductions in lidocaine dosages made based on clinical response and serum concentrations when available.

Hepatic disease
Chronic hepatic disease usually diminishes lidocaine clearance.[68,69] Due to the anticipated reduction in protein binding for this patient population, a continuous infusion should be initiated at 1.3 mg/kg/hr for a lidocaine steady-state concentration of 3 mg/L.[34]

An additional consideration for patients with hepatic dysfunction receiving lidocaine is the potential accumulation of the active metabolite MEGX. This accumulation may increase toxic effects despite "therapeutic" lidocaine concentrations.[11]

Renal disease

Since lidocaine is almost exclusively hepatically eliminated, renal dysfunction has little effect on its disposition and elimination. Therefore, loading and maintenance doses do not require adjustment. Lidocaine therapy may be initiated with a maintenance infusion rate of 3.7 mg/kg/hr to achieve a serum lidocaine steady-state concentration of 4 mg/L.[34]

The active metabolite GX is renally eliminated and, therefore, may accumulate in patients with renal impairment. Significant accumulation of GX appears to occur only with prolonged administration of lidocaine.[18] Nevertheless, it is important to monitor closely for common side effects, including neurological sequelae.

Morbid obesity

The pharmacokinetic parameters describing distribution and elimination of lidocaine in the morbidly obese patient population may vary based on the utilization of ideal versus actual body weight in standardizing these parameters. As a result, IBW should be used for the calculation of bolus dosing, and ABW should be used for the calculation of maintenance rates for continuous intravenous infusion.[33] The exact rate of infusion depends on the particular dosing strategy chosen. (See dosing strategies section.) Particularly in the calculation of infusion rates, the presence of disease states that may further alter lidocaine elimination must also be considered.

Advanced age (elderly)

Advanced age has a gender-specific effect on the distribution and clearance of lidocaine. Compared to young adult control subjects, the elderly have an increased volume of distribution and a decreased total body clearance of lidocaine.[38] Furthermore, both volume of distribution and clearance are increased in elderly females compared to elderly males, although not to a statistically significant degree.

The implications of these alterations in pharmacokinetic parameters on lidocaine dosing are not clear. However, in elderly patients it may be prudent to decrease the maintenance infusion by 10–40% based on individual patient parameters. Maintenance infusions of 2.2–3.4 mg/kg/hr are reasonable for elderly patients without other clearance-altering factors. As with other conditions that may alter clearance, intensive patient monitoring is needed.

In summary, an initial dosage adjustment is warranted in patients with CHF, hepatic dysfunction, morbid obesity, or advanced age. However, an initial dosage reduction is probably not necessary for patients with AMI or renal dysfunction unless other clearance-altering factors are present.

Pregnancy and Lactation

Lidocaine is currently listed as Risk Category C. Lidocaine readily crosses the placenta and is excreted in breast milk. Although the available limited information suggests that the use of lidocaine during pregnancy or in a breast-feeding mother is unlikely to result in harm to the fetus or newborn, its use in this patient population has not been well studied and should only take place when clearly needed.[70]

Dosing Strategies

The optimal dosing strategy for lidocaine should rapidly achieve and consistently maintain total serum concentrations within the therapeutic range. However, the multicompartmental disposition characteristics of lidocaine, the interpatient variability in its pharmacokinetics, and its relatively narrow therapeutic index make designing a dosing strategy difficult.

Loading doses of lidocaine are required to attain adequate serum concentrations quickly within the central compartment. Following equilibration in the central compartment, lidocaine rapidly distributes into the peripheral compartment, so subtherapeutic lidocaine concentrations may be observed. This "therapeutic gap" may require additional dosing interventions to maintain efficacious concentrations. The therapeutic gap may occur during a critical timeframe when adequate drug concentrations are essential for the prevention or treatment of life-threatening ventricular arrhythmias.[71,72] While numerous dosing schemes have been tested for lidocaine, Table 7 and Figures 1–5 focus on seven representative methods for clinical application.[73-75]

Explanation of Method 7: endotracheal administration[2]

During cardiac arrest, it is sometimes difficult to obtain peripheral intravenous access secondary to compensatory peripheral vasoconstriction, which may accompany cardiac arrest. Even when timely intravenous access is possible, drug delivery to the heart may be delayed as a result of a low cardiac output. Therefore, endotracheal administration of lidocaine, as well as other emergent-use medications (e.g., epinephrine, atropine, naloxone, and

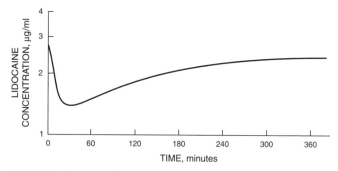

FIGURE 1. Method 1: Time–concentration curve for the single bolus plus infusion technique. (Reproduced, with permission, from Reference 72.)

TABLE 7. Lidocaine Hydrochloride Dosing Methods

Method	Bolus Dose and Timing	Loading Infusion	Maintenance Infusion
1. Single bolus plus infusion technique[71-73]	100 mg initially	—	120 mg/hr
2. Multiple bolus plus infusion technique[71-73]	100 mg initially 50 mg at 20 min	—	120 mg/hr
3. Two-step infusion technique[71,72]	—	200 mg over 25 min	120 mg/hr
4a. Two-step bolus plus infusion technique[72,73]	1.5 mg/kg (100 mg) plus simultaneous loading infusion	0.12 mg/kg/min for 25 min (or 200 mg over 25 min)	1.8 mg/kg/hr (120 mg/hr)
4b. Two-step bolus plus infusion technique[74]	75 mg plus simultaneous loading infusion	150 mg over 20 min	120 mg/hr
5. Exponentially declining infusion technique[73-75]	92 mg	8.3 mg/min exponentially declining to maintenance infusion rate	120 mg/hr
6. ACLS bolus technique[49]	1–1.5 mg/kg followed by 0.5–1.5 mg/kg every 2–10 min up to a total dose of 3 mg/kg	—	120–240 mg/hr
7. Endotracheal administration[2]	1.5 mg/kg repeated every 20–30 min	—	—

diazepam), has been proposed. Although little human data are available regarding this route of administration, the pharmacokinetics of endotracheally administered lidocaine have been examined.

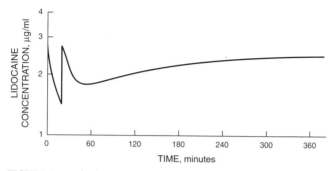

FIGURE 2. Method 2: Time–concentration curve for the multiple bolus plus infusion technique. (Reproduced, with permission, from Reference 72.)

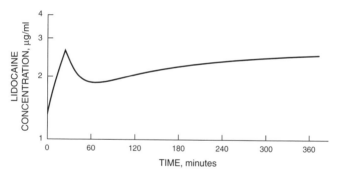

FIGURE 3. Method 3: Time–concentration curve for the two-step infusion technique. (Reproduced, with permission, from Reference 72.)

Following endotracheal administration of 1.5 mg/kg (ABW), serum lidocaine concentrations reach a peak of 2.1 mg/L at an average of 11.7 min. Since distribution and elimination processes rapidly decrease serum concentrations of lidocaine, endotracheal boluses should be given every 20–30 min to maintain therapeutic concentrations. When intravenous access is not possible or feasible, emergent endotracheal lidocaine administration may be a reasonable alternative.

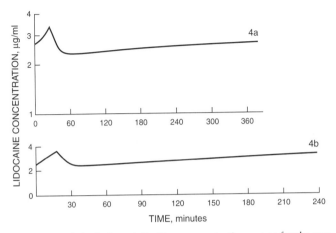

FIGURE 4. Methods 4a and 4b: Time–concentration curves for the two-step bolus plus infusion technique. (Reproduced, with permission, from References 72 and 73.)

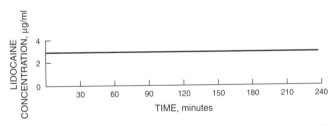

FIGURE 5. Method 5: Time–concentration curve for the exponentially declining infusion technique. (Reproduced, with permission, from Reference 73.)

Comparison of dosing methods

The efficacy of lidocaine as an antiarrhythmic agent is directly linked to the rapid achievement and maintenance of therapeutic lidocaine concentrations.[6] Avoiding the therapeutic gap may be critical during the first few hours following myocardial infarction when the incidence of lethal or potentially lethal arrhythmias is greatest.[42] Salzer et al. reported comparative data for the percentage of time that total lidocaine concentrations were within the therapeutic range (2–4 mg/L) in a small number of patients dosed using Methods 1–4a.[72] They concluded that Method 4a resulted in total lidocaine concentrations within the stated therapeutic range approximately 80% of the time, although two significant outlying patients decreased this percentage from 100%.[72] Riddell et al. reported that all eight of their subjects dosed using Method 5 maintained total concentrations between 1.5 and 5 mg/L 100% of the time.[73]

Of course, all of these dosing regimens serve only as guidelines for lidocaine administration. To achieve optimal efficacy, maintenance infusion rates always must be adjusted according to the patient's underlying clinical condition and other clearance-altering factors.

Each of these methods has both advantages and disadvantages. Although Method 5 requires no human intervention once the drug delivery system is set up, preparation of the delivery system is somewhat complicated and time consuming. The complexity of this system may limit its utility in some hospital settings. Methods 3 and 4 require some intervention to adjust infusion rates but do not require specialized delivery systems. Method 4a provides acceptable concentration–time results that are superior to those achieved with Methods 1–3. Both Methods 4a and 4b are relatively simple to administer and require minimal nursing intervention.

Ultimately, the choice of method should be determined by available personnel, equipment, and facilities in addition to the patient's clinical condition.[72,73,75]

References

1. Lidocaine. In: McEvoy GK, ed. American hospital formulary service drug information 1999. Bethesda, MD: American Society of Health-System Pharmacists; 1999. 1456–9.
2. Raehl CL. Endotracheal drug therapy in cardiopulmonary resuscitation. *Clin Pharm*. 1986; 5:572–9.
3. Huet PM, Lelorier J, Pomier G, et al. Bioavailability of lidocaine in

normal volunteers and cirrhotic patients. *Clin Pharmacol Ther.* 1979; 25:229–30.

4. Cohen LS, Rosenthal JE, Horner DW, et al. Plasma levels of lidocaine after intramuscular injection. *Am J Cardiol.* 1972; 29:520–3.

5. Schwartz ML, Meyer MB, Covino BG, et al. Antiarrhythmic effectiveness of intramuscular lidocaine: influence of different injection sites. *J Clin Pharmacol.* 1974; 15:77–83.

6. Benowitz NL, Meister W. Clinical pharmacokinetics of lidocaine. *Clin Pharmacokinet.* 1978; 3:177–201.

7. Morgan DJ, Horowitz JD, Louis WJ. Prediction of acute myocardial disposition of antiarrhythmic drugs. *J Pharm Sci.* 1989; 78:384–8.

8. Burm AGL, De Boer AG, Van Kleef JW, et al. Pharmacokinetics of lidocaine and bupivacaine and stable isotope labelled analogues: a study in healthy volunteers. *Biopharm Drug Dispos.* 1988; 9:85–95.

9. Ochs HR, Carstens G, Greenblatt DJ. Reduction in lidocaine clearance during continuous infusion and by coadministration of propranolol. *N Engl J Med.* 1980; 303:373–7.

10. Saville BA, Gray MR, Tam YK. Evidence for lidocaine-induced enzyme inactivation. *J Pharm Sci.* 1989; 78:1003–8.

11. Thomson AH, Elliott HL, Kelman AW, et al. The pharmacokinetics and pharmacodynamics for lignocaine and MEGX in healthy subjects. *J Pharmacokinet Biopharm.* 1987; 15:101–15.

12. Bennett PN, Aarons LJ, Bending MR, et al. Pharmacokinetics of lidocaine and its deethylated metabolite: dose and time dependency studies in man. *J Pharmacokinet Biopharm.* 1982; 10:265–81.

13. Wilkinson GR, Shand DG. A physiological approach to hepatic drug clearance. *Clin Pharmacol Ther.* 1975; 18:377–90.

14. Narang PK, Crouthamel WG, Carliner NH, et al. Lidocaine and its active metabolites. *Clin Pharmacol Ther.* 1978; 24:654–62.

15. Collinsworth KA, Strong JM, Atkinson AJ, et al. Pharmacokinetics and metabolism of lidocaine in patients with renal failure. *Clin Pharmacol Ther.* 1975; 18:59–64.

16. Strong JM, Mayfield DE, Atkinson AJ, et al. Pharmacological activity, metabolism, and pharmacokinetics of glycinexylidide. *Clin Pharmacol Ther.* 1975; 17:184–94.

17. Burney RG, DiFazia CA, Peach MJ, et al. Anti-arrhythmic effects of lidocaine metabolites. *N Engl J Med.* 1978; 298:1160–3.

18. Blumer J, Strong JM, Atkinson AJ. The convulsant potency of lidocaine and its N-dealkylated metabolites. *J Pharmacol Exp Ther.* 1973; 186:31–6.

19. Mather LE, Thomas J. Metabolism of lidocaine in man. *Life Sci.* 1972; 11:184–94.

20. Tucker GT, Boyes RN, Bridenbaugh PO, et al. Binding of anilide-type local anesthetics in human plasma. *Anesthesiology.* 1973; 33:287–303.

21. Drayer DE, Lorenzo B, Werns S, et al. Plasma levels, protein binding, and elimination data of lidocaine and active metabolites in cardiac patients of various ages. *Clin Pharmacol Ther.* 1983; 34:14–22.

22. Routledge PA. The plasma protein binding of basic drugs. *Br J Clin Pharmacol.* 1986; 22:499–506.

23. Routledge PA, Stargel WW, Wagner GS, et al. Increased alpha-1-acid glycoprotein and lidocaine disposition in myocardial infarction. *Ann Intern Med.* 1980; 93:701–4.
24. Routledge PA, Barchowsky A, Bjornsson TD, et al. Lidocaine plasma protein binding. *Clin Pharmacol Ther.* 1980; 27:347–51.
25. Gillis AM, Yee YG, Kates RG. Binding of antiarrhythmic drugs to purified human α_1-acid glycoprotein. *Biochem Pharmacol.* 1985; 34:4279–82.
26. Giardina EG, Khether R, Freilich D, et al. Time course of alpha-1-acid glycoprotein and its relation to myocardial enzymes after acute myocardial infarction. *Am J Cardiol.* 1985; 56:262–5.
27. Barry M, Keeling PWN, Weir D, et al. Severity of cirrhosis and the relationship of α_1-acid glycoprotein concentration to plasma protein binding of lidocaine. *Clin Pharmacol Ther.* 1990; 47:366–70.
28. Lerman J, Strong AH, LeDez KM, et al. Effects of age on the serum concentration of α_1-acid glycoprotein and the binding of lidocaine in pediatric patients. *Clin Pharmacol Ther.* 1989; 46:219–25.
29. McNamara PJ, Slaughter RL, Visco JP, et al. Effect of smoking on binding of lidocaine to human serum proteins. *J Pharm Sci.* 1980; 69:749–51.
30. Goolkasian DL, Slaughter RL, Edwards DJ, et al. Displacement of lidocaine from serum α_1-acid glycoprotein binding sites by basic drugs. *Eur J Clin Pharmacol.* 1983; 25:413–7.
31. Burrows FA, Lerman J, LeDez KM, et al. Pharmacokinetics of lidocaine in children with congenital heart disease. *Can J Anaesth.* 1991; 38:196–200.
32. Mihaly GW, Moore RG, Triggs EJ, et al. The pharmacokinetics and metabolism of the anilide local anaesthetic in neonates. *Eur J Clin Pharmacol.* 1978; 13:143–52.
33. Abernethy DR, Greenblatt DJ. Lidocaine disposition in obesity. *Am J Cardiol.* 1984; 53:1183–6.
34. Thomson PD, Melmon KL, Richardson KA, et al. Lidocaine pharmacokinetics in advanced heart failure, liver disease and renal failure in humans. *Ann Intern Med.* 1973; 78:499–508.
35. Zito RA, Reid PR. Lidocaine kinetics predicted by indocyanine green clearance. *N Engl J Med.* 1978; 298:1160–3.
36. Bax NDS, Tucker GT, Woods HF. Lignocaine and indocyanine green kinetics in patients following myocardial infarction. *Br J Clin Pharmacol.* 1980; 10:353–61.
37. Finholt DA, Stirt JA, DiFazio CA, et al. Lidocaine pharmacokinetics in children during general anesthesia. *Anesth Analg.* 1986; 65:279–82.
38. Abernethy DR, Greenblatt DJ. Impairment of lidocaine clearance in elderly male subjects. *J Cardiol Pharmacol.* 1983; 5:1093–6.
39. Lelorier J, Grenon D, Letour Y, et al. Pharmacokinetics of lidocaine after prolonged intravenous infusions in uncomplicated myocardial infarction. *Ann Intern Med.* 1977; 87:700–2.
40. Prescott LF, Yamoah KKA, Talbot RG. Impaired lignocaine metabolism in patients with myocardial infarction. *Br Med J.* 1976; 1:939–41.
41. Bauer LA, Brown T, Gibaldi M, et al. Influence of long-term infusions on lidocaine kinetics. *Clin Pharmacol Ther.* 1982; 31:433–7.

42. Lie KI, Wellens HJ, Van Capelle FJ, et al. Lidocaine in the prevention of primary ventricular fibrillation. *N Engl J Med.* 1974; 291:1324–6.
43. Pieper JA, Johnson KE. Lidocaine. In: Evans WE, Schentag JJ, Jusko WJ, eds. Applied pharmacokinetics: principles of therapeutic drug monitoring. Vancouver, WA: Applied Therapeutics; 1992:21(1–37).
44. ACC/AHA Guidelines for the Management of Patients with Acute Myocardial Infarction. *J Am Coll Cardiol.* 1996; 28:1328–428.
45. Alexander JH, Granger CB, Sadowski Z, et al. Prophylactic lidocaine use in acute myocardial infarction: incidence and outcomes from two international trials. *Am Heart J.* 1999; 137:799–805.
46. Sadowski ZP, Alexander JH, Skrabucha B, et al. Multicenter randomized trial and a systematic overview of lidocaine in acute myocardial infarction. *Am Heart J.* 1999; 137:792–8.
47. MacMahon S, Collins R, Peto R, et al. Effects of prophylactic lidocaine in suspected acute myocardial infarction. *JAMA.* 1988; 260:1910–6.
48. Hine LK, Laird N, Hewitt P, et al. Meta-analytic evidence against prophylactic use of lidocaine in acute myocardial infarction. *Arch Intern Med.* 1989; 149:2694–8.
49. Textbook of Advanced Cardiac Life Support. Dallas, TX: American Heart Association; 1994.
50. Gorgels APM, van den Dool A, Hofs A, et al. Comparison of procainamide and lidocaine in terminating sustained monomorphic ventricular tachycardia. *Am J Cardiol.* 1996; 78:43–6.
51. Nasir N, Taylor A, Doyle TK, et al. Evaluation of intravenous lidocaine for the termination of sustained monomorphic ventricular tachycardia in patients with coronary artery disease with and without healed myocardial infarction. *Am J Cardiol.* 1994; 74:1183–6.
52. Gianelly R. Effect of lidocaine on ventricular arrhythmias in patients with coronary heart disease. *N Engl J Med.* 1967; 277:1215–9.
53. Rademaker AW, Kellen J, Tam YK, et al. Character of adverse effects of prophylactic lidocaine in the coronary care unit. *Clin Pharmacol Ther.* 1986; 40:71–80.
54. Fruncillo RJ, Kozin SH, Digregorio GJ. Effect of amiodarone on the pharmacokinetics of phenytoin, quinidine, and lidocaine in the rat. *Res Commun Chem Pathol Pharmacol.* 1985; 50(3):451–4.
55. Siegmund JB, Wilson JH, Imhoff TE. Amiodarone interaction with lidocaine. *J Cardiovasc Pharmacol.* 1993; 21(4):513–5.
56. Ha HR, Candinas R, Stieger B, et al. Interaction between amiodarone and lidocaine. *J Cardiovasc Pharmacol.* 1996; 28(4):533–9.
57. Stenson RE, Constantino RT, Harrison DC. Interrelationships of hepatic blood flow, cardiac output and blood levels of lidocaine in man. *Circulation.* 1971; 43:205–11.
58. Conrad KA, Byers JM, Finley PR, et al. Lidocaine elimination: effects of metoprolol and of propranolol. *Clin Pharmacol Ther.* 1983; 33:133–8.
59. Bax NDS, Tucker GT, Lennard MS, et al. The impairment of lignocaine clearance by propranolol—major contribution from enzyme inhibition. *Br J Clin Pharmacol.* 1985; 19:597–603.
60. Feely J, Wilkinson GR, McAllister CB, et al. Increased toxicity and

reduced clearance of lidocaine by cimetidine. *Ann Intern Med.* 1982; 96:592–4.

61. Berk SI, Gal P, Bauman JL, et al. The effect of oral cimetidine on total and unbound serum lidocaine concentration in patients with suspected myocardial infarction. *Int J Cardiol.* 1987; 14:91–4.

62. Powell JR, Foster JR, Patterson JH, et al. Effect of duration of lidocaine infusion and route of cimetidine administration on lidocaine pharmacokinetics. *Clin Pharm.* 1986; 5:993–8.

63. Isohanni MH, Neuvonen PJ, Palkama VJ, et al. Effect of erythromycin and itraconazole on the pharmacokinetics of intravenous lignocaine. *Eur J Clin Pharmacol.* 1998; 54(7):561–5.

64. Michalets EL. Update: Clinically significant cytochrome P-450 drug interactions. *Pharmacotherapy.* 1998; 18(1):84–112.

65. Li AP, Rasmussen A, Xu L, et al. Rifampicin induction of lidocaine metabolism in cultured human hepatocytes. *J Pharmacol Exp Ther.* 1995; 274(2):673–7.

66. Bruckner J, Thomas KC Jr, Bikhazi GB, et al. Neuromuscular drug interactions of clinical importance. *Anesth Analg.* 1980; 59(9):678–82.

67. Fukuda S, Wakuta K, Ishikawa T, et al. Lidocaine modifies the effect of succinylcholine on muscle oxygen consumption in dogs. *Anesth Analg.* 1987; 66(4):325–8.

68. Testa R, Campo N, Caglieris S, et al. Lidocaine elimination and monoethylglycinexylidide formation in patients with chronic hepatitis or cirrhosis. *Hepatogastroenterology.* 1998; 45(19):154–9.

69. Shiffman ML, Luketic VA, Sanyal AJ, et al. Hepatic lidocaine metabolism and liver histology in patients with chronic hepatitis and cirrhosis. *Hepatology.* 1994; 19(4):933–40.

70. Briggs GG, Freeman RK, Yaffe SJ. Drugs in pregnancy and lactation. 5th ed. Baltimore, MD: Waverly & Wilkins; 1998:610–2.

71. Greenblatt DJ, Bolognini V, Koch-Weser J, et al. Pharmacokinetic approach to the clinical use of lidocaine intravenously. *JAMA.* 1976; 236:273–7.

72. Salzer LB, Weinreb AB, Marina RJ, et al. A comparison of methods of lidocaine administration in patients. *Clin Pharmacol Ther.* 1981; 29:617–24.

73. Riddell JG, McAllister CB, Wilkinson GR, et al. A new method for constant plasma drug concentration: application to lidocaine. *Ann Intern Med.* 1984; 100:25–8.

74. Stargel WW, Shand DG, Routledge PA, et al. Clinical comparison of rapid infusion and multiple injection methods for lidocaine loading. *Am Heart J.* 1981; 102:873–6.

75. Sebaldt RJ, Nattell S, Kreeft JH, et al. Lidocaine therapy with an exponentially declining infusion. *Ann Intern Med.* 1984; 101:632–4.

Chapter 12
Stanley W. Carson & Sarah H. Roberts

Lithium (AHFS 28:28)

Lithium is a monovalent ion used as a mood stabilizer in the treatment of bipolar (manic-depressive) disorder. It exhibits linear pharmacokinetics that can readily be described with a one-compartment model following oral dosing. The total body clearance of lithium is primarily a function of renal clearance. The volume of distribution approximates total body water (0.8 L/kg). Lithium has an average elimination half-life of approximately 21 hr in normal renal function (range 10–50 hr); therefore, steady-state concentrations are reached in 5–7 days. Acute therapy begins with 600–900 mg of lithium carbonate divided into two or three doses per day. Doses should be individually titrated to concentrations and clinical response of the patient. Twelve-hour trough concentrations should be checked once or twice weekly until the therapeutic range of 0.8–1.2 mEq/L (same as millimoles per liter) is achieved, then every 1–3 months. Maintenance or prophylactic regimens are usually reduced to obtain trough concentrations of approximately 0.6–0.8 mEq/L. Consideration of drug–drug interactions or drug–disease state/condition interactions is also important in monitoring patients on lithium. Any change in either the glomerular filtration rate

(GFR) or renal tubular reabsorption of lithium and/or sodium will likely alter lithium renal clearance and potentially change lithium dosage requirements. Because of a narrow therapeutic index, monitoring of lithium therapy with concentration determinations is essential.

Usual Dosage Range in Absence of Clearance-Altering Factors[1]

These dosages are rough guidelines for the initiation of lithium therapy. Both acute and maintenance dosages should be individualized for all patients and guided by serum lithium concentration determinations. Dosages are listed as milligram equivalents of lithium carbonate (300 mg lithium carbonate = 8.12 mEq of lithium).

Dosage Form	Initial Dosage
Intravenous	None
Oral (tablets, capsules, and syrup)	
Children (<12 years)	Not FDA approved
Adolescents (12–18 years)	600–1200 mg/day (30 mg/kg/day)
Adults (19–59 years)	900–1800 mg/day
Geriatrics (>59 years)	900–1200 mg/day

Warning: Lithium is a monovalent ion, so concentrations are reported as milliequivalents per liter (same as millimoles per liter) rather than in the more familiar concentration term of milligrams per liter.

Dosage Form Availability[2]

Dosage Form	Product
Intravenous	None
Oral tablets: lithium carbonate 300 mg (8.12 mEq)	Lithium Carbonate

	Eskalith
	Lithane
300 mg (8.12 mEq) extended release, film coated	Lithobid
300 mg (8.12 mEq) sustained release	Duralith
450 mg (12.18 mEq) extended release	Eskalith CR
Oral capsules: lithium carbonate	
150 mg (4.06 mEq)	Lithium Carbonate
	Carbolith
	Lithane
300 mg (8.12 mEq)	Lithium Carbonate
	Eskalith
	Carbolith
	Lithane
600 mg (16.24 mEq)	Lithium Carbonate
	Carbolith
Oral syrup: lithium citrate 8 mEq lithium/5 ml	Lithium Citrate

Bioavailability (F) of Dosage Forms[3]

Since an intravenous preparation is not available in the United States, the oral syrup dosage form is usually used as the reference product for other oral dosage forms and is assumed to be 100% bioavailable.

Dosage Form	Relative Bioavailability
Intravenous	Not available
Oral tablets and capsules	95–104%
Lithobid	80%
Eskalith CR	75–85%

General Pharmacokinetic Information

Distribution

The disposition of lithium is classically described by the open, two-compartment model. The volume of the central compartment typically is 0.20–0.25 L/kg, with the peripheral compartment comprising distribution into tissues such as muscle. The apparent volume of distribution (V_β or V_{area}) is approximately 0.8 L/kg with microrate constants of 0.24 hr^{-1} (k_{12}) and 0.19 hr^{-1} (k_{21}) in normal volunteers.[4] This early distribution phase is often obscured by absorption of lithium from tablets and capsules; therefore, lithium disposition usually appears to be monoexponential and can be described with a one compartment model.

Elimination

Lithium is eliminated primarily through the kidneys as the free ion and exhibits no metabolism or protein binding. It is completely filtered across the glomerular membrane, as are sodium and potassium, and is 80% reabsorbed. Therefore, the total body clearance of lithium is primarily a function of renal mechanisms. Any drug–drug interaction or drug–disease state/condition interaction reflects changes in the GFR or changes in the reabsorption of lithium and/or sodium:[3]

Fraction excreted in urine	>95%
Fraction nonrenally excreted	<5%
Active and inactive metabolites	None
Protein binding	None

Clearance (CL)

Determining the renal clearance of lithium is the most important aspect of dosing. Lithium clearance can be estimated from a patient's creatinine clearance (approximately $0.20–0.25 \times CrCl$). Once lithium clearance is determined, the clinician can select the dose (D) and dosage interval (τ) necessary to achieve the target trough (12-hr) steady-state concentration (approximated by Css_{av}; see equation 7 in the introduction). The dose is then adjusted proportionately, based on linear pharmacokinetics (see Figure 1). When body weight is considered in lithium clearance methods, the use of actual body weight (ABW) has been proposed.[8]

Age	Clearance (mean ± SD)
Children and adolescents[5] (9–12 years)	1.58 ± 0.37 L/hr
Adults[4,6] (19–59 years)	1.67 ± 0.32 L/hr
Geriatrics[4,7] (>59 years)	1.07 ± 0.27 L/hr

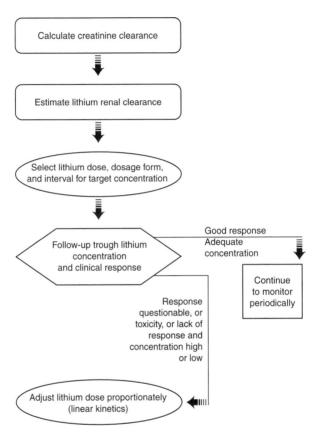

FIGURE 1. General scheme for pharmacokinetic monitoring of lithium therapy in bipolar disorders.

Numerous equations and dosage prediction methods have been proposed to help the clinician identify the appropriate lithium dose for the desired therapeutic concentration. While many methods utilize serum lithium concentrations and a specific pharmacokinetic model, some utilize principles of population pharmacokinetics to tie patient characteristics to changes in lithium clearance.

1. Dosage prediction by a priori demographics

The most common characteristics used for predictions are estimations of renal function, age, and body weight as represented by the method of Zetin et al.:[9]

dose (mg/day) = 486.8 + (746.83 × desired concentration) − (10.08 × age) + [5.95 weight (kg)] + (92.01 × status) + (147.8 × sex) − (74.73 × TCA)

where status is 1 for inpatient, 0 for outpatient; sex is 1 for male, 0 for female; TCA is 1 for concomitant tricyclic antidepressant (TCA) administration, otherwise 0; and age is in years.

Terao et al. proposed another a priori demographic method based on stepwise multiple linear regression and blood urea nitrogen (BUN) as a measurement of renal function:[48]

Dosage (mg/day) = 100.5 + 752.7 × (desired concentration) − [3.6 × age (years)] + [7.2 × weight (kg)] − [13.7 × BUN (mg/dl)]

With concentration in mEq/L, age in years, weight in kg, and BUN in mg/dl.

2. Dosage prediction by lithium renal clearance estimation

Pepin et al.[10] found lithium clearance to be related to the estimated CrCl. However, this method has not been consistently accurate and precise.[11]

$$CL_{lithium} = 0.235 \times CrCl$$

Units for $CL_{lithium}$ will be the same as those used for CrCl.

Perry et al.[12] found a significant ($p < 0.001$) correlation between observed lithium concentrations and predicted steady-state concentrations. The predicted concentrations were calculated using the patient's own elimination half-life from three blood samples and an equation for drug accumulation at steady state (modification of equation 10 in the introduction). Half-life can be estimated from two or three serum samples and the standard monoexponential decay equation (see equation 2 in the introduction) using a hand-held calculator or a pocket nomogram.[13]

3. Dosage prediction by population pharmacokinetics

The classic dosing chart of Cooper et al.[14] is based on population clearance values for lithium and a single 24-hr lithium concentration following a 600-mg lithium carbonate test dose. The utility and limitations of this method were reviewed elsewhere.[2]

The method of Jermain et al.[15] is based on population pharmacokinetics using the NONMEM computer software:

$$CL_{lithium} = [0.0093(L/hr/kg) \times LBW] + (0.0885 \times CrCl)$$

where LBW is the lean body weight in kilograms, and CrCl is the *estimated creatinine clearance in liters per hour.* Age is not directly represented in this model. However, the decline in CrCl and changes in total body water and muscle mass, as reflected in the lean body weight, probably account for the changes in lithium clearance usually attributed to age. This proposed method has not been independently validated.

4. Dosage prediction by Bayesian computer software

Several computer software programs are specifically designed to generate a pharmacokinetic consult for a patient on lithium. These programs generally utilize both a priori patient demographic data and individual lithium concentrations. The advantage is that any serum concentration taken at any known time following any dosage regimen can be modeled to generate patient-specific pharmacokinetic parameters and dosage recommendations.

Volume of Distribution (V)

The volume of distribution is reported to be 20–40% lower in elderly subjects compared to normal healthy, young volunteers. This difference is probably due in part to the decline in total body water and the increase in body fat as a percentage of body weight seen with advanced age.[7]

Age	Volume (mean ± SD)
Children and adolescents[5] (9–12 years)	0.93 ± 0.25 L/kg[a]
Adults[4,6] (19–59 years)	0.85 ± 0.25 L/kg[a]
Geriatrics[4,7] (>59 years)	0.53 ± 0.12 L/kg[a]

[a]Use ideal body weight.

Half-Life and Time to Steady State

Age	Half-Life (mean ± SD)	Time to Steady State (mean ± SD)
Children and adolescents[5] (9–12 years)	17.9 ± 7.4 hr	50–175 hr
Adults[4,6] (19–59 years)	21.5 ± 6.8 hr	85–110 hr
Geriatrics[4,7] (>59 years)	27.1 ± 7.8 hr	110–135 hr

Therapeutic Range[3,16]

Disease or Condition	Therapeutic Range
Acute mania	0.8–1.2 mEq/L
Prophylaxis of mania and/or depression	0.6–0.8 mEq/L

Suggested Sampling Times and Effect on Therapeutic Range

Specific therapeutic ranges for lithium in the treatment of acute mania and prophylaxis of bipolar disorder have not been well defined. Some disagreement undoubtedly is due to a lack of standardized sampling times in past studies and the search for the lowest possible range effective in prophylaxis.

Considerable efforts have been made to standardize the sampling time for lithium. Based on divided daily dosing (bid, tid, or qid), the standard time to draw a lithium concentration is 12 hr after the evening dose and before the morning dose (hold the morning dose if necessary). This time point is arbitrary, but it is usually postabsorption and postdistribution, and it exhibits minimal between-subject variability.

Following once-daily dosing, there will be much greater peak to trough fluctuations around the average steady-state concentration compared to the same daily dosage given as divided doses. Therefore, a 12-hr concentration measurement will be higher and a 24-hr trough lower than the standard 12-hr concentration measurement following divided daily dosing. This is graphically illustrated in Figure 2. The 12-hr concentration measurements were 1.37 versus 1.07, 1.00, and 0.96 mEq/L when the same daily dose was given as a single dose versus divided into two, three, or four doses, respectively. All current therapeutic ranges assume multiple daily doses; no therapeutic range has been established for once-daily dosing. One possible monitoring method for the once-daily dosage patient is to identify the 12-hr lithium concentration that is therapeutic for that individual and to carefully screen for side effects, toxicity, or relapse of manic symptoms.

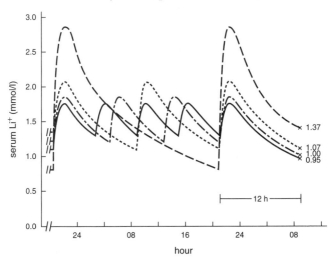

FIGURE 2. Computer-generated steady-state S_{Li} concentration-time profiles of the same total daily dosage of lithium divided into one, two, three, or four doses illustrating the variability of 12-hour S_{Li} concentration due solely to differences in dosage interval.

Source: Reprinted with permission from Reference 3.

Computer software for pharmacokinetic consultations that utilize linear, nonlinear, or Bayesian techniques can be useful when pharmacokinetic parameters are unstable, blood samples are not obtained at standardized time points, dosage regimens are not stable, or steady-state conditions have not been reached.[3] When patients are at steady-state conditions and lithium pharmacokinetic parameters are stable, lithium dosages can be adjusted proportionately to reach the desired concentration.

Pharmacodynamic Monitoring—Concentration-Related Efficacy

The application of pharmacokinetic principles to monitor dynamic responses in clinical practice typically assumes that the response is objective, reversible, and relatively rapid. In psychiatric diseases, response measurements are typically subjective rating scales, the response is delayed for days or weeks, and placebo effects are significant. Sometimes response is expressed as the percent or relative risk of relapse at a particular concentration.

Numerous studies suggest that as lithium concentrations increase from 0.3 to 1.4 mEq/L, the risk of relapse decreases and the incidence of side effects increases.[17-19] The risk of relapse has been reported to increase 2.6 times when median serum lithium concentrations (12-hr postdose) are reduced from 0.83 to 0.53 mEq/L.[19] This finding suggests considerable variation in clinical response within the typical concentration range of 0.4–1.2 mEq/L. The application of pharmacokinetic principles to achieve a more specific lithium concentration may effectively impact lithium therapy.

Pharmacodynamic Monitoring—"Follow-up" Concentrations

Lithium therapy must be monitored with serum concentrations because they are closely related to therapeutic response as well as to lithium toxicity. Generally, steady state is reached 5–7 days following the initiation of therapy or a dosage change.

The current recommendation according to the American Psychiatric Association Practice Guidelines for the Treatment of Patients with Bipolar Disorder[16] is to obtain concentrations every 1–3 months during maintenance therapy. More frequent monitoring is needed if fluid and electrolyte balance changes, if renal function is not stable, or if toxicity is a concern. Other laboratory monitoring parameters and information for patient and family counseling can be found elsewhere.[20]

Pharmacodynamic Monitoring—Concentration-Related Toxicity

Toxicity most often occurs with 12-hr trough concentrations above 1.5 mEq/L. Trough serum concentrations above 3–3.5 mEq/L are usually considered life threatening; hemodialysis, the most effective extrarenal clearance mechanism, should be considered. Since lithium is an ion, activated charcoal is ineffective.

Lithium toxicity is closely related to serum concentrations. Mild and transient effects such as fine tremor, nausea, diarrhea, muscle weakness, polyuria, and polydipsia can be seen at concentrations of less than or equal to 1.5 mEq/L. Moderate toxicity is seen at concentrations above 1.5–2.5 mEq/L and includes coarsening of tremor, confusion, sedation, slurred speech, vomiting, and lethargy. Severe toxicity results in seizures, hyper-reflexia, and cardiovascular collapse and may occur at concentrations above 2.5 mEq/L.[21,22]

Drug–Drug Interactions

Drug–drug interactions with lithium are related to effects on GFR and sodium excretion. Drugs causing a decrease in GFR or a compensatory increase in sodium reabsorption result in reduced lithium clearance and elevated serum concentrations. The major pharmacokinetic interactions are with thiazide diuretics, nonsteroidal anti-inflammatory agents, and angiotensin-converting enzyme inhibitors.

The adjustment factor estimates the change in the kinetic parameter due to the interaction. For example, enalapril may decrease lithium clearance by 50% while caffeine or theophylline may increase it by 20–25%. Because there can be considerable interindividual variation in drug interactions, these adjustment factors should be used with caution.

Drug	Parameter	Adjustment Factor
Thiazide diuretics[23–27]	Renal clearance	0.32–0.74
Indomethacin[28]	Renal clearance	0.70–0.77
Naproxen[29,45]	Renal clearance	0.78–0.88
Flurbiprofen[30]	Renal clearance	0.92
Ibuprofen[3]	Renal clearance	0.8–1.1[a]
Ketorolac[31]	Renal clearance	0.79
Cisplatin/fluids[32,33]	Renal clearance Half-life	1.6[a] 0.25–0.50[a]
Theophylline[34,35]	Renal clearance	1.21
Caffeine[6,36]	Renal clearance	1.2–1.25
ACE inhibitors[37] (lisinopril, enalapril, captopril)	Renal clearance	<50 years 0.87 ≥50 years 0.69
Celecoxib[46,47]	Renal clearance	0.83–0.95
Sodium-containing intravenous fluids[35,38]	Renal clearance	1.2

[a]Not consistent in all studies.

Drug–Disease State or Condition Interactions

Disease state or condition interactions with lithium are related to renal function and usually to GFR and sodium excretion. Thus, disease states and conditions that increase

GFR (e.g., during pregnancy or when fluids are forced) are likely to increase lithium clearance, resulting in lower serum concentrations and shorter half-lives. Conversely, conditions such as aging are associated with decreases in GFR and alterations in total body water and lean muscle mass that also may decrease the volume of distribution, resulting in higher concentrations.

Conditions that result in a compensatory increase in sodium reabsorption, such as dehydration or sodium-restricted diets, also increase the reabsorption of lithium and de-crease lithium clearance. Some reports also indicated a reduction in the amount of lithium excreted in the urine during acute mania, yet the serum concentration-time profile of lithium was essentially the same.[39] This finding suggests a "state"-dependent change in the volume of distribution.

Lithium has been classified as a Category D drug (evidence of human fetal risk, but benefits to the pregnant woman may outweigh the risk) by the Food and Drug Administration (FDA). Current recommendations are to avoid first-trimester exposure if possible. Exposure of the fetus to lithium during the first trimester can lead to a 1/1000 to 1/2000 risk of developing Ebstein's anomaly of the tricuspid valve. The risk in the general population is 1/20,000.[40] Since GFR increases and creatinine clearance can double during pregnancy, dosage requirements will in-crease in the third trimester. Subsequently, lithium dosages that have been increased due to this increase in clearance should be tapered by 25–30% or discontinued altogether just prior to delivery to decrease the risk of neonatal toxicity or toxicity that can be associated with rapid postpartum shifts in plasma volume.[41,42] Diligent monitoring of concentrations is essential. Lithium concentration should be monitored at least monthly, with a thyroid panel and electrolytes during pregnancy.[43] Lithium concentrations in breast milk are approximately 50% of the mother's serum concentrations, and because an infant's renal status is immature, any lithium ingested from breast milk may be cleared more slowly.[42] Therefore, infants should be carefully monitored for hypotonia, lethargy, cyanosis, and hydration status if breast fed.[44]

The adjustment factor estimates the change in lithium clearance. For example, dehydration may decrease lithium clearance to 81% of normal while pregnancy may increase it twofold.

Disease State or Condition	Parameter	Adjustment Factor
Acute mania[39]	Renal clearance	0.6
	Distribution volume	State dependent
Pregnancy[49]	Clearance	2
Aging[4,50]	Renal clearance	0.6–0.7
	Distribution volume	0.62–0.79
Dehydration[51]	Renal clearance	0.81[a]
Low salt diet[52]	Renal clearance	1.2–1.4[a]
Obesity[8]	Renal clearance	1.5
	Distribution volume	0.63
Lithium therapy for >1 year[50]	Half-life	1.29–1.4[b]
Strenuous exercise[53]	Renal clearance	1.19[a]

[a] *Lithium clearance based on single concentration in case reports.*
[b] *Not consistent in all studies.*

References

1. Lithium salts. In: McEvoy GK, ed. American hospital formulary service drug information 93. Bethesda, MD: American Society of Hospital Pharmacists; 1999:2116–24.
2. Lithium salts. In: 1999 Drug topics redbook. Montvale, NJ: Medical Economics Company, Inc.; 1999:406.
3. Carson S. Lithium. In: Evans WE, Schentag JJ, Jusko WJ, eds. Applied pharmacokinetics: principles of therapeutic drug monitoring, 3rd ed. Spokane, WA: Applied Therapeutics; 1992:34-1–34-26.
4. Nielsen-Kudsk F, Amdisen A. Analysis of the pharmacokinetics of lithium in man. *Eur J Clin Pharmacol.* 1979; 16:271–7.
5. Vitiello B, Behar D, Malone R, et al. Pharmacokinetics of lithium carbonate in children. *J Clin Psychopharmacol.* 1988; 8:355–9.
6. Carson SW, Gagnon A, Bahkai Y. Pharmacokinetic and pharmacodynamic effects of caffeine on lithium disposition. *Pharmacotherapy.* 1989; 9:196–7.

7. Karki SD, Carson SW, Gagnon A. Evaluation of total body water and disposition of lithium in elderly patients. *Lithium*. 1992; 3:29–33.

8. Reiss RA, Haas CE, Karki SD, et al. Lithium pharmacokinetics in the obese. *Clin Pharmacol Ther.* 1994; 55:392–8.

9. Zetin M, Garber D, De Antonio M, et al. Prediction of lithium dose: a mathematical alternative to the test-dose method. *J Clin Psychiatry*. 1986; 47(4):175–8.

10. Pepin SM, Bake DE, Nance KS, et al. Lithium dosage calculation from age, sex, height, weight and serum creatinine. Paper presented at 15th Annual ASHP Midyear Clinical Meeting. San Francisco, CA; 1980 Dec 9.

11. Browne JL, Patel RA, Huffman CS, et al. Comparison of pharmacokinetic procedures for dosing lithium based on analysis of prediction error. *Drug Intell Clin Pharm.* 1988; 22:227–31.

12. Perry PJ, Alexander B, Dunner FJ, et al. Pharmacokinetic protocol for predicting serum lithium levels. *J Clin Psychopharmacol*. 1982; 2:114–8.

13. Carson SW, DeVane CL. Estimation of half-life and exponential decay using a nomogram. *Am J Hosp Pharm*. 1983; 40:1696–8.

14. Cooper TB, Bergner P, Simpson GM. The 24-hour serum lithium level as a prognosticator of dosage requirements. *Am J Psychiatry*. 1973; 130:601–3.

15. Jermain DM, Crismon ML, Martin ES III. Population pharmacokinetics of lithium. *Clin Pharm*. 1991; 10:376–81.

16. American Psychiatric Association. Practice guidelines for the treatment of patients with bipolar disorder. *Am J Psychiatry*. 1994 (Supp l); 151:1–36.

17. Prien RF, Caffey EM Jr, Klett CJ. Relationship between serum lithium level and clinical response in acute mania treated with lithium. *Br J Psychiatry*. 1972; 120:409–14.

18. Stokes PE, Kocsis JH, Arcuni OJ. Relationship of lithium chloride dose to treatment response in acute mania. *Arch Gen Psychiatry*. 1976; 33:1080–4.

19. Gelenberg AJ, Kane JM, Keller MB, et al. Comparison of standard and low serum levels of lithium for maintenance treatment of bipolar disorder. *N Engl J Med*. 1989; 321:1489-93.

20. Carson SW, Foslien-Mash C. Lithium pharmacotherapy. *US Pharmacist*. 1990; 15:H1–10.

21. Hansen HE, Amdisen A. Lithium intoxication. *Q J Med*. 1978; 47:123–44.

22. Ereshefsky L, Jann MW. Lithium. In: Mungall D, ed. Applied clinical pharmacokinetics. New York: Raven Press; 1983:245–70.

23. Boer WH, Koomans HA, Beutler JJ, et al. Small intra- and large interindividual variability in lithium clearance in humans. *Kidney Int*. 1989; 35:1183–8.

24. Himmelhoch JM, Proust RI, Mallinger AG, et al. Adjustment of lithium dose during lithium-chlorothiazide therapy. *Clin Pharmacol Ther*. 1977; 22:225–7.

25. Solomon K. Combined use of lithium and diuretics. *South Med J*. 1978; 71(9):1098–9, 1104.

26. Dorevitch A, Baruch E. Lithium toxicity induced by combined amiloride HCl-hydrochlorothiazide administration. *Am J Psychiatry*. 1986; 143:257–8.

27. Chambers G, Kerry RJ, Owen G. Lithium used with a diuretic. *Brit Med J.* 1977; 24:805–6.
28. Frolich JC, Leftwich R, Ragheb M, et al. Indomethacin increases plasma lithium. *Brit Med J.* 1979; 1:1115–6.
29. Ragheb M, Powell AL. Lithium interaction with sulindac and naproxen. *J Clin Psychopharmacol.* 1986; 6:150–4.
30. Hughes BM, Small RE, Brink D, et al. The effect of flurbiprofen on steady-state plasma lithium levels. *Pharmacother.* 1997; 17:113–20.
31. Cold JA, ZumBrunnen TL, Simpson MA, et al. Increased lithium serum and red blood cell concentrations during ketorolac coadministration. *J Clin Psychopharmacol.* 1998; 18:33–7.
32. Pictruszka LJ, Biermann WA, Vlasses PH. Evaluation of cisplatin–lithium interaction. *Drug Intell Clin Pharm.* 1985; 19:31–2.
33. Parfrey PS, Ikeman R, Anglin D, et al. Severe lithium intoxication treated by forced diuresis. *Can Med Assoc J.* 1983; 129:979–80.
34. Cook BL, Smith RE, Perry PJ, et al. Theophylline–lithium interaction. *J Clin Psychiatry.* 1985; 46:278–9.
35. Holstad SG, Perry PJ, Kathol RG, et al. The effects of intravenous theophylline infusion versus intravenous sodium bicarbonate infusion on lithium clearance in normal subjects. *Psychiatry Res.* 1988; 25:203–11.
36. Passmore AP, Kondowe GB, Johnston GD. Renal and cardiovascular effects of caffeine: a dose-response study. *Clin Sci.* 1987; 72:749–56.
37. Finley PR, O'Brien JG, Coleman RW. Lithium and angiotensin-converting enzyme inhibitors: evaluation of a potential interaction. *J Clin Psychopharmacol.* 1996; 16:68–71.
38. Atherton JC, Green R, Hughes S, et al. Lithium clearance in man: effects of dietary salt intake, acute changes in extracellular fluid volume, amiloride and furosemide. *Clin Sci.* 1987; 73:645–51.
39. Almy GL, Taylor MG. Lithium retention in mania. *Arch Gen Psychiatry.* 1973; 29:232–4.
40. Viguera AC, Cohen LS. The course and management of bipolar disorder during pregnancy. *Psychopharmacol Bull.* 1998; 34:339–46.
41. Cohen LS, Rosenbaum JF. Psychotropic drug use during pregnancy: weighing the risks. *J Clin Psychiatry.* 1998; 59(Suppl 2):18–28.
42. Goldberg HL. Psychotropic drugs in pregnancy and lactation. *Int J Psychiatry Med.* 1994; 24:129–47.
43. Llewellyn A, Stowe ZN, Strader JR. The use of lithium and management of women with bipolar disorder during pregnancy and lactation. *J Clin Psychiatry.* 1998; 59(Suppl 6):57–65.
44. Llewellyn A, Stowe ZN. Psychotropic medications in lactation. *J Clin Psychiatry.* 1998; 59(Suppl 2):41–52.
45. Levin GM, Grum C, Eisele G. Effect of over-the-counter dosages of naproxen sodium and acetaminophen on plasma lithium concentrations in normal volunteers. *J Clin Pyschopharmacol.* 1998; 18(3):237–40.
46. Rossat J, Maillard M, Nussberger J, et al. Renal effects of selective cyclooxygenase-2 inhibition in normotensive salt-depleted subjects. *Clin Pharmacol Ther.* 1999; 66(1):76–84.
47. Celebrex Prescribers Information, December 24, 1999.

48. Terao T, Okuno K, Okuno T, et al. A simpler and more accurate equation to predict daily lithium dose. *J Clin Psychopharmacol.* 1999; 19(4):336–40.
49. Schou M, Amdisen A, Steenstrup OR. Lithium and pregnancy-II, hazards to women given lithium during pregnancy and delivery. *Brit Med J.* 1973; 2:137–8.
50. Wallin L, Ailing C, Aurell M. Impairment of renal function in patients on long-term lithium treatment. *Clin Nephrol.* 1982; 18:23–8.
51. Tonks CM. Lithium intoxication induced by dieting and saunas. *Br Med J.* 1977; 2:1396–7.
52. Demers R, Heninger G. Sodium intake and lithium treatment in mania. *Am J Psychiatry.* 1971; 128:132–6.
53. Jefferson JW, Greist JH, Clagnaz PJ, et al. Effect of strenuous exercise on serum lithium level in man. *Am J Psychiatry.* 1982; 139:1593–5.

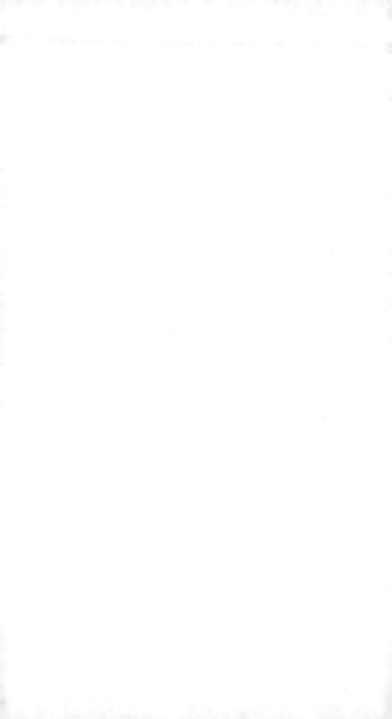

Chapter 13
Mary E. Teresi & John N. McCormick

Methotrexate (AHFS 10:00)

Usual Dosage Range in Absence of Clearance-Altering Factors

Methotrexate (MTX) inhibits several important pathways for folate metabolism. It is approved for treatment of severe forms of psoriasis, rheumatoid arthritis, psoriatic arthritis, systemic dermatomyositis, and various pediatric and adult cancers.[1]

Investigationally, MTX has been used to treat steroid-dependent asthma.[2]

Low doses of methotrexate (LDMTX) are used primarily for immune modulation in chronic diseases or as maintenance therapy for selected cancers. Intermediate and high doses (HDMTX) are used almost exclusively for aggressive cancer chemotherapy, and close monitoring is required to avoid life-threatening toxicity. The intrathecal route is used in the prophylaxis or treatment of meningeal leukemia.

Dose and route selection depends on the disease being treated. The need for leucovorin rescue depends on the MTX dose and the patient's MTX clearance rate. Doses listed are general guidelines; some patients may require more aggressive therapy.

The contributions made by John H. Rodman to this chapter are gratefully acknowledged.

Dosage Form and Amount	Comments and Indications
LDMTX (≤50 mg/m^2): oral (tablets), subcutaneous, intramuscular, and intravenous	Leucovorin rescue generally not required
7.5–15 mg/week	For treatment of rheumatoid arthritis[3] and investigationally for asthma;[2] may be divided into three equal doses given every 12 hr
7.5–30 mg/week	For treatment of psoriasis[4]
15–40 mg/m^2/week	For maintenance therapy of acute lymphocytic leukemia (ALL)
50–60 mg/m^2 intramuscular	For treatment of ectopic pregnancy or nonsurgical abortion (combined with misoprostol)[5,6]
Intermediate dose therapy (>50–500 mg/m^2): intramuscular and intravenous	Leucovorin rescue generally utilized with MTX doses of >100 mg/m^2 but varies with cancer protocols[7]
HDMTX (>500 mg/m^2): intravenous	Preservative-free MTX solution, requires monitoring of plasma MTX concentrations and leucovorin rescue.
1–5 g/m^2	For treatment of ALL
8–12 g/m^2	For treatment of osteosarcoma
Intrathecal[1] <1 year, 6 mg 1–2 years, 8 mg >2–3 years, 10 mg >3–65 years, 12 mg >65 years, may require reduced doses	For prophylaxis or treatment of meningeal leukemia; leucovorin rescue generally not required, but preservative-free MTX solution required

Dosage Form Availability

Dosage Form	Product
Oral tablets: 2.5 mg	Rheumatrex Dose Pack Methotrexate Tablets
Parenteral injection (with preservatives) 2.5 mg/ml 25 mg/ml	 Methotrexate Sodium Injection Methotrexate Sodium Injection Methotrexate Sodium Parenteral

Parenteral injection (preservative free)
25 mg/ml — Folex PFS
Methotrexate LPF Sodium Parenteral
Methotrexate Sodium Injection

20 and 50 mg/vial — Methotrexate Sodium Parenteral

100 mg/vial — Folex
Methotrexate Sodium Parenteral

250 mg/vial — Folex

1 g/vial — Methotrexate Sodium Parenteral

Bioavailability (F) of Dosage Forms

After intramuscular or subcutaneous administration, MTX absorption is relatively complete.[6,8,9] Oral absorption is probably dose dependent and highly variable.[8–11] Low doses (up to 30 mg/m^2) are completely absorbed, whereas higher doses may be affected by many factors.[12]

Dosage Form	Bioavailability Comments
Oral tablets	25–50% with higher bioavailability reported only in seriously flawed studies[8–11] C_{max} = 0.2–10 µM after doses of 10–30 mg/m^2 t_{max} = 1–4 hr
Intramuscular	100% but generally painful and not recommended for doses of >50 mg/m^2
Intravenous	100%
Subcutaneous	100%
Intrathecal	Passes into systemic circulation

Administration of large doses in divided amounts (e.g., 100 mg as 25 mg every 2 hr four times) has been suggested to obviate dose-dependent absorption. However, this method has been evaluated with conflicting results.[10,13,14]

A milky meal before oral administration may reduce C_{max}, the area under the serum concentration–time curve (AUC), and t_{max}.[15] Nonabsorbable antibiotics also may decrease MTX absorption.[16]

With oral administration, the D-isomer achieves only 25% of the AUC of the L-isomer.[17] Most MTX formulations contain less than 5% of the D-isomer.[18] Changes in the small intestinal transit time (optimal of 90–105 min) also alter MTX absorption (decrease if outside range),[19] as does psoriatic enteropathy.[20]

General Pharmacokinetic Information[10,21]

The pharmacokinetics of MTX have been evaluated over a wide range of doses (from 7.5 mg/m^2 to more than 12 g/m^2) and routes of administration.

Protein binding

MTX is approximately 50–60% protein bound. The clinical significance of displacement from albumin binding sites is unclear. Nonsteroidal anti-inflammatory drugs (NSAIDs), salicylates, and probenecid may alter MTX disposition by increasing the free fraction and/or decreasing renal clearance. For LDMTX, concomitant use of these drugs is not contraindicated, but increased monitoring is necessary.[16,22] With HDMTX, the interaction may be pronounced; concomitant administration should be avoided, or renal function and hematologic response should be monitored carefully. The inactive metabolite of MTX, 7-OH MTX, is approximately 90% protein bound.

Distribution

MTX is water soluble and distributes rapidly into extracellular fluids. The primary sites of distribution are listed here.

Distribution Site	Comments
Gut[19,23]	MTX undergoes enterohepatic recycling. GI obstruction or altered transit time delays elimination.
Cerebral spinal fluid (CSF)[10,24]	CSF penetration is dose and administration rate dependent: 1000 mg/m² over 24 hr, CSF = 2.3% of Css 7500 mg/m² bolus, CSF = 10 μM 500 mg/m² over 24 hr, CSF = 0.1 μM Brain tumors as well as cranial radiation may increase CNS penetration and the incidence of MTX-induced leukoencephalopathy.
Synovial fluid[25]	Amount is approximately equal to plasma concentration at 4 and 24 hr after LDMTX.
Saliva[26]	Amount is <7% of plasma concentration. Toxicity (mucositis) may increase if low MTX concentration is maintained for >12 hr.
Effusions[27]	Extravascular effusions (e.g., pleural effusions, "third spacing") may take up significant amounts of drug; MTX slowly reequilibrates into plasma. Influx of drug back into plasma results in apparent prolonged terminal half-life. This may also be important in patients with ascites.
Intracellular transport[10,28]	Cellular transport is active at low concentrations and is saturable. At high concentrations, transport is passive. Intracellular metabolism to polyglutamylated forms is important for efficacy as well as toxicity to normal cells.

Elimination[3,10,21,29–32]

The predominant route of MTX elimination is renal excretion through glomerular filtration, although tubular secretion and reabsorption are clinically important. Renal elimination decreases at increased MTX concentrations due to saturation of tubular secretion.

Renal excretion accounts for 60–85%[21] of MTX elimination as unchanged drug and 1–11%[21,29] as 7-OH MTX (range may increase to 30–40% after HDMTX).[30] Both MTX and 7-OH MTX are unstable in acid environments. Hydration and urinary alkalinization (pH greater than 6.5) are recommended before and after HDMTX to minimize risk of precipitation in renal tubules.[31]

Biliary excretion accounts for less than 10%[32] of MTX elimination. Biliary or GI obstruction may result in delayed terminal elimination.[23]

Metabolism[10,21,30,33]

Three pathways are clinically relevant for MTX metabolism. The significance of each varies with the dose and route of administration.

Pathway	Amount	Comments
Hepatic	≤40%	MTX is metabolized to 7-OH MTX, an inactive metabolite. Percentage formed is related to length of HDMTX intravenous infusion. Less 7-OH MTX is formed with short infusions, possibly due to saturation of aldehyde oxidase at higher plasma MTX concentrations.
Gut	<5%	MTX is metabolized to DAMPA (4-amino-4-deoxy-N-methylpteric acid), an inactive metabolite.
Intracellular	Unknown	Glutamate residues are added to MTX intracellularly; increasing numbers of glutamate residues enhance intracellular retention and cytotoxicity.

Clearance (CL)

MTX clearance is highly variable, even among patients with similar indices (e.g., CrCl) for renal function. Therefore, multiple factors should be assessed prior to and during therapy. Hydration, urinary alkalinization regimens, urine output, emetic episodes, and concurrent intrathecal MTX therapy can influence MTX clearance and plasma concentration profiles.[34] Drugs that interfere with renal tubular secretion or cause nephrotoxicity may reduce MTX clearance (see drug–drug interactions section).

Regimen	Clearance (mean ± SD) (Range)
LDMTX[25]	85 ± 31 (35–189) ml/min/m²
HDMTX	
Adults (≥18 years)[10,21]	57 (35–130) ml/min/m²
Children and adolescents (<18 years)[35]	80 ± 15 (65–106) ml/min/m²
Down, syndrome[35]	64 (45–92) ml/min/m²

Since MTX is predominantly renally eliminated, renal function should be monitored closely. Because MTX solubility is lower at acidic pH, and crystallization in the tubular lumen is an important mechanism for nephrotoxicity, aggressive hydration and urinary alkalinization are important elements of supportive therapy.

With LDMTX, dose modification or leucovorin rescue may be necessary in patients with decreased renal function. A 50% dosage reduction was suggested[21] for patients with a serum creatinine (S_{Cr}) of 1.2–2.0 mg/dl. For patients with a serum creatinine greater than 2.0 mg/dl or a CrCl less than 50 ml/min/m², it was suggested[21] that the MTX dose should be held or the plasma MTX concentration should be monitored and, if necessary, leucovorin should be administered.

Pharmacokinetic data indicate that plasma clearance for MTX in adults with normal renal function is lower than in children.[36] A relationship between the clearance of MTX and CrCl in adults has been reported.[37] However, this finding was based on low doses and may not apply when higher doses saturate renal tubular secretion.[10] A similar study in children reported MTX clearance to be highly variable but significantly correlated with glomerular filtration rate in patients without major renal dysfunction.[38] However, in patients receiving 8–12 g/m² of MTX after various doses of a nephrotoxic agent, cisplatin, serum creatinine and/or CrCl did not correlate well with MTX clearance.[39] However, in general, elevated S_{Cr} and/or decreased CrCl values are indicative of reduced MTX clearance. As in LDMTX therapy, the dose probably should be reduced in patients with a CrCl less than 50 ml/min/m² or held if CrCl decreases dramatically.

In patients with decreased renal function and delayed MTX clearance, high plasma concentrations of the 7-OH MTX metabolite may confound certain analytical methods for measurement of MTX.

Volume of Distribution (V)[10]

The steady-state volume of distribution for MTX in both children and adults is approximately 40–80% of actual body weight.

Half-Life and Time to Steady State

When MTX is given by infusion, biphasic distribution and elimination (i.e., compartment behavior) is apparent, although the distribution half-life ($t\frac{1}{2}$) is often masked during infusions lasting longer than 24 hr. Renal clearance is the primary determinant of half-life during the first 24 hr. Beginning 24 hr after the end of the MTX administration, redistribution from peripheral compartments into the blood determines the rate of MTX clearance from plasma.

The half-life may be prolonged because of prior or concomitant administration of nephrotoxic or renally excreted drugs or because of decreased renal function.

After intravenous bolus MTX administration, triphasic elimination has been reported with the following parameters:

Phase	Half-Life (mean ± SD)	Range[10,21,32,35]
Distribution half-life	0.75 ± 0.11 hr[32]	Not available
Initial half-life (0–24 hr)	1.8 ± 0.5 hr[40]	1.3–3.5 hr
Terminal half-life[a]	10 ± 4 hr	8–27 hr

[a] *May be prolonged secondary to redistribution of MTX from third spaces (see section on drug–disease state or condition interactions).*

LDMTX is usually administered weekly, and the plasma MTX concentration is generally undetectable by 48 hr. Achieving steady state is not an issue. HDMTX is often infused over 4–24 hr, after an initial bolus. Some protocols utilize longer infusions (e.g., 48 hr). Concentrations at 12–24 hr following a loading and maintenance dose regimen will approach steady state.

Therapeutic Range

Both the efficacy and toxicity of MTX are dependent on the concentration obtained and the duration of exposure. MTX is cytotoxic at concentrations greater than 0.05 µM for more than 48 hr.

For psoriasis,[4] asthma,[2] and rheumatoid arthritis,[3,25] when a dose of 7.5–30 mg is administered every week, the expected maximum plasma concentration is 0.25–1.25 µM. The duration of systemic exposure to concentrations greater than 0.05 µM is under 48 hr.

For LDMTX maintenance cancer regimens;[8–10] a weekly dose of 15–40 mg/m^2 yields a maximum plasma concentration of 1–3 µM for oral administration or 7–20 µM for intravenous, intramuscular, or subcutaneous administration. The duration of systemic exposure to concentrations greater than 0.05 µM is under 48 hr.

HDMTX regimens[10,21,29,30] produce maximum concentrations from 10 to greater than 1000 µM, depending on the dose and infusion time. The duration of exposure to MTX concentrations greater than 0.05 µM is generally 72–96 hr or more. Toxicity appears to be related more to the duration of exposure to MTX than to the actual dose or maximum concentration obtained.[41] Leucovorin rescue is required to avoid life-threatening toxicity.

Suggested Sampling Times and Effect on Therapeutic Range

For LDMTX and intermediate dose MTX therapy less than 100 mg/m^2, serum concentration monitoring is generally not necessary. If a patient has a potential drug interaction or reduced renal function or is displaying unexpected toxicity, MTX concentrations should be determined.

For HDMTX and intermediate dose MTX therapy greater than or equal to 100 mg/m^2, sampling times are dependent on the administration schedule. The following concentrations were determined to be risk factors for toxicity at relevant times following an 8–12-g/m^2 dose infused over 4 hr.[10] An initial half-life of longer than 3.5 hr also may indicate a high risk of toxicity.

Hours Postinfusion	Concentrations with High Risk of Toxicity
20 hr	>10 µM
44 hr	>1 µM
68 hr	>0.1 µM
92 hr	>0.05 µM

Leucovorin Rescue[21]

MTX concentrations are indicative of the risk of toxicity and the need for leucovorin rescue. Patients with elevated MTX concentrations require increased leucovorin doses administered for a sufficient period for the MTX concentration to fall below 0.05 µM. Most HDMTX protocols include leucovorin rescue guidelines.

Leucovorin rescue must be initiated within 48 hr after the start of MTX. It is generally begun 24–42 hr after the start of MTX; this schedule allows time for the drug to kill the cancer cells but minimizes damage to normal cells. The risk of toxicity increases the longer leucovorin rescue is held.

Absorption of leucovorin is dose dependent. At absolute doses above 50 mg, the percent absorbed begins to decrease. It is recommended that doses greater than 50 mg be given intravenously. Leucovorin does not reverse MTX toxicity, but it can prevent further cell damage; other supportive care measures also may be required. Since excessive doses of leucovorin may obviate the therapeutic effects of MTX, lower doses are being evaluated.

In some cases, the leucovorin dosage may need to be modified based on the serum MTX concentration and hours postinfusion.[21]

Serum MTX Concentration ≥42 hr after Start of Infusion	Approximate Leucovorin Dose Required
50 µM	1000 mg/m² every 6 hr (intravenous)
5 µM	100 mg/m² every 6 hr (intravenous)
0.5 µM	10 mg/m² every 3 hr (intravenous or oral)
0.1 µM	10 mg/m² every 6 hr (intravenous or oral)
<0.05 µM	No modification

MTX concentration monitoring and leucovorin rescue should be continued until the MTX concentration is less than 0.05 µM.

Pharmacodynamic Monitoring—Concentration-Related Efficacy

The usual concentration–effect relationships are not applicable to MTX because therapeutic response depends on numerous factors. However, because intracellular metabolism is a primary determinant of effect and is poorly correlated to a single measured drug concentration, certain pharmacokinetic parameters that reflect the duration of systemic exposure (e.g., clearance and steady-state concentration) are important.[10,33,42]

Other pharmacodynamic end-points also may be useful in determining the efficacy of MTX therapy.

Psoriasis
- Degree of erythema.
- Scale and elevation of lesions.

Rheumatoid arthritis
- Decrease in joint tenderness.
- Decrease (50% or more) in joint swelling.
- Decrease in erythrocyte sedimentation rate (ESR).
- Decrease in rheumatoid factor.
- Improvement in morning stiffness.
- Improvement in radiologic findings.

Asthma
- Improvement in FEV_1.
- Improvement in pulmonary function tests.
- Decreased inhaler use.

Pregnancy termination
- Decline in hCG levels by ≥15% between 4 and 7 days after MTX administration.
- Absence of gestational sac on vaginal ultrasonographic examination.

Cancer

The pharmacodynamic end-points for efficacy of HDMTX in cancer patients are difficult to assess. However, the feasibility and effectiveness of HDMTX given at 5 g/m^2 have been documented in large numbers of patients treated according to a Cancer Study Group's protocols. In fact, improved outcome of T-cell ALL patients in this group was attributed in part to the use of HDMTX.[43] Another group demonstrated that the level of systemic exposure to HDMTX significantly affected the event-free survival of children with B-lineage ALL.[42] For maintenance therapy of ALL, a WBC count of 2000–4000 has been associated with improved survival,[44] although conflicting reports exist.[45]

Pharmacodynamic Monitoring—Concentration-Related Toxicity

The adverse effects associated with MTX may be acute and transient, as with increased liver function tests (LFTs) after HDMTX, or chronic and subclinical, as with fatty changes in the liver from chronic low dose oral therapy. Adverse effects such as myelosuppression and nephrotoxicity can be severe and potentially life threatening without adequate leucovorin rescue or supportive measures. Although in some cases the adverse effects may or may not be related to MTX concentration, they all are considered toxic effects of MTX therapy.

Severe MTX intoxication may be treated with exchange transfusion, hemodiafiltration, or charcoal hemoperfusion. Rebounds in MTX concentrations may occur after cessation of this therapy, and MTX concentrations should be monitored closely.[46] An investigational agent, carboxypeptidase, may be obtained with permission from the NCI. It works by hydrolyzing MTX to nontoxic metabolites, thereby decreasing MTX concentrations.

The frequency and parameters of monitoring depend on the patient's underlying organ function, the disease being treated, and potential confounding factors such as possible drug interactions, decreased renal function, and other risk factors. The following are general guidelines.

Chronic LDMTX therapy
- LFTs (AST, ALT, Alk Phos, and Alb)—baseline; every 3–4 weeks.
- BUN/S_{Cr}—baseline; every 3–4 weeks.
- CBC with differential—baseline; every 3–4 weeks.

HDMTX (follow protocol guidelines)

- Prior to each dose—Bun/S_{Cr} (plus CrCl); CBC with differential; LFTs (AST, ALT, Alk Phos, and bilirubin).
- During and through 24 hr after MTX administration—urinary output (desired output of 2–3 ml/kg/hr); urine pH (desired pH greater than 6.5).
- After administration—MTX concentration generally every day until less than 0.05 µM; CBC, LFTs, and Bun/S_{Cr} one to three times a week until plasma MTX concentration less than 0.05 µM.

Chronic liver toxicity (cirrhosis and fibrosis)

- Psoriasis—premethotrexate evaluation should include assessment of renal function, liver function tests (ALT, AST, Alk Phos, Bili, and Alb), and hepatitis A, B, and C serology tests. A complete physical exam and medical history should be obtained with emphasis on liver disease, excessive alcohol intake, and/or exposure to hepatotoxic drugs. Liver biopsy is recommended before MTX or during the first 2–4 months of therapy in patients at high risk for liver disease. Otherwise, liver biopsy is not generally necessary until cumulative doses of 1–1.5 g MTX are reached. Renal and liver function tests and CBCs should be repeated at least every 1–2 months during MTX therapy.

- Arthritis[3]—long-term effects of LDMTX in rheumatoid arthritis patients are controversial. Their incidence of hepatotoxicity appears to be lower than that of psoriatic patients. The need for liver biopsies is debatable. Some researchers suggest a pretreatment biopsy, a followup biopsy after a cumulative dose of 1500 mg, and then a biopsy every 2 years during LDMTX therapy. Approximately 50% of patients have exhibited clinically insignificant mild fibrotic changes; whether these changes will evolve into significant fibrosis or cirrhosis is unclear. In high risk patients (see below), liver biopsies

should be performed. However, the risk–benefit ratio is unknown for other rheumatoid arthritis patients.
- Asthma—no current guidelines are available for liver biopsy.
- Cancer—periodic (e.g., monthly) monitoring of liver enzymes is appropriate for patients on maintenance regimens.

Pulmonary fibrosis
- More common in rheumatoid arthritis patients than in psoriatic patients.
- Approximately 40 cases reported in the cancer literature.
- Symptoms of prodromal syndrome headache, malaise, dyspnea, and dry cough.
- Bilateral diffuse patchy infiltrates on chest X-ray.
- Fifty percent of patients present with mild peripheral eosinophilia.
- No current method of predicting or monitoring for this toxicity.

Myelosuppression
- Nadir in counts generally occurs 7–10 days after MTX administration is discontinued.
- Mild suppression (WBC 2000–4000) is desirable for immunosuppression therapy after transplants or during maintenance ALL therapy.
- Significant decrease in WBC or platelets necessitates reduction of LDMTX dose or changes in leucovorin rescue for HDMTX.
- Low grade fevers, frequent infections, easy bruising, or bleeding may indicate myelosuppression.

GI toxicity
- Nausea and vomiting, stomatitis, and mucositis may occur with LDMTX and are common with HDMTX. Changes in dose (LDMTX) or leucovorin rescue, as well as appro-

priate supportive care such as antiemetics, fluids, and/or intravenous nutrition (HDMTX), are often required.

Acute hepatic toxicity
- Generally seen with HDMTX—transient elevation in liver enzymes may occur in 2–3 days. LFTs should return to normal within a week; if enzymes remain elevated, further evaluation is necessary and MTX doses should be held.

Nephrotoxicity
- Generally seen with HDMTX.
- Due to precipitation of MTX or metabolites in renal tubules, generally associated with a low urine pH (prevented with hydration, diuresis, and alkalinization of urine).
- Due to direct cytotoxicity on tubular cells.

Leukoencephalopathy
- A radiographic diagnosis of structural abnormalities (e.g., hypodense areas of white matter) has been reported after intrathecal and HDMTX. The presentation varies from asymptomatic, subclinical dysfunctions to obtundation, cranial nerve abnormalities, confusion, impaired cognition, paraplegia, and, potentially, death. Risk and incidence increase with prior or concomitant cranial radiation or drug therapy.

Miscellaneous
- MTX is considered teratogenic and should not be used in pregnant women.
- MTX may cause abnormal spermatogenesis.
- MTX may cause abortion of pregnancy.
- Other potential side effects are acute dermatitis, radiation recall, and alopecia.

Risk factors for LDMTX-induced hepatotoxicity[4,10]
- Obesity.
- Diabetes.
- Past or present excessive alcohol intake.

- Liver disease.
- Psoriasis.

Risk factors for HDMTX toxicity[10,21,31]
- Decreased renal function—decreases MTX clearance and prolongs initial and terminal half-life. This condition generally requires daily MTX concentration monitoring and leucovorin adjustment (increased dose and duration).
- GI obstruction or third spacing—prolongs terminal half-life by acting as a reservoir of MTX. This condition generally requires prolonged leucovorin administration at standard doses (15–30 mg/m^2).
- Acute and subacute neurotoxicity such as headache, somnolence, or seizure may occur. Prior CNS irradiation may increase chance of neurotoxicity.[47]
- Elevated MTX concentrations at specified sampling times.
- Dehydration, nausea and vomiting, or prior cisplatin therapy—may decrease renal MTX clearance and/or increase risk of drug precipitation in renal tubules, leading to decreased renal function.
- Aciduria—decreases solubility of MTX and 7-OH MTX and may result in precipitation and subsequent renal tubule damage. This condition could create a cycle of decreased renal function, decreased MTX clearance, and increased toxicity.
- Concomitant drugs (see drug–drug interactions).

Drug–Drug Interactions

As the use of MTX increases, more drug interactions are reported. The more frequently encountered interactions are listed here; other references[15,48] provide additional examples.

Cisplatin[39]

As the cumulative dose of cisplatin increases, both clearance and half-life of MTX are affected. With cumulative cisplatin doses greater than 200 mg/m^2, the MTX clearance falls and the half-life increases. With cumulative cisplatin doses greater than 400 mg/m^2, the MTX half-life seems to extend even further. The wide variance in clearance depends on time and underlying renal function. Clearance often improves as more time lapses between cisplatin and MTX therapy. The dose and duration of leucovorin rescue may need to be increased.

Cytosine arabinoside (ARA-C)[48]

MTX enhances the activation of ARA-C if given prior to or concomitantly with ARA-C. If MTX is administered after ARA-C, an antagonistic effect occurs.

Etretinate[49]

The concomitant administration of etretinate and MTX increases the chance of hepatotoxicity.

5-Fluorouracil (5-FU)[48]

MTX enhances the activation of 5-FU if given prior to or concomitantly with 5-FU. If MTX is administered after 5-FU, an antagonistic effect occurs.

Organic acids

Some organic acids (e.g., salicylates, probenecid, and sulfonamides) compete for renal tubular secretion. Other organic acids (e.g., penicillins) can decrease clearance, although the clinical relevance is unknown. This interaction may be more important at low doses when secretory mechanisms are not saturated. Since MTX is 50–60% protein bound, organic acids should be used cautiously in patients receiving MTX because these drugs may displace MTX from plasma proteins.

Nonabsorbable antibiotics[16]

Nonabsorbable antibiotics (e.g., neomycin sulfate) may decrease the bioavailability of MTX tablets by 20–50%.

Omeprazole
MTX secretion by the distal nephron is due to a hydrogen-ion-dependent mechanism. Omeprazole may block active secretion by inhibiting hydrogen–potassium ATPase in the human kidney. This result could cause increased levels of MTX.[50]

NSAIDs[3,16,22]
NSAIDs may increase the MTX half-life by up to 40%. Although the exact mechanism of this interaction is unknown, renal clearance of MTX may be inhibited by NSAIDs. This interaction appears to be more significant with HDMTX and may not be evident during low-dose therapy in patients with normal renal function.[22]

The COX-2 inhibitors have not been found to significantly affect the pharmacokinetics of low-dose methotrexate in patients with rheumatoid arthritis.[51]

Vincristine[10,16]
The toxic effect of vincristine on the GI tract may slow the enterohepatic cycling of MTX, delaying terminal clearance. Vincristine also may increase intracellular accumulation by decreasing MTX efflux out of the cell.

VP-16 and VM-26[10,16]
Both VP-16 and VM-26 many increase intracellular accumulation by decreasing MTX efflux out of the cell.

Miscellaneous
Drugs altering GI transit time and integrity also may affect MTX absorption and clearance. Some nephrotoxic drugs (e.g., acyclovir, aminoglycoside antibiotics, and amphotercin B) may decrease MTX clearance.

Drug–Disease State or Condition Interactions[10,21]

As discussed previously, decreased renal function and GI obstruction can affect both the clearance and half-life of MTX. In addition, dehydration may result in increased nephrotoxicity, delaying MTX clearance.

In conditions such as pleural effusion or ascites, a small percentage (less than 10% of maximum plasma concentration) of MTX accumulates in third spaces.[27] The drug then slowly reequilibrates into the plasma, resulting in a prolonged terminal half-life.

References

1. Methotrexate. In: McEvoy GK, ed. American hospital formulary service drug information 93. Bethesda, MD: American Society of Hospital Pharmacists; 1993:622–8.
2. Mullarkey MF, Blumenstein BA, Andrade WP, et al. Methotrexate in the treatment of corticosteroid-dependent asthma. *N Engl J Med*. 1988; 318:603–7.
3. Bannwarth B, Pehourcq F, Schaeverbeke T, et al. Clinical pharmacokinetics of low-dose pulse methotrexate in rheumatoid arthritis. *Clin Pharmacokinet*. 1996; 30(3):194–210.
4. Roenigk HH, Auerbach R, Maibach H, et al. Methotrexate in psoriasis: consensus conference. *J Am Acad Dermatol*. 1998; 38(3): 478–85.
5. Lipscomb GH, Bran D, McCord MR, et al. Analysis of three hundred fifteen ectopic pregnancies treated with single-dose methotrexate. *Am J Obstet Gynecol*. 1998; 178(6):1354.
6. Creinin MD, Krohn MA. Methotrexate pharmacokinetics and effects in women receiving methotrexate 50 mg per square meter for early abortion. *Am J Obstet Gynecol*. 1997; 177(6): 1444–9.
7. Rodman JH, Crom WR. Selecting an administration route for leucovorin rescue. *Clin Pharm*. 1989; 8:617–21.
8. Teresi ME, Crom WR, Choi KE, et al. Methotrexate bioavailability after oral and intramuscular administration in children. *J Pediatr*. 1987; 110:788–92.
9. Balis FM, Mirro J, Reaman GH, et al. Pharmacokinetics of subcutaneous methotrexate. *J Clin Oncol*. 1988; 6:1882–6.
10. Crom WR, Evans WE. Methotrexate. In: Evans WE, Schentag JJ, Jusko WJ, eds. Applied pharmacokinetics: principles of therapeutic drug monitoring, 3rd ed. Spokane, WA: Applied Therapeutics; 1992; 29-1–42.
11. Chungi VS, Bourne DWA, Dittert LW. Drug absorption VIII: kinetics of GI absorption of methotrexate. *J Pharm Sci*. 1978; 67:560–1.
12. Madden T, Eaton VE. Methotrexate. In: Schomocker GE, ed. Therapeutic drug monitoring, Norwalk, CT: Appleton and Lange; 1995; 527–52.
13. Harvey VJ, Slevin ML, Woollard RC, et al. The bioavailability of oral intermediate-dose methotrexate. Effect of dose subdivision, formulation and timing in the chemotherapy cycle. *Cancer Chemother Pharmacol*. 1984; 13:91–4.

14. Steele WH, Stuart JFB, Lawrence JR, et al. Enhancement of methotrexate absorption by subdivision of dose. *Cancer Chemother Pharmacol.* 1979; 3:235–7.
15. Pinkerton CR, Welshman SG, Glasgow JFT, et al. Can food influence the absorption of methotrexate in children with acute lymphocytic leukemia? *Lancet.* 1980; 944–5.
16. Evans WE, Christensen ML. Drug interactions with methotrexate. *J Rheumatol.* 1985; 12:15–20.
17. Hendel J, Brodthagen H. Entero-hepatic cycling of methotrexate estimated by use of the D-isomer as a reference marker. *Eur J Clin Pharmacol.* 1984; 26:103–7.
18. Cramer SM, Schornagel JH, Kalghatgi KK, et al. Occurrence and significance of D-methotrexate as a contaminant of commercial methotrexate. *Cancer Res.* 1984; 44:1843–6.
19. Pearson ADJ, Craft AW, Eastham EJ, et al. Small Intestinal transit time affects methotrexate absorption in children with acute lymphoblastic leukemia. *Cancer Chemother Pharmacol.* 1985; 14:211–5.
20. Handel L, Hendel J, Johansen A, et al. Intestinal function and methotrexate absorption in psoriatic patients. *Clin Exp Dermatol.* 1982; 7:491–8.
21. Bleyer WA. Clinical pharmacology and therapeutic drug monitoring of methotrexate. *Am Assoc Clin Chem.* 1985; 6:1–14.
22. Iqbal MP, Baig JA, Azra AA, et al. The effects of non-steroidal anti-inflammatory drugs on the disposition of methotrexate in patients with rheumatoid arthritis. *Biopharm. Drug Dispos.* 1998; 19:163–7.
23. Evans WE, Tsiatis A, Crom WR, et al. Pharmacokinetics of sustained serum methotrexate concentrations secondary to gastrointestinal obstruction. *J Pharm Sci.* 1981; 70:1194–8.
24. Evans WE, Hutson PR, Stewart CF, et al. Methotrexate cerebrospinal fluid and serum concentrations after intermediate-dose methotrexate infusion. *Clin Pharmacol Ther.* 1983; 33:301–7.
25. Herman RA, Veng-Pedersen P, Hoffman J, et al. Pharmacokinetics of low-dose methotrexate in rheumatoid arthritis patients. *J Pharm Sci.* 1989; 78:165–71.
26. Ishii E, Yamada S, Higuchi S, et al. Mucositis and salivary methotrexate concentration in intermediate-dose methotrexate therapy for children with acute lymphoblastic leukemia. *Med Pediatr Oncol.* 1989; 17:429–32.
27. Evans WE, Pratt CB. Effect of pleural effusion on high-dose methotrexate kinetics. *Clin Pharmacol Ther.* 1978; 23:68–72.
28. Goldman ID. Membrane transport of methotrexate (NSC-740) and other folate compounds. Relevance to rescue protocols. *Cancer Chemother Rep [3].* 1975; 6:63–72.
29. Slordal L, Kolmannskog S, Prytz PS, et al. Pharmacokinetics of methotrexate and 7-hydroxy-methotrexate after high-dose (33.6 g/m^2) methotrexate therapy. *Pediatr Hematol Oncol.* 1986; 3:127–34.
30. Crom WR, Glynn-Barnhart AM, Rodman JR, et al. Pharmacokinetics of anticancer drugs in children. *Clin Pharmacokinet.* 1987; 12:168–213.

31. Stroller RG, Jacobs SA, Drake JC, et al. Pharmacokinetics of high-dose methotrexate (NSC-740). *Cancer Chemother Rep [3]*. 1975; 6:19–24.
32. Huffman DH, Wan SH, Azarnoff DL, et al. Pharmacokinetics of methotrexate. *Clin Pharmacol Ther.* 1973; 14:572–9.
33. Borsi JD, Sagen E, Ing C, et al. Pharmacokinetics and metabolism of methotrexate: an example for the use of clinical pharmacology in pediatric oncology. *Pediatr Hematol Oncol.* 1990; 7:13–33.
34. Christensen ML, Rivera GK, Crom WR, et al. Effect of hydration on methotrexate plasma concentrations in children with acute lymphocytic leukemia. *J Clin Oncol.* 1988; 6:797–801.
35. Garre ML, Relling MV, Kalwinsky D, et al. Pharmacokinetics and toxicity of methotrexate in children with Downs syndrome and acute lymphocytic leukemia. *J Pediatr.* 1987; 111:606–12.
36. Donelli MG, Zuchetti M, Robatto A, et al. Pharmacokinetics of high-dose methotrexate in infants, children and adolescents with non-B ALL. *Med Pediatr Oncol.* 1995; 24(3):154–9.
37. Bressolle F, Bologna C, Kinowski JM, et al. Effects of moderate renal insufficiency on pharmacokinetics of methotrexate in rheumatoid arthritis patients. *Ann Rheum Dis.* 1998; 57(2):110–3.
38. Murry DJ, Synold T, Pui CH, et al. Renal function and methotrexate clearance in children with newly diagnosed leukemia. *Pharmacotherapy.* 1995; 15(2):144–9.
39. Crom WR, Pratt CB, Green DA, et al. The effect of prior cisplatin therapy on the pharmacokinetics of high-dose methotrexate. *J Clin Oncol.* 1984; 2:655–61.
40. Isacoff WH, Morrison PF, Aroesty J, et al. Pharmacokinetics of high-dose methotrexate with citorum factor rescue. *Cancer Treat Rep.* 1977; 61:1665–74.
41. Goldie JH, Price LA, Harrap KR. Methotrexate toxicity: correlation with duration of administration, plasma levels, dose and excretion pattern. *Eur J Cancer.* 1972; 8:409–14.
42. Evans WE, Crom WR, Abromowitch M, et al. Clinical pharmacodynamics of high-dose methotrexate in acute lymphocytic leukemia. Identification of a relationship between concentration and effect. *N Engl J Med.* 1986; 314:471–7.
43. Reiter A, Schrappe M, Ludwig W-D, et al. Chemotherapy in 998 unselected childhood ALL patients. Results and conclusions of the multicenter trial ALL-BFM 86. *Blood.* 1994; 84:3122–33.
44. Schmiegelow K, Pulczynska MK, Scip M. White cell count during maintenance chemotherapy for standard-risk childhood acute lymphoblastic leukemia: relationship to relapse rate. *Pediatr Hematol Oncol.* 1988; 5:259–67.
45. VanEys J, Berry D, Crist W, et al. Treatment intensity and outcome for children with acute lymphocytic leukemia of standard risk. *Cancer.* 1989; 63:1466–71.
46. Wall SM, Johansen MJ, Molony DA, et al. Effective clearance of methotrexate using high-flux hemodialysis membranes. *Am J Kidney Dis.* 1996; 28(6):846–54.

47. Gokbuget N, Hoelzer D. High-dose methotrexate in the treatment of adult acute lymphoblastic leukemia. *Ann Hematol.* 1996; 72:194–201.
48. Ignoffo RJ. Update of methotrexate drug interactions. *Highlights Antineopl Drugs.* 1986; Nov/Dec:2–17.
49. Larsen FG, Nielsen-Kudsk F, Jakobsen P, et al. Interaction of etretinate with methotrexate pharmacokinetics in psoriatic patients. *J Clin Pharmacol.* 1990; 30:802–7.
50. Reid T, Yuen A, Catolico M, et al. Impact of omeprazole on the plasma clearance of MTX. *Cancer Chemother Pharmacol.* 1993; 33:80–4.
51. Karim A, Tolbert DS, Hunt TL, Hubbard RC, Harper KM. Celecoxib, a specific COX-2 inhibitor, has no significant effect on methotrexate pharmacokinetics in patients with rheumatoid arthritis. *J Rheumatol.* 1999; 26:2539–43.

Chapter 14
Douglas M. Anderson & Kimberly B. Tallian

Phenobarbital
(AHFS 28:12.04 and 28:24.04)

Usual Dosage Range in Absence of Clearance-Altering Factors[1,2]

Phenobarbital exhibits a predictable pharmacokinetic profile with a relatively wide therapeutic window. As a result, dosing protocols are often used with satisfactory results. The dosing recommendations below, based on average pharmacokinetic parameters, should also produce concentrations in the therapeutic range for most patients in each population. However, significant interpatient variation necessitates therapeutic monitoring.

Once-daily dosing at bedtime is preferred to minimize daytime sedation and to increase compliance in ambulatory patients.[3,4] If the clinical situation allows, initial sedation may be minimized by starting therapy with 25% of the recommended maintenance dose and increasing it weekly by another 25% until the full maintenance dose is achieved.[5]

Dosage Form	Loading Dose	Maintenance Dosage
Oral (capsules, tablets, and elixir)		
Neonates (<2 weeks)	15–25 mg/kg	2–4 mg/kg/day

Infants (2 weeks–<1 year)	15–25 mg/kg	5 mg/kg/day
Children		
1–<5 years	10–20 mg/kg	4.5 mg/kg/day
5–<10 years	10–20 mg/kg	3.6 mg/kg/day
10–<15 years	10–20 mg/kg	2.9 mg/kg/day
15–<19 years	10–20 mg/kg	2.5 mg/kg/day
Adults (19–65 years)	10–20 mg/kg	2 mg/kg/day
Geriatrics (>65 years)	10–20 mg/kg	1.1–2 mg/kg/day
Intravenous and intramuscular	Same as oral doses, administered at <50 mg/min[1]	Same as oral doses

For intravenous and intramuscular routes, the sodium salt of phenobarbital is used. The sodium salt fraction (S) equals 0.9. Intravenous phenobarbital loading doses have been reported to cause hypotension, particularly in neonates (possibly due to the propylene glycol content). However, recommended loading doses should be safe if administered at less than 50 mg/min.[1] Phenobarbital's slow elimination precludes the need for continuous intravenous infusions.

Due to phenobarbital's first-order elimination, proportionality may be applied when doses are adjusted during steady-state conditions (i.e., dose increases or decreases result in proportional changes in the phenobarbital concentration).

Dosage Form Availability[6]

Dosage Form	Product
Intravenous and Intramuscular	
30, 60, 65, and 130 mg/ml	Phenobarbital Sodium Injection (Elkins-Sinn, Wyeth-Ayerst)
130 mg/ml	Luminal Sodium (Sanofi Winthrop) Phenobarbital Sodium Injection (Elkins-Sinn, Wyeth-Ayerst)
Oral capsules: 16 mg	Solfoton (Poythress)

Oral elixir	
15 mg/5 ml	Phenobarbital Elixir (Pharmaceutical Associates)
20 mg/5 ml	various manufacturers
Oral tablets: 8, 15, 16, 30, 32, 60, 65, and 100 mg	various manufacturers

Bioavailability (F) of Dosage Forms[2,6,7]

Dosage Form	Bioavailability Comments
Intramuscular	100% with onset of action within 30 min and peak serum concentrations within 3 hr
Intravenous	100% with immediate onset of action
Rectal administration	Faster rate of absorption than either oral or intramuscular route
Oral (capsules, tablets, and elixir)	90–100% with time to peak being highly variable (average of 2 hr)

With the oral dosage forms, large single doses (over 750 mg) may delay or decrease overall absorption in adults due to the insolubility of phenobarbital crystals that form and remain for some time in the stomach. Drugs or diseases that affect GI motility may influence the rate of absorption. However, the effect on the extent of absorption is unclear. The presence of food apparently does not significantly affect the extent of absorption, although the rate may be altered.

General Pharmacokinetic Information

Clearance

Renal excretion of unchanged drug is urine flow and pH dependent (increasing with alkaline urine) but may vary from 20 to 40% in patients with normal renal function. Combined diuresis and alkalosis can increase renal clearance up to fourfold.[2]

Although hepatic disease may decrease phenobarbital clearance,[8] renal excretion apparently increases with impaired hepatic function. Therefore, severe reductions in clearance are averted.[9] Furthermore, renal insufficiency, even in end-stage disease, appears to have little effect on phenobarbital concentrations because of increased hepatic metabolism.[1]

Phenobarbital clearance can be affected, however, by certain drugs, disease states and age. (See sections on drug–drug interactions and drug–disease state or condition interactions.)

Metabolism

Following slow but essentially complete absorption, phenobarbital undergoes extensive non-first-pass, non-dose-dependent biotransformation by hepatic micro-enzymes into inactive metabolites. Phenobarbital is a potent inducer of CYP3A4, CYP1A2, CYP2C, and CYP2D6 hepatic enzymes, requiring approximately 1 week for the effects of induction to be observed.[10] Although some enterohepatic cycling occurs, fecal excretion does not significantly affect clearance.[2]

Protein binding

Phenobarbital binds primarily to albumin in the plasma. Free fractions are affected by albumin concentration; this effect appears to be clinically significant only when combined with renal failure and acidosis.[9,11] In the neonate, the degree of protein binding is affected by postnatal age and serum bilirubin concentration. The free (unbound) phenobarbital concentrations may be as high as 90% of the total concentration at birth, followed by a gradual decline to 70% after 1 week (see volume of distribution).[1]

Clearance (CL)[1,12,13]

The following clearance values can be assumed in the absence of disease or drug interactions.

Age	Clearance (mean ± SD)	Fraction of Parent Drug Excreted in Urine
Neonates and infants (<1 year)	0.0047 ± 0.0002 L/hr/kg	~0.2[a]
Children (1–<19 years)	0.0082 ± 0.0031 L/hr/kg	0.2–0.4
Adults (19–65 years)	0.0056 ± 0.0026 L/hr/kg[b]	0.24–0.5
Geriatrics (>65 years)	0.0024 L/hr/kg	Not available

[a] This value was reported to be greater than or equal to 0.6 during the first week of life.
[b] CL_{renal} and $CL_{nonrenal}$ were reported to be 0.00091 ± 0.00046 and 0.0033 ± 0.0007 L/hr/kg, respectively.

Volume of Distribution (V)

Phenobarbital's volume of distribution ranges from 0.5 to 1 L/kg. Volumes are largest at birth through infancy, decline slightly in childhood, and reach the lowest population values in adults. Significant variation may exist within each age population, due in part to fluctuation of plasma proteins and a correlation with pH.[2] (A weak acid, phenobarbital has a pKa of 7.3, approximating plasma pH. Increases in plasma pH may increase clearance and vice versa.)

Distribution occurs in a biphasic manner, normally reaching the beta phase about 2 hr after administration.[5] At this point, CNS concentrations approximate the serum unbound concentrations after an intravenous dose, ranging from 43 to 60% of serum concentrations.[2] The free fraction increases with hypoalbuminemia and hyperbilirubinemia.[2] As a result of slow distribution into the CNS, phenobarbital has not historically been used for status epilepticus. One study, however, found phenobarbital's efficacy comparable to that of benzodiazepines for status epilepticus.[14]

Readily crossing placental tissue, phenobarbital achieves a fetal concentration approximately equal to that of the mother[1] but may exceed the mother's concentration based on reduced fetal elimination.[15] Data regarding excretion into breast milk varies (1.5–41% of maternal phenobarbital concentrations have been detected).[2,16] Only large doses are reported to produce clinically significant concentrations, with resultant sedation, in nursing infants and neonates.[17]

Age	Volume (mean ± SD)[2,13]	Protein Binding (mean ± SD)
Neonates (<2 weeks)	0.96 ± 0.02 L/kg	36.8 ± 17.2%
Infants and children (2 weeks–19 years)	0.63 ± 0.09 L/kg	51%
Adults and geriatrics (>19 years)	0.61 ± 0.05 L/kg	51%

Half-Life and Time to Steady State[1,2,12]

Phenobarbital's half-life and time to steady state are age group dependent and can be affected by certain drug interactions and disease states. (See sections on drug–drug interactions and drug–disease state or condition interactions.)

Age	Half-Life (mean ± SD)	Time to Steady State
Neonates (<2 weeks)	111 ± 34 hr	2–4 weeks
Infants (2 weeks–<1 year)	63 ± 5 hr	2–4 weeks
Children (1–<19 years)	69 ± 3 hr	1.5–2 weeks
Adults and geriatrics (>19 years)	96 ± 13.2 hr[a]	1.5–7 weeks

[a]*May be higher for patients over 65 years.*

Therapeutic Range

Of the patients whose seizure activity responds to phenobarbital, 84% respond at serum concentrations of 10–40 mg/L.[9] These concentrations are generally considered the therapeutic range. However, patient response should be the definitive guide for dosage adjustment. Behavioral toxicity may occur in the absence of overt signs of clinical toxicity, especially in children.[18] One study showed that 42% of children treated with phenobarbital developed behavioral disturbances, namely hyperactivity and somnolence.[19] Once phenobarbital was discontinued, improvement and resolution of symptoms was observed in 73% of patients.[20] Although the study found no correlation between these disturbances and phenobarbital concentrations, maintaining this population near the lowest effective concentration remains desirable pending further research.

The following condition specific therapeutic ranges also have been suggested.

Clinical Condition	Recommended Therapeutic Range	Comments
Febrile convulsions	16–30 mg/L[8]	A 6-month recurrence rate of <4% was demonstrated at these concentrations versus 21% at ≤15 mg/L or with no drug.[5] Prophylaxis following febrile convulsion may only be necessary when complicated by underlying neurologic disorders, prolonged febrile seizures, or family history of nonfebrile seizures.[8]
Hypoxic ischemic seizures in neonates (perinatal asphyxia)	>30 mg/L initially	20–30 mg/L may be acceptable 24–48 hr after birth; may require lower maintenance doses due to longer than usual half-life.[20]
Generalized tonic–clonic seizures	10–25 mg/L	10 mg/L has improved EEGs (but not necessarily controlled seizures) in 90% of patients.[5] Due to increased incidence of adverse effects, concentrations should generally not exceed 30 mg/L unless required for seizure control.[18]

Refractory status epilepticus	≥70 mg/L	May be employed without consideration of maximum dose or concentration.[21] (ICU required.) This treatment has initiation advantages over high-dose benzodiazepines and phenytoin, as well as a more predictable pharmacokinetic profile.
Cerebral salvage from hypoxic or traumatic brain damage	>75 mg/L[1]	This amount may induce barbiturate coma, particularly in unhabituated patients.[5]

Suggested Sampling Times and Effect on Therapeutic Range[1,5]

Since the peak to trough fluctuation is minimal during dosing intervals, actual sampling times are not usually important. However, sampling times relative to dose administration should be consistent when concentrations are compared. A postloading dose measurement at approximately 2–3 hr following administration is recommended to confirm the therapeutic concentration. If the clinical situation warrants, a concentration may be obtained again in 3–4 days to determine if the maintenance dose is sufficient. (If the loading dose concentration was satisfactory, a decrease from the postload value may indicate the need for a greater maintenance dose, and vice versa. This second concentration may not reflect steady-state conditions.

To document acceptable steady-state values, another concentration may be obtained 3–4 weeks after initiation of therapy, dose changes, or discontinuation or introduction of known enzyme inducers or inhibitors. Concentrations should be determined immediately for any patient in whom seizure control is lost or toxicity is evident. More frequent monitoring may be required during pregnancy and for 8 weeks following delivery.

Pharmacodynamic Monitoring—Concentration-Related Efficacy

The absence of seizures may not be the therapeutic end-point for some conditions. For intracranial hemorrhage or ischemic cerebral lesions in neonates, therapy should be directed by serial EEGs instead of seizure patterns or phenobarbital concentrations.[22]

The efficacy of therapy for seizure disorders is usually determined by seizure frequency. Noncompliance must always be considered with patients receiving anticonvulsants; 25–75% of patients receiving phenobarbital therapy have been reported to be noncompliant.[23]

Pharmacodynamic Monitoring—Concentration-Related Toxicity[1,5,24]

Toxicity with phenobarbital therapy can present as either neurologic or nonneurologic adverse effects. *Neurologic effects* may or may not be concentration related. Table 1 lists several concentration-related neurologic adverse effects. Neurologic adverse effects that may occur without regard to concentration are sedation (in naïve patients), neonatal feeding disorders, sexual dysfunction, and behavioral abnormalities (including lethargy, sleep disorders,

TABLE 1. Phenobarbital Concentration-Related Neurologic Adverse Effects

Adverse Effect	Phenobarbital Concentration
Sedation[a]	≥5 mg/L
Impaired cognition (with or without sedation)[b]	>19 mg/L
Decreased neonatal feeding, respirations, and muscle tone[b]	>30 mg/L
Sedation, slowness, and ataxia[b]	35–80 mg/L
Potential coma[b]	≥65 mg/L
Coma without reflexes (potentially lethal)[b]	≥80 mg/L

[a]*In nonhabituated patients.*
[b]*In habituated or nonhabituated patients.*

TABLE 2. Nonneurological Adverse Effects of Chronic Phenobarbital Therapy[a]

Adverse Effect	Relative Frequency	Monitoring Parameter
Folate deficiency	52%	Folate concentrations
Fetal vitamin K deficit from maternal phenobarbital therapy	<50%	Neonatal coagulation studies
Vitamin D deficiency	10%	Calcium and alkaline phosphatase concentrations
Shoulder–hand syndrome	<6%	If bone joint or bone pain are present, therapy should be reevaluated
Hepatotoxicity	<1%	No monitoring is necessary unless overt signs of toxicity exist

[a]*In general, nonneurologic adverse effects lack a clear relationship to phenobarbital concentration and most often present during chronic therapy.*

hyperactivity in children, irritability, and depression). See Table 2 for nonneurological adverse effects.[25]

Drug–Drug Interactions

Certain drugs may either increase or decrease phenobarbital concentrations (Table 3). Although conflicting studies exist, phenytoin seldom significantly affects phenobarbital concentrations.[26] Importantly, phenobarbital has been shown to induce the metabolism of numerous medications clinically through its effect on various cytochromes (Table 4).

TABLE 3. Drugs Affecting Phenobarbital Concentrations

Increases Phenobarbital Concentrations	Clearance Factor[a]	Mechanism of Interaction
Chloramphenicol[26, b]	0.6	Competitive inhibition of hepatic metabolism
Methsuximide[26, b]	<1	Competitive inhibition of hepatic metabolism
Propoxyphene[26, b]	0.8	Competitive inhibition of hepatic metabolism
Valproic acid[11]	0.7	Competitive inhibition of hepatic metabolism

TABLE 3. (*continued*)

Decreases Phenobarbital Concentrations	Clearance Factor[a]	Mechanism of Interaction
Bicarbonate[1,5,26]	>1	Decreased tubular reabsorption
Charcoal with or without sorbitol[28]	>1	Adsorption of oral phenobarbital
	≥1.5	Adsorption of intravenous phenobarbital during enterohepatic circulation
Cholestyramine[27]	No change	Decreased or delayed absorption of oral phenobarbital from GI tract
Pyridoxine[16,b]	1.4	Unknown
Rifampin[16]	>1	Hepatic induction
Thioridazine and mesoridazine[16,c]	1.3	Hepatic induction

[a] When multiplied by normal phenobarbital clearance, this factor adjusts clearance for the particular drug interaction.
[b] Anecdotal data or from small study populations. Reliability of clearance factor or clinical significance of interaction is not well substantiated.
[c] A similar interaction may exist with other phenothiazines.

TABLE 4. Drugs that May Undergo Hepatic Induction by Phenobarbital

CYP3A4	CYP2D6	CYP2C	CYP1A2
Beta-blockers (except Sotalol)	Methadone	S-Warfarin	Theophylline
Calcium channel blockers	Phenothiazines	Topiramate	
Carbamazepine	Propafenone		
Cimetidine			
Clonazepam			
Corticosteroids			
Cyclosporine			
Digoxin			
Disopyramide			
Etoposide			
Itraconazole			
Ketoconazole			
Nelfinavir			
Oral contraceptives			
Quinidine			
Saquinavir			
Tacrolimus			
Tetracyclines			

TABLE 5. Conditions that Alter Phenobarbital Pharmacokinetics[a]

Clinical Condition	Effect on Clearance	Effect on Half-Life
Hepatic dysfunction[8]		
Cirrhosis[b]	Decrease	Extended
Acute viral hepatitis[b]	No change	No change
Renal failure[1]		
Mild or moderate[b,c]	No change	No change
Severe[b,c]	Decrease	Increase
Hepato–renal[b]	Decrease	Increase
Hemodialysis (4 hr)[d]	~30% of drug removed	Not available
Peritoneal dialysis[e]	~7.5–15% of drug removed[d]	Not available
Pregnancy[1,8,f]	Increase	Decrease
Perinatal asphyxia[20,b] (apgar <5 at 5 min)	Reported to be 0.0048 ± 0.0018 L/hr/kg	Reported to be 148 ± 55 hr
Prolonged starvation[2,b]	Increase	Decrease

[a]Little data exist regarding changes in V in these conditions. However, with perinatal asphyxia, V has been reported to increase by 13%.
[b]A decrease in albumin may cause an increase in free drug.
[c]Studies to date do not suggest that dosage adjustments are necessary for moderate to severe renal failure.[1] Little data exist regarding hepato–renal disease.
[d]One-third of daily phenobarbital dose should be replaced after hemodialysis.[1]
[e]The effect of peritoneal dialysis on phenobarbital clearance is unpredictable. Patients may require more frequent serum concentration monitoring to guide dosing.[1] In phenobarbital toxicity, removal may be increased with 5% albumin dialysate.[29]
[f]Clearance may gradually increase through gestation before returning to baseline within 4–8 weeks following delivery.[1]

Drug–Disease State or Condition Interactions

The effects of certain disease states and clinical conditions on phenobarbital pharmacokinetics are listed in Table 5.

References

1. Gal P. Phenobarbital and primidone. In: Taylor WJ, Diers Caviness MH, eds. A textbook for the clinical application of therapeutic drug monitoring. Irving, TX: Abbott Laboratories Diagnostics Division; 1986: 237–52.

2. Rust SR, Dodson WE. Phenobarbital: absorption, distribution, and excretion. In: Levy RH, Dreifuss FE, Mattson RH, et al., eds. Antiepileptic drugs, 3rd ed. New York: Raven Press; 1989:293–304.
3. Wroblewski BA, Garvin WH Jr. Once-daily administration of phenobarbital in adults: clinical efficacy and benefit. *Arch Neurol.* 1985; 42:699–700.
4. Davis AG, Mutchie KD, Thompson JA, et al. Once daily dosing with phenobarbital in children with seizure disorders. *Pediatrics.* 1981; 68:824–7.
5. Levy RH, Wilenski AJ, Friel PN. Other antiepileptic drugs. In: Evans WE, Schentag JJ, Jusko WJ, eds. Applied pharmacokinetics: principles of therapeutic drug monitoring, 2nd ed. Spokane, WA: Applied Therapeutics; 1986:540–69.
6. Phenobarbital. In: McEvoy GK, ed. American hospital formulary service drug information 93. Bethesda, MD: American Society of Hospital Pharmacists; 1993:1272–3.
7. Maynert EW. Phenobarbital: absorption, distribution, and excretion. In: Woodbury DM, Penry JK, Pippenger CE, eds. Antiepileptic drugs. New York: Raven Press; 1982:309–17.
8. Painter MJ. Phenobarbital: clinical use. In: Levy RH, Dreifuss FE, Mattson RH, et al., eds. Antiepileptic drugs, 3rd ed. New York: Raven Press; 1989:329–40.
9. Booker HE. Phenobarbital: relation of plasma concentration to seizure control. In: Woodbury DM, Penry JK, Pippenger CE, eds. Antiepileptic drugs. New York: Raven Press; 1982:341–50.
10. Landrum-Michalets E. Update: Clinically significant cytochrome P-450 drug interactions. *Pharmacotherapy.* 1998; 18(1):84–112.
11. Pugh CP. Phenytoin and phenobarbital protein binding alterations in a uremic burn patient. *Drug Intell Clin Pharm.* 1987; 21:264–7.
12. Patel IH, Levy RH, Cutler R. Phenobarbital–valproic acid interaction. *Clin Pharmacol Ther.* 1980; 27:515–21.
13. Benet LZ, Williams RL. Design and optimization of dosage regimens; pharmacokinetic data. In: Gilman AG, Rall TW, Nics AS, et al., eds. The pharmacological basis of therapeutics, 8th ed. New York: Pergamon; 1990:1650-735.
14. Shaner MD, McCurdy SR, Hering M, et al. Treatment of status epileptics: a prospective comparison of diazepam and phenytoin versus phenobarbital and optional phenytoin. *Neurology.* 1988; 38:202–7.
15. Nau H, Kuhnz W, Egger HJ, et al. Anticonvulsants during pregnancy and lactation: transplacental, maternal and neonatal pharmacokinetics. *Clin Pharmacokinet.* 1982; 7:508–43.
16. Phenobarbital. In: Drugdex Information System, Micromedex, Inc.; 1992.
17. Fahim MF, King TM. Effect of phenobarbital on lactation in the nursing neonate. *Am J Obstet Gynecol.* 1968; 101:1103.
18. Rall TW, Schleifer LS. Drugs effective in the treatment of epilepsies. In: Gilman AG, Rall TW, Nies AS, et al., eds. The pharmacological basis of therapeutics, 8th ed. New York: Pergamon; 1990:436–62.
19. Wolf S, Forsythe A. Behavior disturbance, phenobarbital, and febrile seizures. *Pediatrics.* 1978; 61:729–31.

20. Donn SM, Crasela TH, Goldstein GW. Safety of a higher loading dose of phenobarbital in the term newborn. *Pediatrics*. 1985; 75:1061–4.

21. Crawford TO, Mitchell WG, Fishman LS, et al. Very-high-dose phenobarbital for refractory status epilepticus in children. *Neurology*. 1998; 38:1035–40.

22. Connell J, Dozeer R, DeVries L, et al. Clinical and EEG response to anticonvulsants in neonatal seizures. *Arch Dis Child*. 1989; 64:459–64.

23. Pugh C, Garnett W. Current issues in the treatment of epilepsy. *Clin Pharm*. 1991; 10:335–58.

24. Mattson RH, Cramer JA. Phenobarbital toxicity. In: Levy RH, Dreifuss FE, Mattson RH, et al., eds. Antiepileptic drugs, 3rd ed. New York: Raven Press; 1989:341–55.

25. Rizack MA, ed. Handbook of adverse drug interactions. New Rochelle, NY: The Medical Letter; 1998:101–7.

26. Kutt H. Phenobarbital: Interactions with other drugs. In: Levy RH, Dreifuss FE, Mattson RH, et al., eds. Antiepileptic drugs, 3rd ed. New York: Raven Press; 1989:313–27.

27. Product information: Questran. In: Physicians' desk reference, 47th ed. Montvale, NJ: Medical Economics Company; 1993:732–33.

28. Berg MS, Rose JQ, Vivister DE, et al. Effect of charcoal and sorbitol–charcoal suspension on the elimination of intravenous phenobarbital. *Ther Drug Monit*. 1987; 9:41–7.

29. Berman LB, Vogelsang P. Removal rates for barbiturates using two types of peritoneal dialysis. *New Engl J Med*. 1964; 270:77–80.

Chapter 15
Michael E. Winter

Phenytoin and Fosphenytoin
(AHFS 28:12.12)

Usual Dosage Range in Absence of Clearance-Altering Factors

Phenytoin, a hydantoin-derivative anticonvulsant, also exhibits antiarrhythmic properties similar to those of lidocaine.

Loading dose[1,2]

When a rapid therapeutic concentration is desired, a loading dose is recommended.

The maximum intravenous infusion rate in neonates, children, and adolescents is 1–3 mg/kg/min. In adults, the maximum infusion rate is 50 mg/min.

For children, adolescents, and adults, the oral loading dose is usually given in 5-mg/kg increments every 2 hr until the total dose has been administered. The usual adult dose is 1000 mg (approximately 15 mg/kg multiplied by 70 kg), given in 400-, 300-, and 300-mg doses, each separated by 2 hr.

Age	Loading Dose
Neonates and infants (<1 year)	15–20 mg/kg
Children (1–<12 years)	15–18 mg/kg
Adolescents (≥12 years), adults, and geriatrics	15–18 mg/kg

Maintenance dose[1-3]

In infants, children, and adolescents, the total daily dose is usually divided into equal doses and given at evenly spaced intervals of 6, 8, or 12 hr. In adults, the usual daily dose is 300 mg given once a day at bedtime (for this schedule, the extended-release product Dilantin Kapseals must be used).

Age	Maintenance Dosage
Neonates (<4 weeks)	3–5 mg/kg/day
Infants (4 weeks–<1 year)	4–8 mg/kg/day
Children (1–<12 years)	4–10 mg/kg/day
Adolescents (12–<18 years)	4–8 mg/kg/day
Adults and geriatrics (≥18 years)	4–7 mg/kg/day

Dosage Form Availability[1,2,4-7]

Phenytoin is available in the acid or sodium salt form and as the phosphate ester prodrug of phenytoin. The sodium salt has a salt fraction (S) of approximately 92% ($S = 0.92$) phenytoin and 8% sodium and is available both intravenously and as a capsule. The acid is available as a suspension or chewable tablet (S is 100%). Fosphenytoin (fosphenytoin ester) is available only as an injectable dosage form that can be administered either intravenously or intramuscularly. Fosphenytoin is labeled as milligrams of phenytoin equivalents (PE) of phenytoin for injection and therefore the S factor for fosphenytoin PE to calculate the milligrams of acid phenytoin is 0.92.

Phenytoin for injection contains propylene glycol, a cardiac depressant. The maximum recommended infusion rate is 50 mg/min for adults and 1–3 mg/kg/min for neonates and pediatrics. Patients receiving phenytoin for injection should be monitored for bradycardia, hypotension, and, if ECG is available, widened PR, QRS, or QT intervals as indications of myocardial depression. Fosphenytoin does not contain propylene glycol and therefore can be administered more rapidly (maximum recommended infusion rate is 150 mg/min). However, bradycardia and hypotension can still occur and transient pruritis is relatively common. Therefore, cardiovascular monitoring is required and infusion rates of less than 150 mg/min should be considered. In addition, fosphenytoin, while requiring refrigeration, is more stable when reconstituted and can be prepared in either dextrose or saline solution.

Daily doses of phenytoin (fosphenytoin and intravenous and oral phenytoin) should be divided, unless Dilantin Kapseals are used. To minimize plasma phenytoin concentration fluctuations, single daily doses of Dilantin Kapseals greater than 6 mg/kg/day also may need to be divided.

The suspension form requires complete dispersion and accurate volume delivery to ensure accurate dose administration. It should be shaken vigorously prior to administration (1–2 min. if the container has not been used for some time).

Intramuscular administration of phenytoin for injection is not recommended. Although absorption following intramuscular administration is probably complete, it is erratic due to precipitation at the injection site. Absorption of fosphenytoin following intramuscular administration is more rapid than either intramuscular phenytoin for injection or oral phenytoin. However, the intravenous route is still preferred when rapid achievement of phenytoin concentration is the goal (e.g., acute seizures or status).

Dosage Form	Product
Phenytoin for injection: 50 mg/ml	Phenytoin Sodium Injection
Fosphenytoin for injection: 50 mg PE/ml	Cerebyx

Oral capsules (extended release): 30 and 100 mg — Dilantin Kapseals

Oral capsules (prompt release) 100 mg — Phenytoin Sodium, Prompt

Oral tablets (chewable): 50 mg — Dilantin Infatabs (Parke-Davis)

Oral suspension 125 mg/5 ml — Dilantin-125
Phenytoin Oral Suspension (UDL, Xactdose)

Bioavailability (*F*) of Dosage Forms[1-3,8,9]

Although all dosage forms of phenytoin are assumed to have a bioavailability of 100%, phenytoin has capacity-limited metabolism; as a result, bioavailability studies are difficult to interpret. Since phenytoin is a weak acid with limited water solubility, its absorption is slow; peak concentrations are delayed for several hours following oral administration.

The time to achieve peak concentration is both product and dose dependent. The suspension and chewable tablets appear to be absorbed more rapidly than capsules. Furthermore, generic capsules are absorbed more rapidly than Dilantin Kapseals. For example, single Dilantin Kapseal doses of 400, 800, and 1600 mg achieve peak concentrations at approximately 8, 13, and 30 hr after administration, respectively. Peak concentrations following these oral doses are only about half of what would be expected following intravenous administration; more likely the result of slow absorption rather than to a reduced extent of absorption.

While data indicate that the phenytoin suspension is completely absorbed in most patients, two notable exceptions are neonates and patients receiving liquid nutritional support (e.g., nasogastric feedings). The reason for the low phenytoin concentrations in these two patient populations following oral administration of the suspension is unclear, and, although debated, the most likely explanation is a decreased bioavailability.

General Pharmacokinetic Information[1-4]

Phenytoin is bound primarily to albumin in the plasma (fraction unbound in plasma equals 0.1). However, less than 5% of the total body phenytoin is bound to albumin. As a result, changes in plasma binding have little impact on the unbound plasma concentration, tissue stores, and pharmacologic response.

Most clinical assays measure the total (total = bound + unbound) phenytoin concentrations. Therefore, alterations in plasma binding require adjustment for the change in the bound concentration. The two factors most commonly associated with altered phenytoin plasma protein binding are hypoalbuminemia and end-stage renal failure (i.e., dialysis patients). Phenytoin concentrations in these patients can be adjusted to represent normal plasma protein binding by using Equations 1 and 2 below.

For low albumin and creatinine clearance greater than 25 ml/min:

$$C_{\text{normal binding}} = \frac{C_{\text{reported}}}{\left[(0.9)\left(\frac{\text{albumin}}{4.4}\right)\right] + 0.1} \quad \text{(Eq. 1)}$$

For normal or low albumin and patient receiving dialysis:

$$C_{\text{normal binding}} = \frac{C_{\text{reported}}}{\left[(0.9)(0.48)\left(\frac{\text{albumin}}{4.4}\right)\right] + 0.1} \quad \text{(Eq. 2)}$$

where

$C_{\text{normal binding}}$ = total phenytoin concentration that would be observed if patient had normal protein binding

C_{reported} = patient's total phenytoin concentration reported by laboratory (represents decreased plasma protein binding)

albumin = patient's albumin concentration in grams per deciliter

These equations should only be used as a guide or approximation because considerable variability has been reported.

Valproic acid in concentrations exceeding 30–40 mg/L displaces phenytoin from plasma albumin. Equation 3 (revised slightly from the original for consistency with similar equations throughout the text) can provide an estimate of the phenytoin concentration assuming plasma binding is normal, i.e., fraction unbound of 0.1:[10]

$$C_{\text{normal binding phenytoin}} = \frac{[0.1 + (0.001 \times C_{\text{valproic acid}})] \times C_{\text{reported phenytoin}}}{0.1} \quad \text{(Eq. 3)}$$

where $C_{\text{valproic acid}}$ and $C_{\text{reported phenytoin}}$ are the measured concentrations of valproic acid and total phenytoin, respectively, obtained at the same time and $C_{\text{normal binding phenytoin}}$ is the total phenytoin concentration that would have been measured if valproic acid was not present.

Clearance (CL)[1,4,11,12]

Renal elimination accounts for less than 5% of phenytoin clearance and is generally considered to be negligible. Phenytoin is cleared primarily (over 95%) by hepatic metabolism, which is capacity limited. Clinically important implications of this clearance include

- Css_{av} is not proportional to the maintenance dose (see Equations 4 and 5).
- Time to steady state (accumulation) is not three to five half-lives. (For a more detailed discussion, refer to the half-life and time to steady state section.)

This capacity-limited clearance is illustrated by

$$CL_{\text{phenytoin}} = \frac{V_{\max}}{K_m + Css_{av}} \quad \text{(Eq. 4)}$$

where $V_{\max}$ is the maximum rate (or velocity) of metabolism, and K_m is the plasma concentration at which metabolism is occurring at half the maximum rate.

This relationship can then be used to calculate maintenance doses and steady-state plasma concentrations:

$$(S)(F)(dose/\tau) = \frac{(V_{max})(Css_{av})}{K_m + Css_{av}} \quad \text{(Eq. 5)}$$

$$Css_{av} = \frac{(K_m)[(S)(F)(dose/\tau)]}{V_{max} - [(S)(F)(dose/\tau)]} \quad \text{(Eq. 6)}$$

Depending on the specific values of V_{max} and K_m used in these equations, a wide range of maintenance doses and steady-state concentrations can be calculated. Since reported values of V_{max} and K_m vary widely, care should be taken that any calculated dose is reasonable for the patient in question. Plasma concentration monitoring is also appropriate to refine or adjust initial dose recommendations.

Age	K_m (mean ± SD)	V_{max} (mean ± SD)[a]
Neonates and infants (<1 year)	[b]	[b]
Children		
6 months–<4 years	6.6 ± 4.2 mg/L	14 ± 4.2 mg/kg/day
4–<7 years	6.8 ± 3.5 mg/L	10.9 ± 3 mg/kg/day
7–<10 years	6.5 ± 3 mg/L	10.1 ± 2.6 mg/kg/day
Adolescents (10–16 years)[c]	5.7 ± 2.7 mg/L	8.3 ± 2.8 mg/kg/day
Adults (18–≤ 59 years)	4.3 ± 3.5 mg/L	7.4 ± 3 mg/kg/day
Geriatrics (>59 years)[d]	5.8 ± 2.3 mg/L	7.4 ± 3 mg/kg/day

[a]*For obese patients, the maximum velocity of drug elimination (V_{max}) for phenytoin probably should be based on ideal body weight (IBW).*
[b]*Estimates for V_{max} and K_m in neonates and infants up to 1 year are uncertain. Some data suggest an initial slow rate of metabolism followed by a rapid increase in the ability to eliminate phenytoin over the first 3 months following birth. The limited data available suggest a K_m of 4–6 mg/L and a V_{max} of 10–13 mg/kg/day.*
[c]*No data are available for the 17 year old.*
[d]*The limited data available suggest that K_m and V_{max} are similar to adult data.*

Volume of Distribution (V)[1,3,4,12–14]

Phenytoin's volume of distribution is calculated in part by using plasma concentrations. Any factor that alters plasma protein binding can alter the concentration and, therefore, the volume of distribution. However, no change in loading dose is generally required (i.e., changes in plasma protein binding result in an equally offsetting decrease in the plasma concentration and an increase in the volume of distribution).

Age	Volume (mean ± SD)
Neonates and infants (<1 year)	1 ± 0.3 L/kg
Children (>1 year), adults, and geriatrics[a]	0.65 ± 0.2 L/kg

[a] *The geriatric population is more likely to have decreased serum albumin.*

Since phenytoin is a relatively lipid-soluble drug, obese patients have a larger volume of distribution (in liters) equal to (0.65 L/kg)[(IBW) + (1.33)(ABW − IBW)], where ABW is actual body weight and IBW is ideal body weight in kilograms.

Half-Life and Time to Steady State[1,4]

The relationship of half-life to a drug's accumulation or decline is applicable only to first-order drugs—those with a constant clearance and volume of distribution. Since phenytoin's elimination is capacity limited and clearance decreases with increasing concentrations (see clearance section), time to achieve steady state is a complex process. Accumulation can be slow but continues for a prolonged period.

Equation 7 can be utilized to determine the time necessary to achieve 90% of the steady-state concentration:

$$t_{90\%} = \frac{(K_m)(V)}{[V_{max} - (S)(F)(\text{dose}/\tau)]^2} [2.3\ V_{max} - (0.9)(S)(F)(\text{dose}/\tau)] \quad \text{(Eq. 7)}$$

where

$$V = \text{L}$$
$$K_m = \text{mg/L}$$
$$V_{max} = \text{mg/day}$$
$$\text{dose}/\tau = \text{mg/day}$$

The accuracy of Equation 7 and the calculated time to steady state depends on the values used for V_{max}, K_m, and V.

When literature estimates or uncertain patient-specific values are used, the actual steady-state concentration and time to achieve 90% of that value may be considerably different than the calculated values. The errors are especially large when the anticipated steady state concentrations are high and the time to 90% of steady state is long. In addition, compliance to the prescribed dosage regimen is an important variable.

The time required for a phenytoin concentration to decline from an initial concentration ($C_{initial}$) to a lower concentration (C) is described by Equation 8 (this equation assumes that no absorption occurs in the time between $C_{initial}$ and C):

$$t = \frac{\left[(K_m)\left(\ln \frac{C_{initial}}{C}\right)\right] + (C_{initial} - C)}{\frac{V_{max}}{V}} \quad \text{(Eq. 8)}$$

where

$$K_m = mg/L$$
$$V_{max} = mg/day$$
$$V = L$$
$$t = days$$

As long as the phenytoin concentrations are much greater than K_m (4 to 5 times higher than K_m), the rate of phenytoin elimination approaches and is only slightly less than V_{max} or the maximum rate of metabolism. Under these conditions, the time required to decline from $C_{initial}$ to C is determined primarily by V_{max} and V. Therefore, at high concentrations the daily decline in the phenytoin concentration can be estimated by using V_{max}/V. Using this approach, the expected maximum decline in phenytoin concentration for the average patient would be approximately 10 mg/L/day, i.e., (V_{max}/V = 6.7 mg/kg/day divided by 0.65 L/kg).

Therapeutic Range[1,15,16]

For *seizure disorders,* the therapeutic range is 10–20 mg/L. Approximately 50% of patients show decreased seizure frequency with phenytoin concentrations equal to or greater than 10 mg/L, and almost 90% respond with concentrations equal to or greater than 15 mg/L.

For *cardiac arrhythmias,* the therapeutic range is 10–20 mg/L. Phenytoin is used infrequently to treat ventricular arrhythmia. However, most arrhythmias amenable to phenytoin therapy respond at concentrations less than 20 mg/L.

Phenytoin also is reported to be effective in some neurologic (nonseizure) disorders. However, most cases are anecdotal, with little or no reference to phenytoin concentrations.

Suggested Sampling Times[1,3,4,17–19]

The time of sampling depends on the clinical situation as well as the route and/or dosage form. As a general rule, intravenous loading doses are reasonably reliable in achieving the desired phenytoin concentrations, but oral loading and oral or intravenous maintenance regimens are less predictable.

When fosphenytoin or phenytoin are administered parenterally sampling should not be performed during the hydrolysis and distribution phase (i.e., within 2 hr after the end of infusion or within 4 hr of an intramuscular fosphenytoin injection).

Administered Dose	Suggested Sampling Time
Loading dose Intravenous	>2 hr after end of infusion (concentration measurements not necessarily recommended but may be useful for assessing V. If V appears to be unusually large, consider potential of decreased protein binding.)
Intravenous (phenytoin for injection or fosphenytoin)	>2 hr after end of infusion
Intramuscular (fosphenytoin)	>4 hr after injection
Oral	About 24 hr after loading dose

Maintenance dose
    Intravenous (divided dose)   Trough
    Oral divided dose   Timing not critical; trough suggested

    Oral single daily dose   Trough recommended (morning sample probably acceptable with bedtime dosing if time after dose is consistent)

After a *regimen is started*, the first sample should be drawn within 3–4 days (not steady state) to ensure that concentrations are not too low or high for a prolonged period. Then, sampling should be performed with decreasing frequency if concentrations are acceptable and stable or every 3–4 days if the maintenance dose must be changed or if phenytoin concentrations are declining or increasing.

At *steady state*, the sampling interval is debatable during stable chronic therapy. Sampling probably should be done every 7–14 days in the acute care setting and every 1–6 months in ambulatory patients.

Following a *change in status* (e.g., change in route, maintenance dose, dosage form or addition of drugs known to alter metabolism or absorption), phenytion concentrations should be monitored in a manner similar to when a regimen is started.

Pharmacodynamic Monitoring—Concentration–Related Efficacy

In the treatment of *seizures*, efficacy directly relates to seizure frequency and improvement of EEG findings.

In the treatment of *cardiac arrythmias*, efficacy directly relates to a normal pulse rate and improvement in ECG findings (normalization in the presence of arrhythmias).

Pharmacodynamic Monitoring—Concentration-Related Toxicity

The concentrations associated with the various side effects listed below are only approximate guidelines;

many patients experience significant side effects at much lower concentrations or no side effects at considerably higher concentrations. These differences may be due to individual susceptibility or sensitivity to phenytoin or, possibly, to alterations in plasma protein binding.

How often a patient should be monitored for concentration-related side effects depends on the course of treatment and the stability of the patient's clinical status and phenytoin concentrations. For example, the patient should be observed continuously and blood pressure and heart rate should be monitored very frequently when intravenous loading doses are administered.

Nystagmus and a simple assessment of mental status (e.g., "How do you feel? Are you tired or sleepy?") are easily checked every time an outpatient is examined or daily in the acute care setting.

Nystagmus

This side effect can be progressive from far lateral at phenytoin concentrations of 15 to over 20 mg/L to straight ahead at concentrations greater than 50 mg/L. Some patients have a baseline nystagmus due to their disease state; others do not develop nystagmus until phenytoin concentrations are well above the usual therapeutic range. Although nystagmus is frequently used to document the presence of phenytoin, it is not generally considered to be a toxic symptom.

CNS depression

This side effect can vary from mild sedation to an inability to concentrate to confusion to coma. Most patients experience relatively mild effects at concentrations of 5–15 mg/L; others tolerate phenytoin concentrations greater than 20 mg/L. Ataxia and impaired motor function are usually observed with phenytoin concentrations greater than 20 mg/L and become more frequent and obvious at concentrations greater than 30 mg/L.

Nonconcentration-related side effects
Some side effects may be more associated with duration of therapy. They include hypertrichosis, coarsening of facial features, folate deficiency, glucose intolerance, gingival hyperplasia, vitamin D deficiency, and osteomalacia.

The presence of propylene glycol in intravenous phenytoin has been reported to cause myocardial depression, hypotension, bradycardia, and widened PR, QRS, and QT intervals. Without propylene glycol, phenytoin has less effect on the myocardium, hence, the more rapid infusion rate for fosphenytoin. However, bradycardia and hypotension still occur but are usually less profound than with phenytoin for injection.

Drug–Drug Interactions

Numerous drugs are reported to interact with phenytoin, but capacity-limited metabolism makes assessment of these interactions difficult. For example, a 10% change in V_{max} would have relatively little impact on a steady-state phenytoin level of 5 mg/L but a significant effect on a steady-state level of 15 mg/L. Likewise, small changes in absorption have similar effects on low and high steady-state phenytoin concentrations. As Css_{av} becomes much greater than K_m, the maintenance dose approaches V_{max}. Under these conditions, a small change in either the maintenance dose or the V_{max} can result in disproportionate changes in the new steady-state concentration.

Because of the potential for very small changes in metabolism or absorption to alter phenytoin concentrations significantly, any regimen change should be closely monitored.

Table 1 is a partial list of drugs that influence phenytoin. Emphasis is given to those drugs most likely to alter phenytoin pharmacokinetics and/or to be encountered in the clinical setting.

TABLE 1. Drugs Influencing Phenytoin Pharmacokinetics

Drug	Effect on Phenytoin Concentration	Mechanism
Amiodarone[20,21]	Increase	Inhibition of metabolism
Antacids[a,22,23]	Decrease	Decreased absorption
Carbamazepine[24]	Decrease	Induction of metabolism
Chloramphenicol[25]	Increase	Inhibition of metabolism
Cimetidine[26]	Increase	Inhibition of metabolism
Ciprofloxacin[27,28]	Decrease	Induction of metabolism
Disulfiram[29]	Increase	Inhibition of metabolism
Fluconazole[30]	Increase	Inhibition of metabolism
Fluoxetine[31]	Increase	Inhibition of metabolism
Isoniazid[32,33]	Increase	Inhibition of metabolism (most significant in phenotypically slow acetylators)
Phenobarbital[b,34,35]	Increase or decrease	Inhibition or induction of metabolism
Phenylbutazone[c,36]	Increase	Inhibition of metabolism; plasma protein displacement
Rifampin[37]	Decrease	Induction of metabolism
Salicylates[d,38]	Decrease	Plasma protein displacement
Sulfonamides[39,40]	Increase	Inhibition of metabolism; plasma protein displacement
Ticlopidine[41]	Increase	Inhibition of metabolism
Trimethoprim[42]	Increase	Inhibition of metabolism
Valproic acid[e,43,44]	Decrease	Plasma protein displacement
Vigabatrin[45]	Decrease	Induction of metabolism?

[a] *A decrease in absorption is not consistently observed. Both drugs should not be administered at the same time; antacid and phenytoin doses should be taken at least 2 hr apart whenever possible.*
[b] *The direction of change (if any) for the phenytoin concentration depends on which phenobarbital effect is predominant (i.e., induction or inhibition of metabolism).*
[c] *The net effect on the total phenytion concentration when there are both displacement from plasma proteins and inhibition of metabolism is complex—a decrease, no change, or an increase in concentration may be observed (also see Footnote d). An inhibition of metabolism increases the unbound phenytoin concentration and the therapeutic effect. The measured or reported phenytoin concentration is a result of both displacement and inhibition of metabolism.*
[d] *Plasma protein displacement results in a decrease in the measured or reported phenytoin concentration but has little effect on the unbound phenytoin concentration or therapeutic effect.*
[e] *Valproic acid displaces phenytoin from its plasma protein binding. It is not clear, however, as to whether valproic acid also inhibits phenytoin metabolism.*

Drug–Disease State or Condition Interactions

As with drug–drug interactions, the effects of disease states on phenytoin therapy are difficult to quantify. In addition, few disease states are known to alter the pharmacokinetics of phenytoin.

Hepatic disease—cirrhosis[46]

Phenytion is eliminated from the body primarily by hepatic metabolism. Therefore, patients with significant hepatic disease may require reduced maintenance doses. These patients frequently also have hypoalbuminemia, which alters the reported or measured phenytion concentration. The reported phenytoin concentration can be "adjusted" by using Equation 1. The altered albumin has little effect on the loading dose required to achieve therapeutic unbound plasma and tissue concentrations (see volume of distribution section).

Renal failure[38]

Patients with end-stage renal failure (i.e., receiving dialysis) have a decreased plasma phenytoin binding affinity for albumin. They also usually have low serum albumin. These factors, which greatly affect the reported concentration, have little influence on the unbound phenytoin concentration and the therapeutic effect. Therefore, patients with renal failure should initially receive normal loading and maintenance doses.

Equation 2 can be used to approximate the total phenytoin concentration that would be observed in renal failure patients if they had normal plasma protein binding ($C_{\text{normal binding}}$). The $C_{\text{normal binding}}$ concentration should be compared to the usual therapeutic range and phenytoin's potential to produce either therapeutic or toxic effects.

Obesity[14]

In obese patients, the ideal or nonobese weight probably best correlates with metabolism and, therefore, maintenance doses. Loading doses, however, do require some adjustment because phenytoin has significant lipid solubility and an increased volume of distribution in obese patients. As stated earlier (see volume of distribution section), the volume of distribution (in liters) in obese patients can be calculated as

$$V_{(obese\ in\ L)} = 0.65\ L/kg\ [(IBW) + 1.33\ (ABW - IBW)]$$

where ABW is actual body weight and IBW is ideal body weight, both in kilograms.

Malabsorption[8,9,47]

There is little direct evidence that phenytion is incompletely absorbed (see bioavailability of dosage forms section). However, patients with diarrhea or rapid GI transit probably have incomplete phenytoin absorption, especially if they take large single doses resulting in prolonged absorption.

AIDS

Although no good studies have been performed, many clinicians believe that AIDS patients achieve low concentrations while receiving normal phenytoin doses. Many patients with AIDS have low serum albumin, GI disorders, and rapid GI transit due to other drug therapy or infectious disease processes. Further studies need to determine if these clinical observations are accurate.

Pregnancy and lactation[48-53]

Most women (>90%) who have epilepsy and continue phenytoin throughout their pregnancy deliver normal babies. However, infants born to women with epilepsy and receiving phenytoin are about two to three times more likely to have some type of congenital defect. The benefits of continuing phenytoin usually outweigh the risks to the fetus if the mother develops uncontrolled seizures.

Decreases in phenytoin concentrations during pregnancy have been reported. The reason for the decrease is unclear but proposed mechanisms include: decreased bioavailability, decreased plasma binding, and increased maternal and/or fetal metabolism. In addition, folate supplementation may also influence phenytoin metabolism. During pregnancy, phenytoin therapy should be monitored closely to ensure optimal therapeutic control of the seizure disorder.

References

1. Tozer TN, Winter ME. Phenytoin. In: Evans WE, Schentag JJ, Jusko WJ, eds. Applied pharmacokinetics: principles of therapeutic drug monitoring, 3rd ed. Vancouver, WA: Applied Therapeutics; 1992: 25.1–25.44.
2. Woodbury DM, Penry JK, Pippenger CE, eds. Antiepileptic drugs. New York: Raven Press; 1982:191–281.
3. Bruni J. Phenytoin. In: Taylor WJ, Diers Caviness MH, eds. A textbook for the clinical application of therapeutic drug monitoring. Irving, TX: Abbott Laboratories Diagnostic Division; 1986:253–67.
4. Phenytoin. In: Winter ME. Basic clinical pharmacokinetics, 2nd ed. Vancouver, WA: Applied Therapeutics; 1988:235–64.
5. Fischer JH, Cwik MJ, Luer MS, et al. Stability of fosphenytoin sodium with intravenous solutions in glass bottles, polyvinyl chloride bags, and polypropylene syringes. *Ann Pharmacother.* 1997; 31:553–9.
6. Knapp LE, Kugler AR. Clinical experience with fosphenytoin in adults: pharmacokinetics, safety, and efficacy. *J Child Neurol.* 1988; 13 (*Suppl 1*):S15–8.
7. Phenytoin. In: McEvoy GK. Amercian Hospital Formulary Service drug information 99. Bethesda, MD: Amercian Society of Health-System Pharmacists; 1999:861–4.
8. Faraji B, Yu PP. Serum phenytoin levels of patients on gastrostomy tube feeding. *J Neuroscience Nurs.* 1998; 30:55–9.
9. Doak KK, Haas CE, Dunnigan KJ, et al. Bioavailability of phenytoin acid and phenytoin sodium with enteral feedings. *Pharmacotherapy.* 1998; 18:637–45.
10. Kerrick JM, Wolff DL, Graves NM. Predicting unbound phenytoin concentrations in patients receiving valproic acid: a comparison of two prediction methods. *Ann Pharmacother.* 1995; 29:470–4.
11. Chiba K, Ishizaki T, Miura H, et al. Michaelis–Menten pharmacokinetics of diphenylhydantion and applications in the pediatric age patient. *J Pediatr.* 1980; 96:479–84.
12. Bauer LA, Blouin RA. Phenytoin Michaelis–Menten pharmacokinetics in caucasian pediatric patients. *Clin Pharmacokinet.* 1983; 8:454–9.
13. Bauer LA, Blouin RA. Age and phenytoin kinetics in adult epileptics. *Clin Pharmacol Ther.* 1982; 31:301–4.
14. Abernethy DR, Greenblatt DJ. Phenytoin disposition in obesity. Determination of loading dose. *Arch Neurol.* 1985; 42:568–71.

15. Buchtal F, Svensmark O, Schiller JP. Clinical and electroencephalographic correlation with serum levels of diphenylhydantion. *Arch Neurol*. 1960; 2:624–30.
16. Reynolds EH, Shorvon SD, Galbraith AW, et al. Phenytoin monotherapy for epilepsy: a long-term prospective study, assisted by serum level monitoring in previously untreated patients. *Epilepsia*. 1981; 22:485–8.
17. Warner A, Privitera M, Bates D. Standards of laboratory practice: antiepileptic drug monitoring. *Clin Chem*. 1998; 44:1085–95.
18. Yukawa E. Optimization of antiepileptic drug therapy. The importance of serum drug concentration monitoring. *Clin Pharmacokinet*. 1996; 31:120–30.
19. Kugler AR, Annesley TM, Nordblom GD, et al. Cross-reactivity of fosphenytoin in two human plasma phenytoin immunoassays. *Clin Chem*. 1998; 44:1474–80.
20. Nolan PE Jr.; Marcus FI, Hoyer GL, et al. Pharmacokinetic interaction between intravenous phenytoin and amiodarone in healthy volunteers. *Clin Pharmacol Ther*. 1989; 46:43–50.
21. Shackleford EJ, Watson FT. Amiodarone–phenytoin interaction. *Drug Intell Clin Pharm*. 1987; 21:921.
22. Garrett WR, Carter BL, Pellock JM. Bioavailability of phenytoin administered with antacids. *Ther Drug Monit*. 1979; 1:435–7.
23. O'Brien WM, Orme ML, Breckenridge AM. Failure of antacids of alter the pharmacokinetics of phenytoin. *Br J Clin Pharmacol*. 1978; 6:276–7.
24. Molholm-Hansen J, Siersbaek-Nielsen K, Skovsted L. Carbamazepine-induced acceleration of diphenylhydantoin and warfarin metabolism in man. *Clin Pharmacol Ther*. 1971; 12:539–43.
25. Harper JM, Yost RL, Stewart RB, et al. Phenytoin–chloramphenicol interaction: a retrospective study. *Drug Intell Clin Pharm*. 1979; 13:425–9.
26. Phillips P, Hansky J. Phenytoin toxicity secondary to cimetidine administration. *Med J Aust*. 1984; 141:602.
27. Pollak PT, Slayter KL. Hazards of doubling phenytoin dose in the face of an unrecognized interaction with ciprofloxacin. *Ann Pharmacother*. 1997; 31:61–4.
28. Dillard ML. Ciprofloxacin-phenytoin interaction. *Ann Pharmacother*. 1992; 26:263.
29. Olesen OV. Disulfiram (Antabuse) as inhibitor of phenytoin metabolism. *Acta Pharmacol Toxicol*. 1966; 24:317–22.
30. Blum RA, Wilton JH, Hilloigoss DM, et al. Effect of fluconazole on the disposition of phenytoin. *Clin Pharmacol Ther*. 1991; 49:420–5.
31. Jalil P. Toxic reaction following the combined administration of fluoxetine and phenytoin: two case reports. *J Neurol Neurosurg Psychiatry*. 1992; 55:412.
32. Miller RR, Porter J, Greenblatt DJ. Clinical importance of the interaction of phenytoin and isoniazid. *Chest*. 1979; 75:356–8.
33. Brennan RW, Dehejia H, Kutt H, et al. Diphenylhydantion intoxication attendant to slow inactivation of isoniazid. *Neurology*. 1970; 20:687–93.
34. Kutt H, Haynes J, Verebely K, et al. The effect of phenobarbital on plasma diphenylhydantoin level and metabolism in man and in rat liver microsomes. *Neurology*. 1969; 19:611–6.

35. Morselli PL, Rizzo M, Garaltini S, et al. Interaction between phenobarbital and diphenylhydantoin in animals and in epileptic patients. *Ann NY Acad Sci.* 1971; 179:88–107.
36. Neuvonen PJ, Lehtovaara R, Bardy A, et al. Antipyretic analgesics in patients on antiepileptic drug therapy. *Eur J Clin Pharmacol.* 1979; 15:263–8.
37. Kay L, Kampmann JP, Svendsen TL, et al. Influence of rifampicin and isoniazid on the kinetics of phenytoin. *Br J Clin Pharmacol.* 1985; 20:323–6.
38. Odar-Cederlof I, Borga O. Impaired plasma protein binding of phenytoin in uremia and displacement effect of salicylic acid. *Clin Pharmacol Ther.* 1976; 20:36–47.
39. Lumholtz B, Siersbaek-Nielsen K, Skovsted L, et al. Sulfamethizole-induced inhibition of diphenylhydantoin, tolbutamide and warfarin metabolism. *Clin Pharmacol Ther.* 1975; 17:731–4.
40. Lunde PKM, Rane A, Yaffe SJ. Plasma protein binding of diphenylhydantoin in man. Interaction with other drugs and the effect of temperature and plasma dilution. *Clin Pharmacol Ther.* 1970; 11:846–55.
41. Privitera M, Welty TE. Acute phenytoin toxicity followed by seizure breakthrough from a ticlopidine-phenytoin interaction. *Arch Neurol.* 1996; 53:1191.
42. Hansen JM, Kampmann JP, Siersbaek-Nielsen K, et al. The effect of different sulfonamides on phenytoin metabolism in man. *Acta Med Scand Suppl.* 1979; 624:106–10.
43. Mattson RH, Cramer JA, Williamson PD, et al. Valproic acid in epilepsy: clinical and pharmacological effects. *Ann Neurol.* 1978; 3:20–5.
44. Monks A, Richens A. Effect of single doses of sodium valproate on serum phenytoin levels and protein binding in epileptic patients. *Clin Pharmacol Ther.* 1980; 27:89–95.
45. Rambeck B, Pecht U, Wolf P. Pharmacokinetic interactions of the new antiepileptic drugs. *Clin Pharmacokinet.* 1996; 31:309–24.
46. Wallace S, Brodle MJ. Decreased drug binding in serum from patients with chronic hepatic disease. *Eur J Clin Pharmacol.* 1976; 9:429–32.
47. Bauer LA. Interference of oral phenytoin absorption by continuous nasogastric feedings. *Neurology.* 1982; 32:570–2.
48. Briggs GG, Freeman RK, Yaffe SJ. Drugs in pregnancy and lactation. 5th ed. Baltimore, MD: Williams & Wilkins; 1998:859–63.
49. Chen SS, Perucca E, Lee JN, et al. Serum protein binding and free concentrations of phenytoin and phenobarbitone in pregnancy. *Br J Clin Pharmacol.* 1982; 13:547–52.
50. van der Klign E, Schobben F, Bree TB. Clinical pharmacokinetics of antiepileptic drugs. *Drug Intell Clin Pharm.* 1980; 14:647–85.
51. Nau H, Kuhnz W, Egger HJ, et al. Anticonvulsants during pregnancy and lactation: transplacental, maternal and neonatal pharmacokinetics. *Clin Pharmacokinet.* 1982; 7:508–43.
52. Horning MG, Stillwell WG, Nowling J, et al. Identification and quantification of drugs and drug metabolites in human breast milk using GC-MS-COM methods. *Mod Probl Pediatr.* 1975; 15:73–9.
53. Committee on Drugs, American Academy of Pediatrics. The transfer of drugs and other chemicals into human milk. *Pediatrics.* 1994; 93:137–50.

Chapter 16
John A. Pieper

Procainamide
(AHFS 24:04)

Usual Dosage Range in Absence of Clearance-Altering Factors

Procainamide, a class IA antiarrhythmic agent, is approved for the treatment of life-threatening ventricular arrhythmias and less severe but symptomatic ventricular arrhythmias in carefully selected patients. An unapproved but common use for procainamide is as prophylactic therapy to maintain normal sinus rhythm after conversion of atrial fibrillation and/or flutter by other methods. As a class IA antiarrhythmic agent, procainamide decreases myocardial excitability, contractility, and conduction velocity.

Procainamide clearance is dependent on both renal and nonrenal (metabolic) routes of elimination. Approximately 40–60% of procainamide clearance is mediated by renal mechanisms, with contributions from both glomerular filtration and active tubular secretion. Hepatic metabolism is responsible for 40–60% of procainamide clearance. The primary pathway is the conversion of procainamide to N-acetylprocainamide (NAPA), a class III

The contributions made by Donna J. Carroll to this chapter are gratefully acknowledged.

antiarrhythmic, via the polymorphically expressed *N*-acetyltransferase 2 (NAT2) enzyme system. Due to the complexities of procainamide pharmacokinetics, the suggested dosages should be considered as initial guides. Doses should be individualized based on patient response and appropriate monitoring.

Procainamide can be administered orally, intramuscularly, or intravenously in the acute setting. All dosage forms are procainamide hydrochloride, which is 87% procainamide base ($S = 0.87$). Oral therapy should begin with conventional tablets or capsules. Extended-release forms of procainamide should be used for maintenance therapy only and should not be chewed or crushed.[1]

Dosage Form	Dosage
Oral (tablets and capsules)	
Neonates and infants (<1 year)	Not available
Children[a] (1–12 years)[1,2]	15–50 mg/kg/day divided equally every 3–6 hr
Adolescents (13–≤18 years)	Not available
Adults (>18–75 years)[3–8]	Up to 50 mg/kg/day (ABW[c]) divided equally every 3–6 hr (regular and sustained release)
	8–12 hr (extended release)
Older geriatrics[b] (>75 years)[9,10]	<50 mg/kg/day (ABW[c]) divided equally every 3–6 hr (regular and sustained release)
	8–12 hr (extended release)
Intramuscular	
Neonates and infants (<1 year)	Not available
Children (1–12 years)[1,2]	20–30 mg/kg/day (ABW[c]) divided equally every 3–6 hr
Adolescents (13–≤18 years)	Not available
Adults (>18–75 years)[3–8]	50 mg/kg/day (ABW[c]) divided equally every 3–6 hr
Older geriatrics (>75 years)	Not available
Intravenous	
Neonates and infants (<1 year)	Not available

Children (1–12 years)[1,2]	Load: 3–6 mg/kg (IBW[c]) over 5 min Continuous infusion: 0.02–0.08 mg/kg/min (ABW[c])
Adolescents (13–≤18 years)	Not available
Adults (>18–75 years)[3–8]	Load: 12–17 mg/kg (IBW[c]) or 100 mg every 5 min (until control of arrhythmia or toxicity) at maximum rate of 50 mg/min Continuous infusion: 1–6 mg/min Intermittent infusion: 50 mg/kg/day (ABW[c]) divided equally every 3–6 hr at maximum rate of 50 mg/min
Older geriatrics (>75 years)	Not available

[a]Limited data are available. Dosing should begin at lower end of range with titration based on clinical response and procainamide concentrations up to a maximum of 4 g/day.
[b]Maintenance doses appear to be lower than adult doses; therefore, the dose should be based on clinical response and procainamide concentrations.
[c]ABW = actual body weight; IBW = ideal body weight

Dosage Form Availability[1,7]

Dosage Form[a]	Product
Parenteral:[b] 100 and 500 mg/ml	Pronestyl
Oral capsules: 250, 375, and 500 mg (immediate release)	Pronestyl
Oral tablets (film coated)	
250, 375, and 500 mg (immediate release)	Pronestyl Filmlok
250, 500, 750, and 1000 mg (extended release)	Procan SR[c]
500 mg (extended release)	Pronestyl-SR Filmlok
Oral tablets 500 and 1000 mg (sustained release)	Procanbid

[a]All dosage forms are procainamide hydrochloride. The fraction of dose (S) that is procainamide is 0.87.
[b]This product should be diluted with dextrose 5% or normal saline prior to intravenous administration to facilitate control of administration rate.
[c]Procan SR is formulated with a wax matrix which may be detected in the feces after all of the drug is released. This wax matrix shell does not represent incomplete absorption.

Bioavailability (*F*) of Dosage Forms[3–6,9]

Dosage Form	Bioavailability Comments
Intravenous	100% with peak serum concentrations achieved at end of infusion
Intramuscular	100% with peak serum concentrations achieved within 45–60 min; absorption rate half-life of 10–17 min
Oral capsules and film-coated tablets (immediate release)	83% (±16%) with peak serum concentrations achieved within 45–75 min; absorption rate half-life of 20 min
Oral film-coated tablets (extended release)	85% with peak serum concentrations achieved within 3–4 hr; absorption rate half-life of 3 hr

General Pharmacokinetic Information[3–10]

Clearance

The fraction of procainamide excreted unchanged in patients with normal renal function ranges from 40 to 60%. Renal clearance is approximately three times CrCl; therefore, proximal tubular secretion as well as glomerular filtration appears to be involved in the renal elimination process. Distal tubular reabsorption is clinically insignificant.

Metabolism

The fraction of procainamide metabolized in normal subjects is 40–60%. The majority of procainamide's metabolism results from hepatic acetylation, leading to the formation of NAPA. Other metabolites include para-aminobenzoic acid (PABA) and desethylprocainamide (DEPA).

Protein binding

Protein binding of procainamide is approximately 15%.

Clearance (CL)[3-5,9,11,12]

Procainamide is cleared by renal and metabolic mechanisms as illustrated by the equation

$$CL_{total} = CL_{renal} + CL_{metabolism}$$

In adult patients with normal renal function, approximately half of the clearance is renal while half is due to nonrenal metabolism. A normal CL_{renal} can be assumed to be approximately 0.27 L/hr/kg or three times the CrCl. The $CL_{metabolism}$ value consists of both acetylation clearance and a nonrenal, nonacetylated metabolic clearance. The $CL_{acetylation}$ value is based on the acetylation phenotype. For fast acetylators, $CL_{acetylation}$ is approximately 0.19 L/hr/kg. For slow acetylators, it is approximately 0.07 L/hr/kg. Therefore, an average $CL_{acetylation}$ can be assumed to be approximately 0.13 L/hr/kg. Approximately 50% of the black and white population in the United States are fast acetylators while the other 50% are slow acetylators. Asian patients tend to be fast acetylators (80–90%). The nonrenal, nonacetylated metabolic clearance appears to be 0.1 L/hr/kg. The average $CL_{metabolism}$ in fast and slow acetylators is 0.29 L/hr/kg and 0.17 L/hr/kg, respectively. The total procainamide clearance, then, in fast acetylators is 0.56 L/hr/kg and 0.44 L/hr/kg in slow acetylators.

The above information then can be translated as

$$CL_{total} = 3(CrCl) + [(CL_{acetylation} + 0.1\ L/hr/kg)(ABW)]$$

where CrCl is expressed in L/hr and $CL_{acetylation}$ in L/hr/kg.

The steady-state average concentration equation also can be rearranged to calculate a patient's CL_{total}:

$$CL_{total} = \frac{(S)(F)(dose/\tau)}{Css_{av}}$$

In patients with New York Heart Association Class II-III CHF on digoxin, diuretics, and ACE inhibitors, CL_{total} appears to be similar to controls (0.61

L/hr/kg versus 0.53 L/hr/kg),[11] although earlier studies suggested a 25–50% decrease in the metabolic clearance of procainamide in nonoptimally treated heart failure patients.[9,12] In obese patients, clearance appears to correlate best with actual body weight (ABW).

The following clearance values are offered as guidelines in patients with normal renal function for age when the above equations cannot be used.[5,9,13]

Age	Total Clearance[a] (mean ± SD)
Neonates and infants (<1 year)	Pharmacokinetic data are lacking
Children (1–12 years)	1.16 ± 0.12 L/hr/kg Pharmacokinetic data are lacking, but available data suggest increased clearance in comparison to adults. One study[13] ($n = 6$) documented a clearance of 0.56 ± 0.12 L/hr/kg.
Adolescents (13–18 years)	Pharmacokinetic data are lacking
Adults (19–75 years)	Fast acetylators 0.56 L/hr/kg Slow acetylators 0.44 L/hr/kg

[a]*Values will be significantly lower in patients with renal dysfunction.*

Volume of Distribution (V_{SS})[4,11]

Procainamide distributes extensively into lean body tissue and poorly into adipose tissue. In obese patients, the volume of distribution at steady state appears to correlate best with IBW. The volume of distribution in medically treated heart failure patients and controls are similar.

Age	Volume (mean ± SD)
Neonates and infants (<1 year)	Pharmacokinetic data are lacking
All other age groups	2 ± 0.42 L/kg (IBW)

Half-Life and Time to Steady State[3-8,12,14]

Age	Distribution Half-Life	Terminal Half-Life	Time to Steady State
Neonates and infants (<1 year)	Pharmacokinetic data are lacking		
Children[a] (1–12 years)	5 min	<3 hr	<12 hr
Adolescents (13–≤18 years)	Pharmacokinetic data are lacking		
Adults (>18–75 years)	5 min	3 hr	12–18 hr
Older geriatrics (>75 years)	>5 min	>3 hr	>12–18 hr

[a]*The small amount of data available suggests that the procainamide half-life in children is significantly shorter than adult estimates.*

N-Acetylprocainamide (NAPA) Predictions[4,5,13,15]

The contribution of NAPA to the overall antiarrhythmic activity of procainamide is usually of limited clinical importance, although in some patients (e.g., those with renal impairment) it may be appropriate to monitor NAPA concentrations. Although no guidelines exist to quantify toxic concentrations for NAPA, cardiac toxicity may result when NAPA concentrations exceed 30 mg/L. NAPA concentrations above 30 mg/L were reported to have little additional antiarrhythmic effect.

The following predictions are useful for estimating NAPA production in an adult population. There is limited information on NAPA production in children.

NAPA production (the "dose" of NAPA)

$$\text{rate of conversion} = (Css_{\text{av procainamide}})(CL_{\text{acetylation}})$$

where $CL_{\text{acetylation}} = 0.07$ L/hr/kg (slow), 0.13 L/hr/kg (average), 0.19 L/hr/kg (fast).

Clearance (CL)

The clearance of NAPA is based primarily on renal function, but in part on nonrenal paths. This can be represented by the equation

$$CL_{total} = CL_{renal} + CL_{nonrenal}$$

Average renal and nonrenal clearance values in patients with normal renal function is

$$CL_{total} = 2.8 \text{ ml/min/kg (ABW)} + 0.5 \text{ ml/min/kg (ABW)}$$
$$= 3.3 \text{ ml/min/kg}$$

For patients with reduced renal function, the following method may be used to predict NAPA clearance:

$$CL_{total} = 1.6 \text{ (CrCl L/hr)} + (0.025 \text{ L/hr/kg)(ABW)}$$

Volume (V)

$$V = 1.5 \text{ L/kg}$$

Half-life (t½)

$$t½ = 6.2 \text{ hr}$$

Both the procainamide concentration and acetylation clearance determine the NAPA production. The acetylation clearance of procainamide is based on the acetylation phenotype (see clearance section). NAPA concentrations may accumulate dramatically in patients with poor renal function. NAPA clearance is 77–87% renal and 13–23% nonrenal. A 6-hr half-life is based on normal renal function. Patients with poor renal function may have a half-life of 30 hr or more.

Therapeutic Range[3–5,15]

The therapeutic range for procainamide is 4–10 mg/L. In the reported studies, therapy was effective in 85% of cardiac patients with premature ventricular beats with concentrations of 4–8 mg/L. Concentrations of 8–12 mg/L increased the percentage of patients effectively treated by 10%, although 5% of the patients had serious toxicities. These higher concentrations may be needed in patients with sustained ventricular tachycardia. Procainamide concentrations of 15–20 mg/L may be appropriate in some patients in controlled situations. The suggested therapeutic range for the sum of procainamide and NAPA is 5–30 mg/L.

Suggested Sampling Times and Effect on Therapeutic Range[3-5]

With *immediate-release tablets and capsules*, trough concentrations are more reproducible than peak concentrations. Therefore, trough samples are recommended.

With *extended-release tablets*, the sampling time is less significant because the concentrations vary less. Consistency of sampling time relative to dosing time is, however, strongly recommended. If the dosing interval exceeds 6 hr, significant peak-to-trough variations may be observed in patients with short half-lives. In this case, a trough concentration may be most useful.

With *continuous infusion*, sampling at any time during the infusion is appropriate once steady state is achieved.

Careful clinical monitoring for efficacy and toxicity is always required. In addition, procainamide concentrations can provide useful information, especially when obtained at steady state. Steady-state procainamide concentrations are achieved within 12–24 hr of therapy. Steady-state NAPA concentrations are not reached for at least 24 hr and may require up to 1 week if the patient has significant renal dysfunction. Furthermore, procainamide concentrations probably should be obtained following changes in a patient's clinical status, changes in the dosage regimen, or signs of toxicity or inadequate response.

Pharmacodynamic Monitoring—Concentration-Related Efficacy

The following are useful indicators of procainamide efficacy:

- Conversion of atrial arrhythmia to normal sinus rhythm.
- Heart rate normalization.
- ECG normalization.
- Suppression of sustained ventricular arrhythmias.

Pharmacodynamic Monitoring—Concentration-Related Toxicity[4-8,16]

The exact relationship between NAPA concentrations and toxicity is not clearly established. Individuals with NAPA concentrations that are greater than 30 mg/L may experience serious cardiac toxicity. Therefore, these concentrations should be monitored in patients with renal dysfunction. Both minor and major procainamide concentration-related toxicities can occur.

Minor Toxicities	Major Toxicities
GI disturbances	≥20% decrease in arterial pressure[a]
Malaise, weakness	>30% prolongation of PR, QRS, and QT intervals[b]
Dizziness, giddiness	
<20% decrease in arterial pressure[a]	Development of new arrhythmias
	Cardiac arrest
10–30% prolongation of PR, QRS, and QT intervals[b]	Drug-induced systemic lupus erythematosus (SLE)[c]

[a]*Frequent blood pressure monitoring is needed when therapy is initiated (especially intravenous therapy); monitoring can be less frequent when maintenance therapy is established.*
[b]*Continuous ECG monitoring is needed with intravenous dosing, and frequent monitoring is required during initiation of oral therapy; occasional monitoring is required during maintenance therapy.*
[c]*Drug-induced SLE appears to occur during maintenance therapy, primarily in slow acetylators. About 60–70% of patients on procainamide develop antinuclear antibody (ANA) titers after 1–12 months of therapy, and 20–30% of these patients develop signs and symptoms of SLE. Common symptoms include polyarthralgia, arthritis, and pleuritic pain. Fever, myalgia, skin lesions, and pericarditis as well as*

cardiac tamponade also occur. ANA titers should be monitored regularly in patients on long-term therapy or when lupus-like reactions occur. The clinical signs and symptoms of drug-induced SLE usually diminish several days to weeks after procainamide therapy is discontinued. One study[16] suggested that the presence of antiguanosine antibodies may indicate patients at risk for developing procainamide-induced SLE.

Toxicities related to the intravenous infusion rate of procainamide are hypotension and bradycardia. However, these toxicities generally can be avoided if procainamide is infused at a rate of less than or equal to 50 mg/min.

Idiosyncratic reactions are rare but include

- Angioneurotic edema.
- Maculopapular rash.
- Granulomatous hepatitis.
- Agranulocytosis.
- Leukopenia.
- Thrombocytopenia.

The patient should know the signs and symptoms of neutropenia, including sore throat, fever, malaise, and other symptoms of infection. Routine blood counts should be performed frequently during the first 3 months of therapy due to the increased incidence of neutropenia during this time. Periodic blood counts also should be performed throughout maintenance therapy. A drop in the neutrophil count to less than 2000 cells/mm^3 requires immediate attention.

Important Drug–Drug Interactions[4,11,17–19]

Drug	Effect	Mechanism
Amiodarone[a]	Increase in procainamide concentration by 40–60%	Inhibition of both hepatic and renal clearance of procainamide
Cimetidine[b]	Increase in procainamide concentration and NAPA concentration by 20–40% each	Reduced tubular secretion of procainamide and NAPA

Ethanol (chronic use)	Increase in NAPA concentration and decrease in procainamide concentration	Enhanced acetylation of procainamide in liver
Ofloxacin	Increase in procainamide AUC and peak concentration by 20–25%	Decreased renal clearance of procainamide
Para-aminobenzoic acid	Increase in NAPA concentration and $t_{1/2}$	Decreased NAPA renal clearance
Quinidine	Increase in procainamide concentration	Unknown; possible reduced renal clearance of procainamide
Ranitidine	Increase in procainamide and NAPA concentrations by 10–20%	Decreased renal clearance
Trimethoprim[d]	Increase in procainamide concentration by 50–60% and NAPA concentration by 50%	Interference with renal secretion of procainamide and NAPA; inhibition of metabolism of procainamide

[a]*Procainamide concentrations should be monitored when amiodarone is added to therapy. Procainamide dose may need to be reduced 25%.*
[b]*The procainamide dose may need to be reduced if the response to procainamide and NAPA is enhanced.*
[c]*Clinical importance not known.*
[d]*Procainamide and NAPA concentrations should be monitored when trimethoprim is coadministered.*

Drug–Disease State or Condition Interactions[3–8]

Disease State or Condition	Adjustment Factors		
	Clearance	Volume of Distribution	Half-Life
Renal disease[a]	Decreased[b]	Same	Increased[b]
Obesity[c]	Use ABW	Use IBW	Not available

| Geriatric age (>70 years)[d] | Decreased | Not available | Increased |

[a] Renal disease decreases procainamide clearance with no notable change in the volume of distribution; therefore, an increase in the procainamide half-life is expected. The renal clearance value must be reduced in proportion to renal function. One study[4] suggested a one-third reduction for patients with moderate cardiac or renal impairment. An additional one-third reduction is suggested for patients with severe renal impairment. Since 85% of NAPA's total body clearance is due to renal clearance, NAPA appears to accumulate to a greater extent than procainamide in patients with renal failure.
[b] Magnitude depends on degree of renal dysfunction
[c] Obese patients apparently have increased renal clearance of procainamide. Therefore, the patient's ABW should be used to predict clearance. The volume of distribution in obese patients appears to correlate best with IBW.
[d] Data suggest that renal clearance declines to a greater extent than expected based on the age-related decrease in glomerular filtration rate. (Refer to clearance section.)

References

1. Procainamide hydrochloride. In: McEvoy GK, ed. American hospital formulary service drug information 99. Bethesda, MD: American Society of Health-System Pharmacists; 1999:1480–5.
2. Taketomo CK, Hodding JH, Kraus DM, eds. Pediatric dosage handbook, 5th ed. Cleveland, OH: Lexi-Comp; 1998–99:913–6.
3. Koch-Weser J, Klein SW. Procainamide dosage schedules, plasma concentrations and clinical effects. *JAMA*. 1971; 215:1454–60.
4. Coyle JD, Lima JJ. Procainamide. In: Evans WE, Schentag JJ, Jusko WJ, eds. Applied pharmacokinetics: principles of therapeutic drug monitoring, 3rd ed. Vancouver, WA: Applied Therapeutics; 1992:22-1–22-33.
5. Procainamide. In: Winter ME. Basic clinical pharmacokinetics, 4th ed. Spokane, WA: Applied Therapeutics, 1994:356–78.
6. Roden DM. Antiarrhythmic drugs. In: Hardman JG, Limbird LE, Molinoff PB, et al., eds. The pharmacological basis of therapeutics, 9th ed, New York: McGraw-Hill; 1996:839–79.
7. Burnham RM, Scott JA, Short RM, eds. Facts and comparisons. St. Louis, MO: Facts and Comparisons; 1999:145g-146.
8. Bauman JL, Schoen MD. The arrhythmias. In: Pharmacotherapy: a pathophysiologic approach, 3rd ed., Stamford, CT: Appleton and Lange; 1997:323–59.
9. Bauer LA, Black D, Genjiler A, et al. Influence of age, renal function and heart failure on procainamide clearance and N-acetylprocainamide serum concentrations. *Int J Clin Pharmacol Ther Toxicol*. 1989; 27:213–6.
10. Koup JR, Abel RB, Smithers JA, et al. Effect of age, gender and race on steady state procainamide pharmacokinetics after administration of Procanbid sustained-release tablets. *Ther Drug Monit*. 1998; 20:73–7.
11. Tisdale JE, Rudis MI, Padhi ID, et al. Disposition of procainamide in patients with chronic congestive heart failure receiving medical therapy. *J*

Clin Pharmacol. 1996; 36:35–41.

12. Grasela TH, Sheiner LB. Population pharmacokinetics of procainamide from routine clinical data. *Clin Pharmacokinet.* 1984; 9:545–54.

13. Singh S, Gelband H, Mehtra AV, et al. Procainamide elimination kinetics in pediatric patients. *Clin Pharmacol Ther.* 1982; 32:607–11.

14. Giardina E-GV, Dreyfuss J, Bigger JT, et al. Metabolism of procainamide in normal and cardiac subjects. *Clin Pharmacol Ther.* 1976; 19:339–51.

15. Dutcher JS, Strong JM, Lucas SV, et al. Procainamide and N-acetylprocainamide kinetics investigated simultaneously with stable isotope methodology. *Clin Pharmacol Ther.* 1977; 22:447–57.

16. Weisbert RH, Yee WS, Colburn KK, et al. Antiguanosine antibodies: a new marker for procainamide-induced systemic lupus erythematosus. *Ann Intern Med.* 1986; 104:310–3.

17. Hansten PD, Horn JR, eds. Drug interactions analysis and management. Vancouver, WA: Applied Therapeutics: 1997; 445–7.

18. Martin DE, Shen J, Griener J, et al. Effects of ofloxacin on the pharmacokinetics and pharmacodynamics of procainamide. *J Clin Pharmacol.* 1996; 36:85–91.

19. Tisdale JE, Rudis MI, Padhi ID, et al. Inhibition of N-acetylation of procainamide and renal clearance of N-acetyl procainamide by para-aminobenzoic acid in humans. *J Clin Pharmacol.* 1995; 35:902–10.

20. Christoff PB, Conti Dr, et al. Procainamide disposition in obesity. *Drug Intell Clin Pharm.* 1983; 17:516–22.

Chapter 17
Paul E. Nolan, Jr. & Christy M. Evans

Quinidine (AHFS 24:04)

Usual Dosage Range in Absence of Clearance-Altering Factors

Quinidine, an antiarrhythmic agent with cardiac actions similar to those of procainamide, is used primarily as prophylactic therapy to maintain normal sinus rhythm after conversion of atrial fibrillation and/or flutter by other methods. It also is used to prevent recurrence of paroxysmal atrial fibrillation, paroxysmal atrial tachycardia, paroxysmal AV junctional rhythm, paroxysmal ventricular tachycardia, and atrial or ventricular premature contractions.[1,2]

Although the use of quinidine seemed to fall out of favor in the 1980's, a recent retrospective analysis cites quinidine as one of the most commonly used sinus rhythm agents over the past decade.[2]

Quinidine is available in three salt forms with differing salt fractions (S): gluconate ($S = 0.62$), polygalacturonate ($S = 0.6$), and sulfate ($S = 0.83$). Dosages are usually expressed in terms of their particular salt.[1]

Dosage Form	Route/Dose	Quinidine Equivalent, mg	Product
Quinidine gluconate	Intravenous and intramuscular: 80 mg/ml	50	Quinidine Gluconate Injection
	Oral tablet: 324 mg extended-release	202	Quinaglute Dura-Tabs, Quinatime
	Oral tablet: 330 mg extended-release	206	Duraquin
Quinidine polygalacturonate	Oral tablet: 275 mg	165	Cardioquin
Quinidine sulfate	Oral tablet: 200 and 300 mg	166 and 249	Quintora
	Oral tablet: 300 mg	249	Quinidex Extentabs

Bioavailability (F) of Dosage Forms

Irrespective of the specific formulation or salt form, the bioavailability of quinidine is less than 100% as a result of first-pass hepatic metabolism.[3] Quinidine can be administered orally as either a conventional-release or sustained-release formulation.

Dosage Form	% Quinidine Base (S)	Route	Comment
Quinidine gluconate	62%	Intramuscular	77% by fluorometry in healthy volunteers[4]
		Oral (extended release)	71% (range 54–88%) by non-specific fluorometry in healthy volunteers
Quinidine polygalacturonate	60%	Oral tablet	70% by HPLC in healthy volunteers[5]

Quinidine sulfate	83%	Oral (immediate release)	87% by HPLC in arrhythmia patients[6]; 70% (range 51–106%) by specific HPLC in healthy volunteers[7]
		Oral (extended release)	85% by nonspecific fluorometry in healthy volunteers[8a]

[a]The less specific assay used in this study may explain the increased bioavailability of the sulfate preparation relative to previous studies in healthy humans.

General Pharmacokinetic Information

Accurate estimation of the clinical pharmacokinetic parameters of quinidine is highly dependent upon the analytical methods utilized to quantitate quinidine concentrations.[9] Specific assays such as HPLC can separate and/or distinguish quinidine from dihydroquinidine, a contaminant found in all quinidine preparations, and the various metabolites of quinidine.[9] Therefore, relative to the pharmacokinetic parameters obtained from studies using nonspecific assays, the use of a specific quinidine assay should result in

- Diminished estimates of quinidine concentrations, bioavailability, area under the curve (AUC), and the amount of quinidine excreted unchanged in the urine.
- Shorter estimates of the terminal elimination half-life.
- Increased estimates of total body clearance.[9]

Controversy exists regarding whether the pharmacokinetics of quinidine are nondose dependent or dose dependent. In two of the three investigations reporting no change in mean pharmacokinetic characteristics, only single intravenous[10] or oral[11] doses of quinidine were administered. However, two of the four subjects in a third study exhibited a greater than proportional increase in

AUC and steady-state quinidine concentrations relative to the increase in dose.[12]

Two other studies demonstrated dose-dependent pharmacokinetics for quinidine and both administered quinidine to steady state.[13,14] The cause of the dose-dependent pharmacokinetics may be either saturable first-pass hepatic removal[13] or saturable renal secretion.[14]

Clinicians should therefore anticipate greater than proportional increases in quinidine concentrations in some patients as quinidine doses are increased.

Absorption

Quinidine, a weak base, is principally absorbed in the small intestine.[3] The rate and extent of absorption varies among the quinidine formulations and salt forms and among study populations. The intersubject and interpatient variability in the extent of absorption of quinidine can, in part, be attributed to differences in assay methodology (see section on bioavailability [*F*] of dosage forms).

The extent of absorption is equivalent between commercially available quinidine sulfate tablets and the quinidine sulfate solution.[15] For healthy volunteers, the average time to peak plasma quinidine concentrations for the tablets is achieved within 1.5 hr.

In patients with arrhythmias, but without clinical evidence of heart failure, hepatic disease, or renal dysfunction, peak plasma quinidine sulfate concentrations occur within 2 hr following dosage administration.[6] Increased bioavailability in these patients may result from previous disease-mediated reductions either in hepatic blood flow or in hepatic microsomal activity and a subsequent decrease in hepatic first-pass metabolism.

The extent of absorption from a sustained-release formulation of quinidine sulfate has been shown equivalent to that from a conventional-release formulation.[8] However, maximum quinidine concentrations occur at

3.3 hr for the sustained-release formulation as compared to about 1 hr for the conventional-release preparation.

Quinidine gluconate sustained-release tablets are more slowly absorbed than quinidine sulfate conventional-release tablets.[16] Comparisons between extended-release sulfate and gluconate products suggest that the sulfate product produces less peak-to-trough fluctuations with an every 12-hr dosage schedule.[17]

The bioavailability (rate and extent) of quinidine polygalacturonate is analogous to that of quinidine sulfate tablets in healthy subjects.[5]

The co-ingestion of either conventional-release or sustained-release oral quinidine products with food generally results in some alterations in the absorption of quinidine.[18,19] The protein binding of quinidine significantly increases in the postprandial state. The frequency of nausea may be reduced when quinidine is taken with food.

Relative to the fasting state, the extent of quinidine absorption from a sustained-release quinidine gluconate tablet is significantly enhanced when coadministered with either a low fat or high fat meal.[19] The rate of quinidine absorption is significantly increased following a low fat meal.

Distribution

The distribution of quinidine within the body is predominantly extravascular.[20] Following either intravenous or oral administration, the disposition is most often described by an open two-compartment model.[20] However, the pharmacokinetics of quinidine also may be described by a three-compartment model.[21] For this chapter, a two-compartment model is assumed.

Elimination

Renal excretion of unchanged quinidine accounts for only 13–18% of an administered dose.[3,6] The renal elimination of quinidine occurs in part via glomerular filtration and is positively correlated with creatinine clearance.[22] Quinidine also undergoes active renal tubular secretion.[23] The renal excretion of quinidine varies inversely with urine pH.[24] Neither hemodialysis[25] nor peritoneal dialysis[26] has a clinically significant impact upon the systemic removal of quinidine. However, hemodialysis may remove some of the polar metabolites of quinidine.[6]

Metabolism

Quinidine is eliminated from the body primarily by oxidative hepatic metabolism.[3] The hepatic microsomal P450 isoenzyme responsible for quinidine oxidation is CYP3A4.[27] The metabolites of quinidine produce electrophysiologic effects which are qualitatively similar to, but quantitatively less than or equal to, quinidine.[28–31] Given the pharmacodynamic and pharmacokinetic properties, it is likely that the metabolites and contaminant of quinidine contribute to both the therapeutic and proarrhythmic effects of the parent drug.

Metabolites/Other[28,32,33]	Activity	Ratio[a]	$t\frac{1}{2}$
3-Hydroxyquinidine	++[b]	[c]	12.4 hr[30]
2'-Oxoquinidinone	?[d]	[c]	—
Quinidine 10,11-dihydrodiol	?	0.25[29,32]	—
Quinidine N-oxide	none	[c]	2.5 hr[31]
O-Desmethylquinidine	?	<0.25[29,32]	—
Dihydroquinidine[e,f]	+?[31]	<0.5[32]	11–24 hr[34]

[a]*Concentration relative to quinidine concentration.*
[b]*++ = ~ equivalent to quinidine.*
[c]*The sum of these three metabolites may equal or exceed that of quinidine.*[28,32]
[d]*? = activity unknown.*
[e]*Dihydroquinidine is a contaminant found in all commercial preparations.*[32]
[f]*Competes with quinidine for binding sites on plasma proteins.*[35]

Protein binding

In general, quinidine is extensively protein bound. However, the protein binding of quinidine is variable[36] and highly dependent upon the experimental conditions including temperature,[27] the presence of heparin, and blood collection techniques.[37] Quinidine binds principally to albumin but mostly to alpha$_1$-acid glycoprotein (AAG); therefore, variations in circulating lipoproteins should not alter the unbound serum concentrations. Quinidine does not appear to bind significantly to circulating lipoproteins. Protein binding averages 87% in normal subjects and is concentration independent over a range of total quinidine concentrations of 1–5 mg/L.[38] The protein binding of quinidine increases in trauma patients, following acute myocardial infarction or cardiac surgery, in atrial fibrillation and flutter, and in prehospital cardiac arrest, because these situations cause an increase in AAG.[38-41] The protein binding of quinidine is decreased in chronic liver disease and with the coadministration of heparin.[38-45] Renal impairment in patients not undergoing hemodialysis may demonstrate either similar, decreased, or increased protein binding relative to normal subjects.[43]

Protein Binding	Condition	Quinidine Bound, %
Normal		87
Increase	Trauma	92.5
	Following cardiac surgery	97
	Following myocardial infarction	95
	Prehospital cardiac arrest	94
Decrease	Chronic liver disease	64–82
	Cardiac catherization	69
	Collection by vacutainer	60–88

Clearance (CL)

In healthy volunteers, the mean total body clearance averages 0.29 L/hr/kg with a range of 0.14–0.43 L/hr/kg.[7] In patients with arrhythmias but without cardiac, renal, or hepatic dysfunction, the mean total body clearance is 0.29 L/hr/kg (range of 0.10–0.50 L/hr/kg).[6] Several factors including disease states and concomitantly administered drugs can affect the elimination kinetics of quinidine. These are specifically addressed in subsequent sections.

Volume of Distribution (V)

The following values for the volume of distribution of the central compartment (V_c) and the apparent volume of distribution (V_β) have been found for select patient populations.

Population	Central Volume	Apparent Volume
Healthy volunteers	0.40 ± 0.34 L/kg[10]	2.53 ± 0.72 L/kg[10]
Patients with arrhythmias (without congestive heart failure)	0.91 ± 0.35 L/kg[7]	3 ± 0.52 L/kg[12]
Patients with hepatic dysfunction	0.44 ± 0.12 L/kg[24]	3.8 ± 0.4 L/kg[25]
Patients with CHF		1.81 ± 0.49 L/kg[24]

Half-Life and Time to Steady State

In healthy volunteers, the mean elimination half-life of quinidine is 5.7 hr (range of 4.5–7.2 hr; time to steady state 22–35 hr).[7] In patients with arrhythmias but without cardiac, renal, or hepatic dysfunction, the half-life averages 7.8 hr (range of 4.8–11.8 hr; time to steady state 25–60 hr).[6] Several factors including disease states and concomitantly administered drugs can affect the half-life (see drug–drug interactions and drug–disease state or condition interaction sections).

Therapeutic Range

Analogous to determining the pharmacokinetic parameters for quinidine, defining the therapeutic range for quinidine is dependent upon the assay methodology used to measure quinidine concentrations.[9] Therefore, the therapeutic range for quinidine is broader for a nonspecific quinidine assay because of the inability to separate quinidine from both dihydroquinidine and several metabolites. Utilizing a nonspecific assay, Sokolow and Ball reported a therapeutic range for quinidine of 1–16 mg/L in order to successfully convert either chronic atrial fibrillation or flutter to normal sinus rhythm.[46]

Several studies also attempted to determine a therapeutic range for quinidine in atrial fibrillation, one of which used a relatively specific assay (i.e., modified Cramér and Isaksson assay consisting of double extraction plus fluorescence).[47] The mean (± SD) serum quinidine concentration for patients who remained in sinus rhythm was 2.2 ± 0.8 mg/L. This value is consistent with that reported for other ventricular and supraventricular tachyarrhythmias for which serum quinidine concentrations were measured by a specific or relatively specific assay.

An investigation using a specific HPLC procedure to quantitate quinidine concentrations in patients with either unifocal, multifocal, or paired ventricular premature beats (VPBs) or unsustained ventricular tachycardia suggested a therapeutic range of 2–6 mg/L.[48] Some patients responded at concentrations of less than 2 mg/L. Conversely, in the treatment of either supraventricular or ventricular tachycardia, some patients required quinidine concentrations (as determined by a relatively specific enzyme immunoassay procedure) as high as 8 or 9 mg/L, respectively.[49]

In summary, as a general guideline for patient monitoring, quinidine concentrations within the range of 2–6 mg/L should be considered therapeutic, given an adequate clinical response.

Dosing Strategies

When selecting quinidine for a patient with an arrhythmia, the clinician must consider the following:
1. Be sure of the therapeutic goal. Depending upon the arrhythmia and accompanying symptoms, the therapeutic

goal may be conversion to and maintenance of normal sinus rhythm[47]; reduction of the baseline ectopy by some percentage (e.g., 63–95% reduction in baseline arrhythmia frequency)[50]; or prevention of induction of the arrhythmia by programmed electrophysiologic studies.[51]
2. Be aware of the patient's entire clinical condition. Specifically, determine if the patient has associated clinical conditions (e.g., advanced age or hypokalemia) or disease states (e.g., CHF or hepatic disease), or is receiving drugs (e.g., amiodarone or phenytoin) which may affect the kinetics or dynamics of quinidine.
3. Be aware that quinidine modifies the pharmacokinetics and pharmacodynamics of other drugs (e.g., digoxin and propafenone).
4. Accurately determine baseline PR, QRS, and QT intervals.
5. Be aware of the cardiovascular and noncardiovascular adverse effects associated with quinidine therapy (see pharmacodynamic monitoring—concentration-related toxicity section).
6. Be familiar with the quinidine assay used by the reference laboratory to quantitate quinidine concentrations.

Quinidine therapy is initiated either with maintenance or "loading" doses to produce estimated concentrations of 3–4 mg/L.

Maintenance doses of quinidine are administered either orally or intravenously. The hypotension which can accompany intravenous administration of quinidine appears related to the rate at which the dose is administered.[52] If the intravenous dose of quinidine is administered at a rate not greater than 0.3–0.5 mg/kg/min, the severity of the hypotension is generally minimal. The total intravenous loading dose administered at this rate should be 6–10 mg/kg. Oral loading doses of quinidine may consist of a single dose of 600–1000 mg of conventional-release quinidine sulfate.[53] Alternatively, other investigators utilize 200–400 mg every 2 hr for a total of five doses.[46]

Prior to initiating quinidine therapy for the management of atrial fibrillation or atrial flutter, it is critical to administer an agent such as digoxin, diltiazem, verapamil, or a beta-blocker to control ventricular rate response. An individualized pharmacokinetic approach could consist of

- An initial determination of the total, daily steady-state dose of oral, conventional-release quinidine sulfate, sustained-release quinidine sulfate, sustained-release quinidine gluconate (or intravenous quinidine gluconate) using the C steady-state equation (see Introduction).
- Division of this total daily dose into two to four equal doses depending upon formulation and patient clinical characteristics.

Regardless of the approach used, it is advisable to initiate quinidine therapy in a hospitalized, monitored setting for 2–3 days.[54]

Suggested Sampling Times and Effect on Therapeutic Range

Monitoring of concentrations of quinidine may be indicated in a number of clinical situations:

- To establish baseline dose–concentration relationships in patients begun on quinidine therapy.
- During quantitative evaluation of a patient's arrhythmia with Holter monitoring or during programmed electrophysiologic studies (PES) so that steady-state quinidine concentrations can be targeted to those at which the arrhythmia was rendered either suppressed or noninducible, respectively.
- During or following recurrence of the arrhythmia after initial successful suppression.
- In the presence of CHF or hepatic dysfunction because these conditions alter the pharmacokinetics of quinidine.
- Following initiation of concomitant therapy with a drug known or suspected to have a pharmacokinetic interaction

Salt Form	Route	Indication	Load	Maintenance
Quinidine Gluconate	Intravenous	Conversion	800 mg diluted in 40 ml of dextrose–5% water (50 ml total volume). To be infused at 16 mg/min (1 ml/min); larger doses may be used after evaluation of patient (i.e., ECG and BP)	N/A
	Intramuscular	Conversion	600 mg followed by an additional dose of 400 mg every 2 hr; dosage adjusted to patient response and tolerance	N/A
	Oral (extended release)	Maintenance of normal sinus rhythm		324–660 mg/8–12 hr; larger doses or more frequent administration only after evaluation with ECG and concentration.
Quinidine polygalacturonate	Oral tablets	Conversion	275–825 mg/3–4 hr; if normal rhythm not restored following third or fourth dose, increase in increments of 137.5–275 mg	275 mg 2–3 times a day

Quinidine sulfate	Oral tablets (regular or extended release)	Conversion of AF or maintenance of normal sinus rhythm	Regular release: 200 mg/2–3 hr for 5–8 doses	Regular release: 200–400 mg/3–4 times a day ER: 600 mg/8–12 hr; larger doses or more frequent administration only after EKG and conc. (maximum dose: 3–4 g/day)
		Termination of paroxysmal ventricular tachycardia	Regular release: 400–600 mg/2–3 hr until arrhythmia is terminated	N/A
		Decrease of atrial or ventricular premature contraction[a]	Regular release: 200–300 mg three or four times daily	N/A

[a] *In patients with structural heart disease, data indicate that quinidine actually increases mortality and should only be used for life-threatening arrhythmias.*

with quinidine, potentially resulting in changes in plasma quinidine concentrations.
- During the appearance of suspected quinidine cardiac or systemic toxicity.
- For suspected patient noncompliance.
- Following a change in dose or dosage forms or commercial brands of quinidine.
- When a patient's response to quinidine at usual doses is abnormal or difficult to evaluate.

Pharmacokinetic steady state is generally achieved within 2 days for most patients taking quinidine. Therefore, a trough blood sample following 48 hr of continuous quinidine therapy would be an appropriate time to evaluate steady-state dose–concentration relationships.

Pharmacodynamic Monitoring— Concentration-Related Efficacy

Utilizing a nonspecific assay, an early concentration-response relationship for quinidine was reported by Sokolow and Ball for patients with chronic atrial fibrillation or flutter.[46] Normal sinus rhythm was achieved in 153 out of 214 attempts (71.5%). The average (and range) quinidine concentrations at which conversion resulted were 6.1 mg/L (1–16 mg/L), and 85% of the successful conversions occurred at concentrations of 8 mg/L or less.

In a study examining the relationship between serum quinidine concentrations and maintenance of sinus rhythm in patients with atrial fibrillation, the mean (± SD) serum quinidine concentration in responders was 2.2 ± 0.8 mg/L.[47] This value, however, was not different from nonresponders.

Twelve of fourteen (86%) patients with ventricular arrhythmias (i.e., unifocal, multifocal, or paired VPBs or unsustained ventricular tachycardia) evaluated by

Holter monitoring demonstrated a therapeutic response at steady-state quinidine concentrations ranging from 0.7 to 5.9 mg/L.[48] However, all but three responders required quinidine concentrations greater than 2.0 mg/L. A specific HPLC assay was utilized in this investigation.

Thirty-eight patients with supraventricular tachycardia and 43 patients with ventricular tachycardia were administered quinidine and evaluated by PES.[49] Twenty-five of the 38 (66%) patients with supraventricular tachycardia responded to quinidine. The mean (and range) quinidine concentration was 2.9 mg/L (1.0–8.3 mg/L) for the responders. Only eight of the 43 (19%) patients with ventricular tachycardia responded to quinidine. The mean (and range) quinidine concentration for these responders was 3.9 mg/L (2.0–9.1 mg/L). However, for both groups of responders, the quinidine concentrations were not significantly different than those reported for the nonresponders. Therefore, quinidine concentrations must be evaluated in conjunction with careful clinical evaluation of the patient. Enzyme immunoassay (EMIT®, Syva Co., Palo Alto, CA), a relatively specific method, was utilized to quantitate quinidine concentrations.

Pharmacodynamic Monitoring— Concentration-Related Toxicity

Quinidine produces concentration-dependent changes in the ECG.[55] With increasing quinidine concentrations there are decreases in intraventricular conduction and delays in ventricular repolarization as evidenced by widening of the QRS interval and an increase in the QT interval, respectively. However, lengthening of the QT interval generally occurs at usual therapeutic quinidine concentrations and occasionally below the lower limit of the therapeutic range. Increases in the QRS interval infrequently occur at therapeutic quinidine concentrations.

Prolongation of the QT interval beyond 0.55 second, especially in the presence of either hypokalemia, hypomagnesemia, sinus bradycardia (<50 beats/minute), or other drugs which prolong ventricular repolarization or a pre-quinidine prolonged QT interval, may predispose a patient to developing quinidine-induced torsades de pointes ventricular tachycardia (i.e., quinidine syncope).[56,57] Torsades de pointes is a potentially life-threatening ventricular tachycardia characterized by a polymorphous QRS morphology at a rate of 150–300 beats/minute with sinusoidal rotation of the QRS axis around the isoelectric line on the ECG.[58]

This arrhythmia develops in patients with either congenital or acquired prolongation of the QT interval. Although episodes of torsades de pointes may occur after months of uneventful treatment, most episodes occur within the first few days of quinidine therapy.[55] Therefore, initiation of quinidine therapy should occur on an inpatient basis, if possible.[54]

Other concentration- or dose-related effects of quinidine may involve CNS toxicity and GI effects.[55] These effects occur at all serum concentrations but most frequently at concentrations above the therapeutic range. Elevated quinidine concentrations are associated with the syndrome of cinchonism. Symptoms of cinchonism include tinnitus, vertigo, blurred vision, headache, and other CNS effects.

Quinidine-induced diarrhea, nausea, and anorexia appear to be dose related. Therefore, initiation of quinidine therapy without a loading dose and the use of sustained-release quinidine preparations may reduce the frequency of these adverse effects.

Most of the other adverse effects of quinidine appear unrelated to quinidine concentrations.[55] These include hypersensitivity reactions such as hepatitis, fever, rash, and thrombocytopenia. Quinidine may also induce systemic lupus erythematosus.

Drug–Drug Interactions

Many drug-drug interactions that occur are not clinically significant (e.g., dose reductions and increases are not required). Some interactions occur and a dose

Object Drug	Interacting Drug	Change in Object Drug	Impact
Quinidine	Amiodarone[59,60]	↑	Increased concentrations and cardiac dysrhythmia may result; decrease quinidine dose by 30–50%
Quinidine	Cimetidine[61,62]	↑	Increase quinidine concentration by 50%, decrease dose by 33%
Quinidine	Verapamil[63,66]	↑	Decreased hepatic clearance; decrease dose of quinidine by 20–50%
Quinidine	Ketoconazole fluconazole, and itraconazole[67,68]	↑	30-fold increase in concentration after 7 days; monitor concentrations and adjust dose accordingly
Quinidine	Grapefruit juice[66]	↑	Delayed absorption and CYP 3A4 inhibition; the effects are variable in each subject; grapefruit juice should be avoided
Quinidine	Hydantoin and barbituate anticonvulsants[70]	↓	CYP 3A4 induction
Quinidine	Rifampin[71]	↓	CYP 3A4 induction; the change in $t^{1/2}$ is not predictive of the change in quinidine concentration
Quinidine	Nifedipine[72,73]	↑, ↓, or ↔	CYP 3A4 enzyme induction, inhibition, or no effect

Quinidine	Macrolides[68]	↑	Presumed CYP 3A4 inhibition; monitor QT; if corrected QT interval prolongation occurs, discontinuation of the macrolide may be required
Quinidine	Magnesium antacids[74] and kaolin-pectin	↑	Monitor concentration and signs of toxicity of quinidine; adjust dose as required
Warfarin[68]	*Quinidine*	↑	Anticoagulation is increased and bleeding may occur; monitor PT/INR and adjust warfarin as needed
Neuromuscular blocking agents[75]	*Quinidine*	↑	Effects of neuromuscular blocker can be enhanced, lower doses of blockers may be required
Digoxin[60,65,66,76–78]	*Quinidine*	↑	Increased effects of digoxin and increased concentrations; decrease digoxin dose according to concentration
Procainamide[79,80]	*Quinidine*	↑	Increase N-acetylprocainamide (NAPA) concentrations with toxicity; monitor procainamide and NAPA concentrations
Propafenone[81]	*Quinidine*	↑	Concentration can be enhanced in CYP2D6 extensive metabolizers; monitor ECG
Beta blockers[68]	*Quinidine*	↑	In CYP2D6 extensive metabolizers, heart rate and blood pressure effects increase
Tricyclic antidepressants[68]	*Quinidine*	↑	In CYP2D6 extensive metabolizers

reduction or increase cannot be recommended because the extent of the interaction may differ from one patient to another. Therefore, dosing recommendations are provided where available. Otherwise, clinical judgment and serum concentrations must dictate the change in dose.

Pharmacodynamic Interactions

As previously discussed, quinidine has been implicated in causing torsades de pointes ventricular tachycardia.[57] The likelihood of torsades de pointes occurring in a patient may be enhanced if quinidine is concurrently prescribed with other drugs or in clinical situations which have been described to induce torsades de pointes. Examples of other drugs which have induced torsades de pointes include procainamide, disopyramide, sotalol, amiodarone, bepridil, lithium, erythromycin, and terfenadine.[57] The coadministration of digoxin and diuretics may also increase the risk of developing quinidine-induced proarrhythmic effects.[78]

Clinical conditions which predispose patients to the development of drug-induced torsades de pointes include hypokalemia, hypomagnesemia, sinus bradycardia (<50 beats/minute), and prequinidine QT prolongation.[57] Therefore, careful monitoring of a patient's entire drug regimen, electrolytes, and ECG is critical to minimize the risk of developing quinidine-induced torsades de pointes. Discontinuing quinidine, if the corrected QT interval is prolonged greater than 0.55 second, should reduce the likelihood of propagating torsades de pointes.[56]

Drug–Disease State or Condition Interactions

Condition	Interaction
Elderly[22,82,83]	Elderly patients have a longer half-life (9.7 hr) and diminished total body and renal clearances (0.16 and 0.06 L/hr/kg, respectively). There is an inverse relationship between age and clearance. There may be an accumula-

	tion of active metabolite. No changes in protein binding.
Pediatrics[84]	Elimination in children is inversely proportional to age (clearance decreases with increasing age).
CHF[85-88]	Total body clearance (0.19 L/hr/kg), volume (0.44 L/kg), rate of absorption, and renal CL are decreased. There is no change in half-life because volume and clearance are decreased by the same proportion. When the ejection fraction (EF) is less than 30%, the efficacy of quinidine is diminished (<30%), and the risk of proarrhythmia is increased.
Hepatic disease[43,44]	Increased half-life and volume (3.8 L/kg), and decreased clearance (0.31 L/hr/kg). Unbound concentrations tend to be higher (36%) due to decreased available protein binding.
Renal disease[22,32,88,89]	Metabolites accumulate and increase the half-life (11.7 hr); therefore, dosing intervals should increase to 12 hr.
Pregnancy[90,91]	Can be used safely in pregnancy, readily crosses the placenta. Pregnant patients can have alterations in protein binding; therefore, monitoring of concentrations are indicated. Fetal concentration–maternal concentration ranges from 0.2 to 0.9, though the fetus will have higher unbound portion of drug. Dose 200–300 mg three or four times a day. After delivery, the maternal concentration may increase by as much as 50%.

References

1. McEvoy GK, ed. Quinidine. In: American Hospital Formulary Service Drug Information 99. Bethesda, MD: American Society of Health-System Pharmacists; 2000:1589–94.

2. Stafford RS, Robson DC, Misra B, et al. Rate control and sinus rhythm maintenance in atrial fibrillation. *Arch Intern Med.* 1998; 158:2144–8.

3. Ueda CT, Williamson BJ, Dzindzio BS. Absolute quinidine bioavailability. *Clin Pharmacol Ther.* 1976; 20:260–5.

4. Mason WD, Covinsky JO, Velentine JL, et al. Comparative plasma concentrations of quinidine following administration of one intramuscu-

lar and three oral formulations to 13 human subjects. *J Pharm Sci.* 1976; 65:1325–9.
5. McGilveray IJ, Midha KK, Rowe M, et al. Bioavailability of 11 quinidine formulations and pharmacokinetic variation in humans. *J Pharm Sci.* 1981; 70:524–9.
6. Conrad KA, Molk BL, Chidsey CA. Pharmacokinetic studies of quinidine in patients with arrhythmias. *Circulation.* 1977; 55:1–7.
7. Guentert TW, Holford NHG, Coates PE, et al. Quinidine pharmacokinetics in man: choice of a disposition model and absolute bioavailability studies. *J Pharmacokinet Biopharm.* 1979b; 7:315–30.
8. Gibson DL, Smith GH, Koup JR, et al. Relative bioavailability of a standard and a sustained-release quinidine tablet. *Clin Pharm.* 1982; 1:366–8.
9. Guentert TW, Upton RA, Holford NHG, et al. Divergence in pharmacokinetic parameters of quinidine obtained by specific and nonspecific assay methods. *J Pharmacokinet Biopharm.* 1979a; 7:303–11.
10. Fremstad D, Nilsen OG, Storstein L, et al. Pharmacokinetics of quinidine related to plasma protein binding in man. *Eur J Clin Pharmacol.* 1979; 15:187–92.
11. Gey GO, Levy RH, Pettet G, et al. Quinidine plasma concentrations and exertional arrhythmia. *Am Heart J.* 1975; 90:19–24.
12. Russo J, Russo ME, Smith RA, et al. Assessment of quinidine gluconate for nonlinear kinetics following chronic dosing. *J Clin Pharmacol.* 1982; 22:264–70.
13. Bolme P, Otto U. Dose-dependence of the pharmacokinetics of quinidine. *Eur J Clin Pharmacol.* 1977; 12:73–6.
14. Wooding-Scott RA, Smalley J, Visco J, et al. The pharmacokinetics and pharmacodynamics of quinidine and 3-hydroxyquinidine. *Br J Clin Pharmacol.* 1988; 6:415–21.
15. Guentert TW, Upton RA, Holford NHG, et al. Gastrointestinal absorption of quinidine from some solutions and commercial tablets. *J Pharmacokinet Biopharm.* 1980; 8:243–55.
16. Greenblatt DJ, Pfeifer HJ, Ochs H, et al. Pharmacokinetics of quinidine in humans after intravenous, intramuscular and oral administration. *J Pharmacol Exp Ther.* 1977; 202:365–78.
17. Wright GJ, Melikian AP, Pitts JE, et al. Comparative quinidine plasma profiles at steady state of two controlled-release products and quinidine sulfate in solution. *Biopharm Drug Dispos.* 1987; 8:159–72.
18. Woo E, Greenblatt DJ. Effect of food on enteral absorption of quinidine. *Clin Pharmacol Ther.* 1980; 27:188–93.
19. Martinez MN, Pelsor FR, Shah VP, et al. Effect of dietary fat content on the bioavailability of a sustained release quinidine gluconate tablet. *Biopharm Drug Dispos.* 1990; 11:17–29.
20. Ueda CT, Hirschfeld DS, Scheinman MM, et al. Disposition kinetics of quinidine. *Clin Pharmacol Ther.* 1976b; 19:30–36.
21. Ochs HR, Greenblatt DJ, Woo E. Clinical pharmacokinetics of quinidine. *Clin Pharmacokinet.* 1980; 5:150–68.
22. Ochs HR, Greenblatt DJ, Woo E, et al. Reduced quinidine clearance in elderly persons. *Am J Cardiol.* 1978b; 42:481–5.
23. Notterman DA, Drayer DE, Metakis L, et al. Stereoselective renal

tubular secretion of quinidine and quinine. *Clin Pharmacol Ther.* 1986; 40:511–17.

24. Gerhardt RE, Knouss RF, Thyrum PT, et al. Quinidine excretion in aciduria and alkaluria. *Ann Intern Med.* 1969; 71:927–33.

25. Woie L, Oyri A. Quinidine intoxication treated with hemodialysis. *Acta Med Scand.* 1974; 195:237–9.

26. Hall K, Meatherall B, Krahn J, et al. Clearance of quinidine during peritoneal dialysis. *Am Heart J.* 1982; 104:646–7.

27. Guengerich FP, Muller-Enoch D, Blair IA. Oxidation of quinidine by human liver cytochrome P-450. *Mol Pharmacol.* 1986; 30:287–95.

28. Thompson KA, Murray JJ, Blair IA, et al. Plasma concentrations of quinidine, its major metabolites, and dihydroquinidine in patients with torsades de pointes. *Clin Pharmacol Ther.* 1988; 43:636–42.

29. Thompson KA, Blair IA, Woosley RL, et al. Comparative in vitro electrophysiology of quinidine, its major metabolites and dihydroquinidine. *J Pharmacol Exp Ther.* 1987; 241:84–90.

30. Vozeh S, Uematsu T, Guentert TW, et al. Kinetics and electrocardiographic changes after oral 3-OH-quinidine in healthy subjects. *Clin Pharmacol Ther.* 1985; 37:575–81.

31. Ha H-R, Vozeh S, Uematsu T, et al. Kinetics and dynamics of quinidine-N-oxide in healthy subjects. *Clin Pharmacol Ther.* 1987; 42:341–5.

32. Drayer DE, Lowenthal DT, Restivo KM, et al. Steady-state serum levels of quinidine and active metabolites in cardiac patients with varying degrees of renal function. *Clin Pharmacol Ther.* 1978; 24:31–9.

33. Rakhit A, Holford NHG, Guentert TW, et al. Pharmacokinetics of quinidine and three of its metabolites in man. *J Pharmacokinet Biopharm.* 1984; 12:1–21.

34. Ackerman BH, Olsen KM, Pappas AA. Disposition of dihydroquinidine among patients receiving parenteral quinidine. *Pharmacother.* 1990; 10:245 (abstr).

35. Ueda CT, Makoid MC. Quinidine and dihydroquinidine interactions in human plasma. *J Pharm Sci.* 1979; 68:448–50.

36. Kates RE. Therapeutic monitoring of antiarrhythmic drugs. *Ther Drug Monit.* 1980; 2:119–26.

37. Kessler KM, Leech RC, Spann JF. Blood collection techniques, heparin and quinidine protein binding. *Clin Pharmacol Ther.* 1979; 25:204–10.

38. Edwards DJ, Axelson JE, Slaughter RL, et al. Factors affecting quinidine protein binding in humans. *J Pharm Sci.* 1984; 73:1264–7.

39. Garfinkel D, Mamelok RD, Blaschke TF. Altered therapeutic range for quinidine after myocardial infarction and cardiac surgery. *Ann Intern Med.* 1987; 107:48–50.

40. Kessler KM, Lisker B, Conde C, et al. Abnormal quinidine binding in survivors of prehospital cardiac arrest. *Am Heart J.* 1984; 107:665–9.

41. McCollum PL, Crouch MA, Watson SE. Altered protein binding of quinidine in patients with atrial fibrillation and flutter. *Pharmacother.* 1997; 17:753–9.

42. Kessler KM, Humphries WC, Black M, et al. Quinidine pharmacokinetics in patients with cirrhosis or receiving propranolol. *Am Heart J.* 1978; 96:627–35.

43. Perez-Mateo M, Erill S. Protein binding of salicylate and quinidine in plasma from patients with renal failure, chronic liver disease and chronic respiratory insufficiency. *Eur J Clin Pharmacol.* 1977; 11:225–31.
44. Kessler KM, Perez GO. Decreased quinidine plasma protein binding during hemodialysis. *Clin Pharmacol Ther.* 1981; 30:122–26.
45. Kessler KM, Wozniak PM, McAuliffe D, et al. The clinical implication of changing unbound quinidine levels. *Am Heart J.* 1989; 118:63–9.
46. Sokolow M, Ball RE. Factors influencing conversion of chronic atrial fibrillation with special reference to serum quinidine concentration. *Circulation.* 1956; 14:568–83.
47. Byrne-Quinn E, Wing AJ. Maintenance of sinus rhythm after DC reversion of atrial fibrillation. A double-blind controlled trial of long-acting quinidine bisulphate. *Br Heart J.* 1970; 32:370–6.
48. Carliner NH, Fisher ML, Crouthamel WG, et al. Relation of ventricular premature beat suppression to serum quinidine concentration determined by a new and specific assay. *Am Heart J.* 1980; 100:483–9.
49. Berry NS, Bauman JL, Gallastegui JL, et al. Analysis of antiarrhythmic drug concentrations determined during electrophysiologic drug testing in patients with inducible tachycardias. *Am J Cardiol.* 1988; 61:922–4.
50. Crawford MH, Bernstein SJ, Deedwania PC, et al. ACC/AHA Guidelines for Ambulatory electrocardiography. *J Am Coll Cardiol.* 1999; 34:912–48.
51. Mason JW. A comparison of seven antiarrhythmic drugs in patients with ventricular tachyarrhythmias. *N Engl J Med.* 1993; 329(7):452–8.
52. Woo E, Greenblatt DJ. A reevaluation of intravenous quinidine. *Am Heart J.* 1978; 96:829–32.
53. Gaughan CE, Lown B, Lanigan J. Acute oral testing for determining antiarrhythmic drug efficacy. *Am J Cardiol.* 1976; 38:677–84.
54. Roden DM, Woosley RL, Primm RK. Incidence and clinical features of the quinidine-associated long QT syndrome: implications for patient care. *Am Heart J.* 1986; 111:1088–93.
55. Kim SY, Benowitz NL. Poisoning due to class IA antiarrhythmic drugs. Quinidine, procainamide and disopyramide. *Drug Safety.* 1990; 5:393–420.
56. Tzivoni D, Keren A, Banai S, et al. Terminology of torsades de pointes. *Cardiovasc Drugs Ther.* 1991; 5:505–8.
57. Zehender M, Hohnloser S, Just H. QT-interval prolonging drugs: mechanisms and clinical relevance of their arrhythmogenic hazards. *Cardiovasc Drugs Ther.* 1991; 5:515–30.
58. Keren A, Tzivoni D. Torsades de pointes: prevention and therapy. *Cardiovasc Drugs Ther.* 1991; 5:509–14.
59. Saal AK, Werner JA, Greene HL, et al. Effect of amiodarone on serum quinidine and procainamide levels. *Am J Cardiol.* 1984; 53:1264–7.
60. Frietag D, Bebee R, Sunderland B. Digoxin-quinidine and digoxin-amiodarone interactions. *J Clin Pharm Ther.* 1995; 20:179–83.
61. Hardy BG, Schentag JJ. Lack of effect of cimetidine on the metabolism of quinidine: effect on renal clearance. *Int J Clin Pharmacol Ther Toxicol.* 1988; 26:388–91.
62. Hardy BG, Zador IT, Golden L, et al. Effect of cimetidine on the

pharmacokinetics and pharmacodynamics of quinidine. *Am J Cardiol.* 1983; 52:172–5.
63. Edwards DJ, Lavoie R, Beckman H, et al. The effects of coadministration of verapamil on the pharmacokinetics and metabolism of quinidine. *Clin Pharmacol Ther.* 1987; 41:68–73.
64. Maisel AS, Motulsky HJ, Insel PA. Hypotension after quinidine plus verapamil. Possible additive competition at alpha-adrenergic receptors. *N Engl J Med.* 1985; 312:167–70.
65. Shibata K, Hirasawa A, Foglar R, et al. Effects of quinidine and verapamil on human cardiovascular alpha receptors. *Circulation.* 1998; 97:1227–30.
66. Bauer LA, Horn JR, Pettit H. Mixed effect modeling for detection and evaluation of drug interactions. *Ther Drug Monit.* 1996; 18:46–52.
67. McNulty RM, Lazor JA, Sketch M. Transient increase in plasma quinidine concentrations during ketoconazole-quinidine therapy. *Clin Pharm.* 1989; 8:222–5.
68. Michelats EL. Update: clinically significant cytochrome p-450 drug interactions. *Pharmacother.* 1998; 18:84–112.
69. Min DI, Ku YM, Geraets DR. Effect of grapefruit juice on the pharmacokinetics of quinidine in healthy volunteers. *J Clin Pharm.* 1996; 36:469–76.
70. Data JL, Wilkinson GR, Nies AS. Interaction of quinidine with anticonvulsant drugs. *N Engl J Med.* 1976; 294:699–702.
71. Twum-Barima Y, Carruthers SG. Quinidine-rifampin interaction. *N Engl J Med.* 1981; 304:1466–9.
72. Farringer JA, Green JA, O'Rourke RA, et al. Nifedipine-induced alterations in serum quinidine concentrations. *Am Heart J.* 1984; 108:1570–2.
73. Munger MA, Jarvis RC, Nair R, et al. Elucidation of the nifedipine-quinidine interaction. *Clin Pharmacol Ther.* 1989; 45:411–6.
74. Zin MB. Quinidine intoxication from alkali ingestion. *Tex Med.* 1970; 66(12)64–6.
75. Feldman S, Karalliedde L. Drug interactions with neuromuscular blockers. *Drug Safety.* 1996; 15:261–73.
76. Rodin SM, Johnson BJ. Pharmacokinetic interactions with digoxin. *Clin Pharmacokinet.* 1988; 15:227–44.
77. Hager WD, Fenster P, Mayersohn M, et al. Digoxin-quinidine interaction. Pharmacokinetic evaluation. *N Engl J Med.* 1979; 300:1238–41.
78. Minardo JD, Heger JJ, Miles WM, et al. Clinical characteristics of patients with ventricular fibrillation during antiarrhythmic drug therapy. *N Engl J Med.* 1988; 319:257–62.
79. Kim S, Seiden S, Matos J, et al. Combination of procainamide and quinidine for better tolerance and additive effects for ventricular arrhythmias. *Am J Cardiol.* 1985; 56:84–8.
80. Hughes B, Dyer JE, Schwartz AB. Increased procainamide plasma concentrations caused by quinidine: a new drug interaction. *Am Heart J.* 1987; 114:908–9.
81. Funck-Brentano C, Kroemer HK, Pavlou H, et al. Genetically-

determined interaction between propafenone and low dose quinidine: role of active metabolites in modulating net drug effect. *Br J Clin Pharmacol.* 1989; 27:435–44.
82. Drayer DE, Hughes M, Lorenzo B, et al. Prevalence of high (3S)-3-hydroxyquinidine/quinidine ratios in serum, and clearance of quinidine in cardiac patients with age. *Clin Pharmacol Ther.* 1980; 27:72–5.
83. Ackerman BH, Olsen KM. Accumulation of 3-hydroxyquinidine following chronic quinidine therapy. *DICP Ann Pharmacother.* 1991; 25:867–9.
84. Szefler SJ, Pieroni DR, Gingell RL, et al. Rapid elimination of quinidine in pediatric patients. *Pediatrics.* 1982; 70:370–5.
85. Ueda CT, Dzindzio BS. Quinidine kinetics in congestive heart failure. *Clin Pharmacol The.* 1978; 23:158–64.
86. Ueda CT, Dzindzio BS. Bioavailability of quinidine in congestive heart failure. *Br J Clin Pharmacol.* 1981; 11:571–7.
87. Meissner MD, Kay HR, Horowitz LN, et al. Relation of acute antiarrhythmic drug efficacy to left ventricular function in coronary artery disease. *Am J Cardiol.* 1988; 61:1050–5.
88. Kessler KM, Lowenthal DT, Warner H, et al. Quinidine elimination in patients with congestive heart failure or poor renal function. *N Engl J Med.* 1974; 290:706–9.
89. Fattinger K, Vozeh S, Ha HR, et al. Population pharmacokinetics of quinidine. *Br J Clin Pharmacol.* 1991; 31:279–286.
90. Ito S, Magee L, Smallhorn J. Drug therapy for fetal arrhythmias. *Clin Perinatol.* 1994; 21:543–72.
91. Rotmensh HH, Elkayam U, Frishman W, et al. Antiarrhythmic drug therapy during pregnancy. *Ann Intern Med.* 1983; 98:487–97.

Chapter 18
Edress H. Darsey

Theophylline (AHFS 86:16)

Usual Dosage Range in Absence of Clearance-Altering Factors[1]

Theophylline is a bronchial smooth muscle relaxant used in the treatment of asthma and other respiratory diseases. It is also used to treat apnea, bradycardia, and ventilator weaning in neonates.

Caution is required when dosing patients who are unhealthy, smokers, and/or on other medications that alter theophylline clearance (refer to drug–drug interactions and drug–disease state or condition interactions sections).

Theophylline products are available in different salt forms with a wide range of bioavailabilities. The following dose recommendations are suggested to achieve serum theophylline concentrations of 5–10 mg/L in the neonate and 10 mg/L in all other patient populations. All doses are expressed in terms of anhydrous theophylline; dosage adjustments then can be made for the other salt forms (see bioavailability of dosage forms section).

Loading dose[2]

The suggested loading dose of theophylline for patients without a history of theophylline use is 4.8 mg/kg (6mg/kg of aminophylline). If the patient has been receiving theophylline, it is advisable to draw a stat serum concentration and to base the loading dose on it using

$$LD = \frac{(C_D - C_O)V}{SF}$$

where
- LD = loading dose in mg/kg
- C_D = concentration desired
- C_O = concentration obtained
- V = volume of distribution
- S = fraction of salt form
- F = bioavailability

Only rapid release products should be used for oral loading doses.

Maintenance dose[1,3,4]

All doses are expressed in terms of *anhydrous theophylline* and should be converted to the proper dosage if *aminophylline* is administered. The following theophylline dosing chart represents the recommended starting dose. Further dosing should be individualized based on the patient's measured theophylline concentration and therapeutic response. A patient's theophylline clearance should be calculated. Next, a patient-specific dose should be calculated based on the patient's clearance of the drug. If an additional bolus is needed, the loading dose equation may be used to calculate an appropriate patient-specific dose. Ideal body weight should be used to calculate maintenance doses for obese patients.

Population	Intravenous Maintenance Dose, Continuous Infusion	Oral/Intravenous Maintenance Dose
Neonates	N/A	
Postnatal age (PNA) ≤24 days		1 mg/kg every 12 hr
PNA >24–<28 days)		1.5 mg/kg every 12 hr

Infants (4–52 weeks)		total daily dose (mg) = [(0.2 × age in weeks) + 5] × (weight in kg)
		PNA up to 26 weeks: administer total daily dose divided every 8 hr[a]
		PNA >26 weeks: administer total daily dose divided every 6 hr[a]
1–9 years	0.8–1 mg/kg/hr	20–24 mg/kg/day[b]
9–12 years	0.7 mg/kg/hr	16 mg/kg/day[b]
12–16 years	0.6 mg/kg/hr	14 mg/kg/day[b]
Adults	0.4 mg/kg/hr	10 mg/kg/day (do not exceed 900 mg/day)[b]
Young adult smokers	0.7 mg/kg/hr	16 mg/kg/day[b]
Older patients and patients with cor pulmonale, congestive heart failure, or liver failure	0.25 mg/kg/hr	6 mg/kg/day (do not exceed 400 mg/day)[b]

[a]*Dosing interval refers to use of fast release oral product.*
[b]*Dosing interval in children and healthy adults can be divided every 8–12 hr with use of slow-release products.*

Dosage Form Availability[1,6]

Theophylline is available in different salt forms with different theophylline equivalence. In the conversion from one product to another, both bioavailability and theophylline salt equivalence are important. For this reason, theophylline dosage forms are presented here by their salt categories.

Dosage Form	Product
Aminophylline (anhydrous) (86 ± 2% theophylline)	
Oral liquid: 105 mg/5 ml	Aminophylline DF
Aminophylline (hydrous) (79 ± 2% theophylline)	

Oral tablets: 100 and 200 mg	Aminophylline
Oral tablets (extended release): 225 mg	Phyllocontin
Parenteral Injection 25 mg/ml	Aminophylline
Rectal suppositories	
250 mg	Truphylline
500 mg	Truphylline

Oxtriphylline (64 ± 2% theophylline)

Oral elixir: 100 mg/5 ml	Choledyl Elixir
Oral syrup: 50 mg/5 ml	Choledyl Pediatric Syrup
Oral tablets: 100 and 200 mg	Choledyl
Oral tablets (extended release, film coated): 400 and 600 mg	Choledyl SA

Theophylline (anhydrous)

Oral capsules: 100 and 200 mg	Bronkodyl Elixophyllin
Oral capsules (extended release):	
50 and 75 mg	Slo-bid Gyrocaps Theo-Dur Sprinkle
60 mg	Slo-Phyllin 60 Gyrocaps
65 mg	Aerolate III
100 and 300 mg	Slo-bid Gyrocaps Theo-24
125 mg	Slo-bid Gyrocaps Slo-Phyllin 125 Gyrocaps Theo-Dur Sprinkle Theovent
130 mg	Aerolate JR Theobid Jr. Duracap Theoclear L.A.-130 Theospan-SR
200 mg	Slo-bid Gyrocaps Theo-24 Theo-Dur Sprinkle
250 mg	Elixophyllin SR Slo-Phyllin 250 Gyrocaps Theovent
260 mg	Aerolate SR Theobid Duracap Theoclear L.A.-260

300 mg	Theospan-SR Theo-24
Oral solution 26.7 mg/5 ml	Theolair
Oral syrup 80 mg/15 ml	Aquaphyllin Slo-Phyllin Theoclear–80 Theostat 80
Oral elixir 80 mg/15 ml	Theophylline Asmalia Elixomin Elixophyllin Lanophyllin

Oral tablets
  100 and 200 mg
  125 and 250 mg
  300 mg
	Slo-Phyllin
	Theolair
	Quibron-T Dividose

Oral tablets (extended release) 100 mg	Sustaire Theo-Dur Theo-Sav Theox
200 mg	Constant-T Theo-Dur Theolair-SR Theo-Sav Theox T-Phyl
250 and 500 mg	Respbid Theolair-SR
300 mg	Constant-T Quibron-T/SR Sustaire Theo-Dur Theolair-SR Theo-Sav Theox
400 and 600 mg	Uni-Dur Uniphyl
450 mg	Theo-Dur
Parenteral injection (for infusion) 0.4–4 mg/ml in dextrose (6.4, 0.8, 1.6, 2, 3.2, and 4 mg/ml)	Theophylline and 5% Dextrose Injection

Bioavailability (F) of Dosage Forms[1,6-8]

The bioavailability of theophylline depends on its formulation and route of administration. When a patient is changed from intravenous to oral therapy, the maintenance infusion should be stopped and oral therapy should be begun immediately.[8] The theophylline equivalence of each salt form should be considered when this conversion is made.

Dosage Form	Bioavailability Comments
Intravenous aminophylline	100%
Oral liquids	100%
Oral tablets and capsules (immediate release)	100%; rate of absorption may be slowed when ingested with food or antacids
Oral tablets and capsules (enteric coated)	Incomplete and unpredictable, with no clinical indication for use
Oral tablets and capsules (extended release)	90–100% with extent and rate of absorption dependent on particular product[a]
Suppositories (cocoa butter)	Slow and erratic
Suppositories (PEG)	90–100%
Rectal solution	90–100%

[a] *Generally, products taken once a day exhibit incomplete absorption when ingested with food. Theo-Dur Sprinkle absorption is markedly impaired. Theo-24 has resulted in rapid release of a potentially toxic amount of theophylline.*

Along with the route, form, and particular product of theophylline, its salt equivalence must be considered. The theophylline salt equivalence (S) for each salt, compared to anhydrous theophylline, is

Drug	Anhydrous Theophylline Content (mean ± SD)
Aminophylline anhydrous	86 ± 2%
Aminophylline hydrous	79 ± 2%

Oxtriphylline　　　　　　　　　　64 ± 2%
Theophylline monohydrate　　　　91 ± 1%

General Pharmacokinetic Information

Clearance and metabolism

In adults, theophylline is 85–90% metabolized by hepatic biotransformation into relatively inactive metabolites (demethylation by the P450 1A2 and hydroxylation by the P450 2E1 and P450 3A3). The only active metabolite, 3-methylxanthine, forms slower than the rate of excretion and, therefore, exhibits no pharmacologic effects. Dosing adjustments are not required for renal dysfunction.[2,3]

In neonates, the N-demethylation pathway is absent, fully maturing by 1 year of age. Approximately 50% of the theophylline dose is excreted unchanged in the urine, and 7–10% of the dose is converted to the active metabolite caffeine in neonates. Caffeine has an extremely long half-life of approximately 100 hr, and concentrations are approximately 30% or more of theophylline concentrations. The cytochrome P450 pathway appears to be almost absent in neonates. Dosing adjustments for renal dysfunction (urine output less than 2 ml/kg/hr) are necessary in the neonate.[2,3]

Protein binding

Theophylline is approximately 40% bound to plasma proteins in adults and 36% bound in neonates.[1,2] Due to the low percentage of protein binding, changes in protein binding should not affect theophylline clearance.

Clearance (CL)[3]

The following clearance values are for neonates and healthy, nonsmoking adults and children. Refer to the drug–disease state or condition interactions section for clearance values of other patient populations.

Population	Mean (Range) Total Body Clearance[a], L/hr/kg
Premature neonates	
PNA 3–15 days	0.017 (0.005–0.029)
PNA 25–57 days	0.038 (0.002–0.072)
Term infants	
PNA 1–2 days	NR[b]
PNA 3–30 weeks	NR
Children	
1–4 years	0.102 (0.03–0.174)
4–12 years	0.096 (0.048–0.138)
6–17 years	0.084 (0.012–0.156)
13–15 years	0.054 (0.024–0.084)
Adults (16–60 years) healthy, nonsmoking asthmatics	0.039 (0.016–0.062)
Elderly (>60 years) nonsmokers with normal cardiac, liver, and renal function	0.025 (0.013–0.037)

[a]Adapted with permission from reference 3.
[b]NR = Not reported or not reported in a comparable format.

Volume of Distribution (V)[6,9]

In patients with reduced protein binding, the volume of distribution will be slightly larger than the values listed below. Altered theophylline clearance does not affect this theophylline parameter.

Age	Volume
Neonates (0 –<4 weeks)	0.8 L/kg
Infants (4 weeks–<1 year)	0.5–0.7 L/kg
Children (≥1 year), adolescents, adults, and geriatrics	0.5 L/kg

Half-Life and Time to Steady State[3]

The half-lives and estimated times to steady state for theophylline in neonates and healthy, nonsmoking adults and children are listed below. The time to steady state is between three and five half-lives.

Population	Mean (Range) Half-Life[a], hr	Mean (Range) Time to Steady State, hr
Premature neonates		
PNA 3–15 days	30(17–43)	150(85–215)
PNA 25–57 days	20(9–31)	100(47–153)
Term infants		
PNA 1–2 days	25–27	125–132.5
PNA 3–30 weeks	11(6–29)	55(30–145)
Children		
1–4 years	3.4(1.2–5.6)	17(6–28)
4–12 years	NR[b]	
6–17 years	3.7(1.5–5.9)	19(3–30)
13–15 years	NR	
Adults (16–60 years) healthy, nonsmoking asthmatics	8(6–13)	41(31–64)
Elderly (>60 years) nonsmokers with normal cardiac, liver, and renal function	10(2–18)	49(8–90)

[a]Adapted with permission from reference 3.
[b]NR = Not reported or not reported in a comparable format.

Therapeutic Range[1,2,10–12]

For *asthma*, the therapeutic range was traditionally considered to be 10–20 mg/L. Literature now indicates that ranges of 5–15 mg/L enhances safety, giving up little, if any, therapeutic benefit.

For *chronic obstructive pulmonary disease* (COPD), the therapeutic range is also 5–15 mg/L. Since it is debatable whether theophylline increases diaphragmatic contractility in these patients, its efficacy is questionable. Because these patients are usually elderly (and/or may be on multiple medications) and their clinical status often changes in a manner that affects theophylline concentrations, serum concentrations should be monitored often.

For *apnea or bradycardia in neonates*, the therapeutic range is 5–10 mg/L. Although a wide range of doses has been suggested, many neonates respond with low concentrations. Therapy should be started at low concentrations and increased by 3 mg/L as necessary.

For *ventilator weaning of neonates*, the therapeutic range is 5–20 mg/L. However, studies supporting the desired theophylline concentration for ventilator weaning are limited. Some authors suggest that concentrations greater than 8 mg/L are required to enhance diaphragmatic contractility and promote relaxation of respiratory muscles.

Suggested Sampling Times and Effect on Therapeutic Range

Therapeutic reference ranges often refer to concentrations drawn as peaks.[2] If a trough concentration is preferred, it is important to be consistent with the timing of sampling.

Sampling times for the various age groups, along with the reasons for the timing, are listed below.

Neonates
- 2 hr after the first loading dose to calculate the volume of distribution, if necessary.
- Every 4–7 days to calculate clearance and evaluate need for dosage adjustment.

Infants, children, adults, and geriatrics
- 30 min after the first loading dose, if administered intravenously, to calculate the volume of distribution and additional loading doses.

- 12–24 hr after initiation of maintenance dose to determine if adequate concentrations are being maintained or if the drug is accumulating rapidly, if determined necessary.
- 72 hr after initial dosing and then every 24–72 hr as needed to calculate clearance and evaluate need for dosage adjustment.
- Every 4–7 days once hospitalized patient is stabilized, unless otherwise indicated, to calculate clearance and evaluate need for dosage adjustment.
- Every 1–6 months in ambulatory patients.

Pharmacodynamic Monitoring—Concentration-Related Efficacy[7]

The following are useful indicators of theophylline efficacy.

Asthma or COPD
- Decrease in severity of wheezing and rales.
- Decrease in amount of ventilator support.
- Heart rate normalization.
- Respiration rate normalization.
- Improvement of FEV_1.

Apnea or bradycardia in neonates
- Decrease in number and depth of apneic and bradycardic episodes.
- Decrease in amount of ventilator support.
- Heart rate normalization.

Pharmacodynamic Monitoring—Concentration-Related Toxicity[5,7]

To reduce the potential for concentration-related toxicity, the following should be monitored whenever theophylline is used.

- Liver function in patients receiving theophylline for asthma or COPD.
- Renal function in neonates receiving theophylline for apnea or bradycardia. (Urine output should be 2 ml/kg/hr or more.)[5]
- Drugs or disease states that may decrease theophylline clearance.

Seizures and death induced by theophylline can occur in the absence of any other adverse effect; therefore, theophylline concentrations should be monitored.

The following concentration-related adverse effects have been documented in adults.

Serum Concentration	Adverse Effect
>20 mg/L	Nausea, vomiting, and diarrhea Headache Irritability Insomnia Tremor
>35 mg/L	Hyperglycemia Hyperkalemia Hypotension[a] Cardiac arrhythmias Hyperthermia Seizures, brain damage, and death

[a]*May also occur due to too rapid an infusion; infusion rate should not exceed 20 mg/min.*

In neonates receiving theophylline for apnea, bradycardia, or ventilator weaning, the following adverse effects may indicate toxicity: tachycardia (heart rate of more than 180 beats/min), irritability, seizures, and vomiting (vomitus "coffee ground" like in appearance).

Drug–Drug Interactions[3,13,14]

The following selected drugs, when given concomitantly with theophylline, *decrease* its clearance:

- Allopurinol
- Cimetidine
- Ciprofloxacin
- Diltiazem
- Disulfiram
- Erythromycin
- Nifedipine
- Norfloxacin
- Oral contraceptives
- Propranolol
- Trivalent influenza vaccine
- Troleadomycin
- Verapamil

The following selected drugs, when given concomitantly with theophylline, *increase* its clearance:

- Albuterol
- Carbamazepine
- Isoproterenol
- Ketoconazole
- Loop diuretics
- Nevirapine
- Phenobarbital
- Phenytoin
- Rifampin
- Sulfinpyrazone
- Sympathomimetics

Drug–Disease State or Condition Interactions[3,16]

Condition[a]	Mean (Range) Theophylline Clearance, L/hr/kg	Mean (Range) Theophylline Half-Life, hr
Acute pulmonary edema	0.02 (0.004–0.141)[a]	19 (3–82)[a]
COPD, >60 years, stable nonsmoker >1year	0.032 (0.026–0.038)	11 (9–13)
COPD with cor pulmonale	0.029 (0.005–0.053)	NR[b]

	Theophylline Clearance (mean ± SD), L/hr/kg	Theophylline Half-Life (mean ± SD), hr
Cystic fibrosis (14–28 years)	0.075 (0.019–0.132)	60 (2–10)
Fever associated with acute viral respiratory illness (children 9–15 years)	NR[b]	7 (1–13)
Liver disease		
Acute hepatitis	0.021 (0.015–0.027)	19 (17–22)
Cholestasis	0.039 (0.015–0.087)	14 (6–32)
Cirrhosis	0.019 (0.006–0.042)[c]	32 (10–56)[c]
Pregnancy		
1st trimester	NR	9 (3–14)
2nd trimester	NR	9 (4–14)
3rd trimester	NR	13 (8–18)
Sepsis with multiorgan failure	0.028 (0.011–0.114)	19 (6–24)
Thyroid disease		
Hypothyroid	0.023 (0.008–0.034)	12 (8–25)
Hyperthyroid	0.048 (0.041–0.058)	5 (4–6)
	NR	4.1 ± 1

	Theophylline Clearance (mean ± SD), L/hr/kg	Theophylline Half-Life (mean ± SD), hr
Smoking[e]		
Moderate cigarette use	0.063 ± 0.019	5.4 ± 1
Heavy cigarette use	0.072 ± 0.03	4.3 ± 1
Marijuana use	0.09 ± 0.024	4.3 ± 1
Cigarette and marijuana use	0.051 ± 0.001	6.4 ± 1
Past cigarette use (≥2 years ago)	0.043 ± 0.012	5.9 ± 0.8
Elderly smokers	4.54 ± 0.27 L/hr[d]	5.2 ± 1
Diet[e]		
Low carbohydrate and high protein	0.048 ± 0.016	NR
High carbohydrate and low protein		
Charcoal-broiled beef (heavy consumption)	5.45 ± 0.56 L/hr[d]	4.7 ± 0.4

Caffeine	NR	Increased
Cabbage or brussels sprouts (heavy consumption)	NR	Decreased

^aAdapted with permission from references 3 and 16.
^bNR = Not reported or not reported in a comparable format.
^cReported range or estimated range (mean ± 2SD) where actual range not reported.
^dNote different units
^eValues are mean ±SD.

References

1. Theophyllines. In: McEvoy GK, ed. American hospital formulary service drug information 98. Bethesda, MD: American Society of Health-System Pharmacists; 1998:2986–93.
2. Edwards DJ, Zarowitz BJ, Slaughter RL. Theophylline. In: Evans WE, Schentag JJ, Jusko WJ, eds. Applied pharmacokinetics:principles of therapeutic drug monitoring, 3rd ed. Spokane, WA: Applied Therapeutics; 1992:13-1–13-38.
3. Hendeles L, Jenkins J, Temple R. Revised FDA labeling guideline for theophylline oral dosage forms. *Pharmacother*. 1995;15(4):409–27.
4. Taketomo CK, Hodding JH, Kraus DM. Pediatric dosage handbook, 5th ed. Hudson, OH: Lexi-comp; 1998-99:61–4,1046–52.
5. Traub SL, Johnson CE. Comparisons of methods of estimating creatinine clearance in children. *Am J Hosp Pharm*. 1980;37(2):195–201.
6. Kastrup EK, ed. Facts and comparisons drug information. St. Louis, MO: J.B. Lippincott; 1999.
7. Winter ME. Theophylline. In: Winter ME, ed. Basic clinical pharmacokinetics. Spokane, WA: Applied Therapeutics; 1994:405–45.
8. Hendeles L, Weinberger M. Theophylline, a state of the art review. *Pharmacother*. 1983; 3:2–24.
9. Jonkman JHG. Food interactions with sustained-released preparations, a review. *Clin Pharmacokinet*. 1989; 16:162–79.
10. Moore ES, Faix RG, Banagale RC, et al. The population pharmacokinetics of theophylline in neonates and young infants. *J Pharmacokinet Biopharm*. 1989; 17:47–66.
11. Self TH, Heilker GM, Alloway RR, et al. Reassessing therapeutic range for theophylline for laboratory report forms: the importance of 5–15 mg/L. *Pharmacother*. 1993; 13(6):590–4.
12. National Institutes of Health. Guidelines for the diagnosis and management of asthma. National asthma education program expert panel report, 1991; DHHS publication No. 91-3042.
13. Milsap RL, Krauss AN, Auld PA. Oxygen consumption in apneic premature infants after low-dose theophylline. *Clin Pharmacol Ther*. 1980; 28(4):536–40.

14. Upton RA. Pharmacokinetic interactions between theophylline and other medication (part I). *Clin Pharmacokinet.* 1991; 20:66–80.
15. Upton RA. Pharmacokinetic interactions between theophylline and other medication (part II). *Clin Pharmacokinet.* 1991; 20:135–50.
16. Hendeles L, Massanari M, Weinberger M. Theophylline. In: Evans WE, Schentag JJ, Jusko WJ, eds. Applied pharmacokinetics:principles of therapeutic drug monitoring, 2nd ed. Spokane, WA: Applied Therapeutics; 1986:1105–209.

Chapter 19
Barry E. Gidal & Nina M. Graves

Valproic Acid
(AHFS 28:12.92)

Usual Dosage Range in Absence of Clearance-Altering Factors

Valproic acid is a carboxylic acid-derivative anticonvulsant used in the management of partial and generalized seizures including absence, tonic-clonic, and myoclonic seizures. Valproic acid may be used as monotherapy or in combination with other antiepileptic drugs.

Valproic acid is available in two other salts, valproate sodium and divalproex sodium. Dosages of all salt forms are expressed in terms of valproic acid (mw = 144.2 g mol^{-1} $S = 1$).[1]

Dosage Form	Dosage (mean ± SD)[a]
Oral (capsules, tablets, and solution)	
Neonates (<4 weeks)[2]	19.8 mg/kg/day
Infants (4 weeks–<1 year)[2]	34.2 ± 14.4 mg/kg/day
Children	
1–<5 years	Not available
5–<10 years[3,4]	25 ± 9 mg/kg/day
10–<15 years[3]	17.6 ± 2.5 mg/kg/day
Adolescents (15–18 years)	Not available
Adults (18–<60 years)[5]	13 ± 5 mg/kg/day
Geriatrics (≥60 years)[6]	11 ± 4 mg/kg/day

[a]*Doses are for monotherapy to achieve mean Css$_{av}$ of 75 mg/L.*

Dosage Form Availability[1]

Dosage Form	Product
Valproic acid	
Oral capsules: 250 mg	Depakene
Divalproex sodium	
Oral capsules (coated particles): 125 mg	Depakote Sprinkle
Oral tablets (enteric coated, delayed release): 125, 250, and 500 mg	Depakote
Valproate sodium	
Valproate sodium Injection: 500 mg/5 ml	Depacon
Oral solution: 250 mg/5 ml	Depakene Syrup Valproic Acid Syrup

A rectal solution made with equal parts of valproate sodium solution and water also has been used.[7] Current administration guidelines suggest that intravenous valproic acid be administered slowly (maximum rate = 20 mg/min); however, faster rates of administration have been safely employed (3–6 mg/kg/min).[8] The parenteral formulation may be given intravenously only; intramuscular administration may result in tissue necrosis.

Bioavailability (*F*) of Dosage Forms

Valproic acid is almost completely (90–100%) absorbed.[6,9–11] The bioavailability of capsules and enteric-coated tablets is similar, although more variability apparently exists with the enteric-coated form.[12] The rate of absorption depends on the dosage form.

Depakene capsules and syrup are absorbed quickly. Depakote products, however, due to their coatings, result not only in improved GI tolerability but also in delayed absorption, thus resulting in a shift of the area under the serum concentration–time curve to the right.[11–14] Depakote tablets are not sustained release but rather are delayed release. Depakote Sprinkles do exhibit a sustained-release profile and may be better tolerated due to a decreased peak–trough variability.

The delay in Depakote absorption may be 1–6 hr, with no change in the extent of absorption. This delay is dependent on gastric-emptying time and gastric pH; the lag phase for absorption differs significantly between fed and fasted patients. For both regular and coated preparations, food decreases the rate of absorption but not its extent. The time to achieve peak concentrations may be delayed 3–8 hr. Once absorption starts, however, it is usually complete within 1–1.5 hr.[14]

General Pharmacokinetic Information

Clearance

Clearance depends primarily on the age of the patient and concomitant medications. The diurnal fluctuation in valproic acid concentration–time profiles is great.[15] Nighttime concentrations show little peak–trough variability following Depakote administration. Morning trough concentrations can be significantly lower or higher than the trough concentrations obtained during the day. The lower apparent oral clearance of valproic acid at higher concentrations may reflect either saturable protein binding or partial saturation of intrinsic clearance. It is not removed efficiently by hemodialysis (<20%).

Metabolism

Valproic acid is primarily eliminated by the liver, with no first-pass metabolism. Since valproic acid is a low extraction drug, clearance is independent of blood flow. Only 3–7% of a dose is excreted unchanged in the urine.

The metabolism of valproic acid in the liver is extensive. The three main metabolic pathways, in order of importance, are conjugation with glucuronic acid, β-oxidation, and Ω-oxidation.[12] Valproic acid–glucuronide accounts for approximately 60% of the recovered dose in the urine; valproic acid may competitively inhibit the metabolism of other drugs that form glucuronide conjugates. One of valproic acid's potentially hepatotoxic metabolites, 4-ene, may be produced in larger quantities in patients on concomitant enzyme inducers, leading, in part, to the higher hepatotoxicity seen in children on polytherapy.[16]

Protein binding

Valproic acid is 90–95% protein bound to albumin.[5,9,17,18] Its protein binding is saturable.[5,19,20] This effect may be magnified in patients with significant hypoalbuminemia.[21] Therefore, although unbound concentrations may increase proportionally with dose, total concentrations may exhibit curvilinear kinetics (i.e., less than proportional increases in concentrations with dose changes).[22] The free fraction fluctuates more than the total concentrations due to fluctuations in free fatty acid concentrations in the morning and diurnal differences in unbound concentrations and total clearance.[5,23]

Valproic acid distributes into breast milk, with a plasma–milk ratio of about 5.1 ± 2.7%, approximately equal to the unbound valproic acid concentration.[24]

Clearance (CL)

The following clearance values can be assumed in the absence of disease or drug interactions when valproic acid is used in monotherapy.

Age	Multiple-Dose Clearance (mean ± SD)
Neonates (<4 weeks)[2,50]	0.011–0.018 L/hr/kg
Infants (4 weeks –<1 year)[2,25,26]	0.019 ± 0.008 L/hr/kg
Children (3–16 years)[3,25,27]	0.018 ± 0.006 L/hr/kg
Adults (18–<60 years)[5,28]	0.009 ± 0.005 L/hr/kg
Geriatrics (>60 years)[12,29]	0.007 ± 0.005 L/hr/kg

Volume of Distribution (V)

The following volume of distribution values can be assumed in the absence of disease or drug interactions when valproic acid is used in monotherapy.

Age	Single-Dose Volume (mean ± SD)	Multiple-Dose Volume (mean ± SD)
Neonates (<4 weeks)[2]	0.28 L/kg	Not available
Infants (4 weeks–<1 year)[25,26]	Not available	0.32 L/kg
Children (3–16 years)[3,19,27]	Not available	0.22 ± 0.05 L/kg
Adults (18–<60 years)[5,28]	0.12 ± 0.028 L/kg	0.15 ± 0.10 L/kg
Geriatrics (≥60 years)[30]	0.16 ± 0.02 L/kg	Not available

Half-Life and Time to Steady State

The following half-life ($t\frac{1}{2}$) values can be assumed in the absence of disease or drug interactions when valproic acid is used in monotherapy. Steady-state values are based on five half-lives.

Age	Half-Life (mean ± SD)
Neonates (<4 weeks)[2]	17.2 hr
Infants (4 weeks–<1 year)[2,26]	12.5 ± 2.8 hr
Children (3–16 years)[3,4,27,31]	11 ± 4 hr
Adults (18–<60 years)[5,28]	11.9 ± 5.7 hr
Geriatrics (≥60 years)[30]	15.3 ± 1.7 hr

Therapeutic Range

Response to valproic acid is highly variable and dependent on the type and severity of seizure and an individual's pharmacokinetic parameters. Various seizure disorders or epileptic syndromes may require higher or lower average concentrations.

In general, studies correlating valproic acid concentrations with clinical response have found that 40–50 mg/L is the minimum effective concentration for optimal seizure control. Seizure control tends to improve as the serum concentration increases from 40 to 120 mg/L. Monotherapy trials suggest that higher concentrations (>80 mg/L) may be more effective than lower concentrations in treating complex-partial seizures.[32] Whether a different optimal or therapeutic concentration range exists for conditions such as migraine headache or bipolar-effective disorder has not been established firmly. In addition, seizure control may improve with prolonged therapy, independent of changes in serum concentrations.

Some patients may benefit from trough concentrations greater than 120 mg/L without adverse effects. However, the incidence of adverse effects such as tremor and thrombocytopenia may increase at higher concentrations.[33] Increased CNS toxicity is generally seen with 175–200 mg/L concentrations. An unbound valproic acid concentration range has likewise not been established, although, in some cases, markedly elevated unbound concentrations have been associated with neurotoxicity. Determination of unbound valproic acid concentrations should be considered in patients with hypoalbuminemia.[21]

Typical adverse events include tremor, weight gain, hair loss, hyperammonemia, GI distress, and decreased cognitive functioning.[16] Patients with these reactions must be followed closely. Adverse reactions associated with elevated concentrations of valproic acid, such as thrombocytopenia and platelet dysfunction, may not be readily detectable by patient histories or physical assessment. Thus, potentially toxic concentrations may be present but not apparent.

Effect of age
　　Elderly patients may display an increased free fraction as a result of lower serum albumin concentrations. Elderly patients have been observed to have a reduced unbound clearance (~40%) as compared to younger subjects.[29]

Dosing
　　The recommended starting dose for valproic acid is 15 mg/kg/day, typically given as a starting dose of 250 mg once or twice daily. Dosage is gradually titrated upward (5–10 mg/kg/day) every 3–5 days. Eventual maintenance dosage depends upon concomitant medications and, most importantly, clinical response (efficacy versus toxicity). Maintenance dosages typically range between 15 and 60 mg/kg/day. Oral loading doses of valproic acid may produce unacceptable GI side effects. Loading doses of intravenous valproic acid of 25 mg/kg have been reported to result in peak concentrations of 100–200 mg/L.[8]

Suggested Sampling Times and Effect on Therapeutic Range

Timing of sample collections
　　To determine the trough value, valproic acid concentrations should be obtained prior to a morning dose, as these are the most consistent day-to-day values. Determination of peak concentrations is not typically employed. Timing of the peak concentration depends on the dosage form and the circumstances under which valproic acid is ingested. The absorption of Depakote is highly dependent on administration in the fed or fasted state.[14] Depakene potentially produces large differences between peak and trough concentrations.
　　The diurnal fluctuation in valproic acid concentration–time profiles is great.[15] Nighttime concentrations show little peak–trough variability following Depakote

administration. Morning trough concentrations can be significantly lower or higher than the trough concentrations obtained during the day.

Resampling guidelines

Valproic acid concentrations should be obtained 3–5 days after any change in dosage or dosing interval. Other indications for monitoring serum concentrations include signs of toxicity, decreased seizure control, addition or withdrawal of other antiepileptic or interacting drugs, and suspected noncompliance.

Initial monitoring guidelines

Since valproic acid clearance at low concentrations may be significantly different than at higher steady-state concentrations, valproic acid concentrations generally should not be determined following the first dose.[14] This difference is probably due to an increase in the free fraction as the valproic acid concentration increases. The most cost-efficient strategy involves achieving steady-state conditions before determining valproic acid concentrations.

Dosage adjustment

The simplest approach to dosage adjustment is based on the measurement of a trough concentration at steady state during a dosing interval. Once this concentration is determined, valproic acid dosages may be adjusted by a desired proportion. One must keep in mind that as concentrations increase, a curvilinear relationship between total concentration and dose is observed. Thus, at higher concentrations, any given increase in the valproic acid dose results in proportional increases in the unbound concentration but *less than* proportional increases in the total serum concentration. Therefore, a given total concentration may represent an unexpected degree of response or toxicity.

Pharmacodynamic Monitoring— Concentration-Related Efficacy

Efficacy of valproic acid therapy is judged by a decrease in seizure activity. It may take several days to more than 1 week to achieve the full therapeutic effect at a given serum concentration.[1] Little clinical or animal data exist to indicate specific synergistic or antagonistic pharmacodynamic interactions with other agents.

Pharmacodynamic Monitoring— Concentration-Related Toxicity

The more common dose-related adverse effects of valproic acid therapy are GI in nature (e.g., nausea, vomiting, and diarrhea). Although hepatotoxicity also has been reported in patients receiving valproic acid, a clear dose relationship is not established. Severe hepatotoxicity may be preceded by nonspecific symptoms such as loss of seizure control, malaise, and weakness.[1] Thrombocytopenia, platelet aggregation defects, and tremor also appear to be concentration related. Evidence from clinical trials with the antiepileptic drug lamotrigine do suggest that pharmacodynamic interactions between this agent and valproic acid exist and may lead to an increased incidence of tremor and rash.

Drug–Drug Interactions[4,25,34–37]

Pharmacokinetic interactions with valproic acid are common and clinically important. Valproic acid is an enzyme inhibitor and is subject to enzyme induction. The concomitant administration of drugs that utilize enzyme metabolism may affect the actions of these drugs and of valproic acid.

For example, valproic acid decreases the elimination of *carbamazepine* epoxide,[38–41] (via inhibition of epoxide hydrolase) *phenobarbital* (30–50%),[42,43] and *ethosux-*

imide.[44] Because of protein binding displacement, *phenytoin* total concentrations can decline during comedication with valproic acid, while unbound concentrations can increase secondary to inhibition of intrinsic clearance. Clearance of *lamotrigine* is also markedly inhibited by valproic acid, resulting in significant prolongations in lamotrigine $t\frac{1}{2}$.[45] The combination of valproic acid and lamotrigine increases the risk for potentially serious rash. The mechanism for this apparent interaction is still unknown. Valproic acid also significantly reduces the clearance of *lorazepam*.[46] These interactions are presumably mediated via inhibition of glucuronyl transferase. These effects can lead to clinically significant increases in serum concentrations of these compounds, with possible associated clinical toxicity. Enzyme inducers such as *rifampin*, phenytoin, carbamazepine, *primidone*, and phenobarbital increase the elimination of valproic acid, often requiring higher doses.[31,38,47,48]

Co-administration of *felbamate* can reduce valproic acid clearance, possibly via inhibition of beta-oxidation. Through a similar mechanism, *aspirin* may also inhibit valproic acid metabolism.[49] *Cimetidine* and *ranitidine* do not affect the clearance of valproic acid. Caution also should be used when administering valproic acid concomitantly with *CNS depressants*, other *anticonvulsants, monoamine oxidase inhibitors*, and *anticoagulants*. Valproic acid does not appear to alter the pharmacokinetics of *oral contraceptive agents*.

Drug–Disease State or Condition Interactions

In both *hepatic disease* and *renal impairment*, an increase in the volume of distribution and free fraction can be expected. With hepatic cirrhosis, the free fraction increases to 29%; in renal failure, the free fraction increases to 18%.[7,50] There is also a reported increase in the free fraction of approximately 10% during the last 2–3 weeks of *pregnancy*.[51] *Head trauma* can also transiently increase valproic acid free fraction and total clearance.[52]

References

1. Valproate sodium. In: McEvoy GK, ed. AHFS drug information 2000. Bethesda, MD: American Society of Hospital Pharmacists; 2000; 2001–7.
2. Irvine-Meek JM, Hall KW, Otten NH, et al. Pharmacokinetic study of valproic acid in a neonate. *Pediatr Pharmacol*. 1982; 2:317–21.
3. Chiba K, Suganuma T, Ishizaki T, et al. Comparison of steady-state pharmacokinetics of valproic acid in children between monotherapy and multiple antiepileptic drug treatment. *J Pediatr*. 1985; 106:653.
4. Cloyd JC, Kriel RL, Fischer JH. Valproic acid pharmacokinetics in children. II. Discontinuation of concomitant antiepileptic drug therapy. *Neurology*. 1985; 35:1623–7.
5. Bowdle TA, Patel IH, Levy RH, et al. Valproic acid dosage and plasma protein binding and clearance. *Clin Pharmacol Ther*. 1980; 28:486–92.
6. Perucca E, Gatti G, Frigo GM, et al. Pharmacokinetics of valproic acid after oral and intravenous administration. *Br J Clin Pharmacol*. 1978; 5:313–8.
7. Holle L, Gidal BE, Collins DM. Valproate in status epilepticus. *Ann Pharmacother*. 1995; 29:1042–4.
8. Venkataraman V, Wheless JW. Safety of rapid intravenous infusion of valproate loading doses in epilepsy patients. *Epilepsy Res*. 1999 (in press).
9. Klotz U, Antonin KG. Pharmacokinetics and bioavailability of sodium valproate. *Clin Pharmacol Ther*. 1977; 21:736–43.
10. Chun AHC, Hoffman DJ, Friedmann N, et al. Bioavailability of valproic acid under fasting/nonfasting regimens. *J Clin Pharmacol*. 1980; 20:30–6.
11. Wilder BJ, Karas BJ, Hammond EJ, et al. Twice daily dosing of valproate with divalproex. *Clin Pharmacol Ther*. 1983; 34:501–4.
12. Baillie TA, Sheffels PR. Valproic acid. Chemistry and biotransformation. In: Antiepileptic drugs, 4th ed. Levy RH, Mattson RH, Meldrum BS, eds. New York, NY: Raven Press; 1995:589–604.
13. Levy RH, Cenraud B, Loiseau P, et al. Meal-dependent absorption of enteric coated sodium valproate. *Epilepsia*. 1980; 21:273–80.
14. Fischer JH, Barr AN, Paloucek FP, et al. Effect of food on the serum concentration profile of enteric-coated valproic acid. *Neurology*. 1988; 38(8):1319–22.
15. Riva R, Albani F, Franzoni E, et al. Valproic acid free fraction in epileptic children under chronic monotherapy. *Ther Drug Monit*. 1983; 5:197–200.
16. Dreifuss FE. Valproate: toxicity. In: Levy RH, Dreifuss FE, Mattson RH, et al., eds. Antiepileptic drugs, 4th ed. New York: Raven Press; 1995; 641–8.
17. Gugler R, Schell A, Eichelbaum M, et al. Disposition of valproic acid in man. *Eur J Clin Pharmacol*. 1977; 12:125–32.

18. Patel IH, Levy RH. Valproic acid binding to human serum albumin and determination of free fraction in presence of antiepileptics and free fatty acids. *Epilepsia*. 1979; 20:85–90.
19. Otten N, Hall K, Irvine-Meek J, et al. Free valproic acid: steady-state pharmacokinetics in patients with intractable epilepsy. *Can J Neurol Sci*. 1984; 11:457–60.
20. Cramer JA, Mattson RH. Valproic acid: in vitro plasma protein binding and interactions with phenytoin. *Ther Drug Monit*. 1979; 1:105–16.
21. Gidal BE, Collins DM, Deinlich B. Valproic acid neurotoxicity in a hypoalbuminemic patient. *Ann Pharmacother*. 1993; 27:32–4.
22. Gidal BE, Maly MM, Spencer NM, et al. Relationship between valproic acid dosage, plasma concentration and clearance in adult monotherapy patients with epilepsy. *J Clin Pharm Ther* 1995; 20:215–9.
23. Bauer LA, Davis R, Wilensky A, et al. Diurnal variation in valproic acid clearance. *Clin Pharmacol Ther*. 1984; 35:505–9.
24. von Unruh GE, Froescher W, Hoffmann F, et al. Valproic acid in breast milk: how much is really there? *Ther Drug Monit*. 1984; 6:272–6.
25. Hall K, Otten N, Irvine-Meek J, et al. First dose and steady state pharmacokinetics of valproic acid in children with seizures. *Clin Pharmacokinet*. 1983; 8:447–55.
26. Herngren L, Lundberg B, Negardh A. Pharmacokinetics of total and free valproic acid during monotherapy in infants. *J Neurol*. 1991; 238:315–9.
27. Cloyd JC, Fischer JH, Kriel RL, et al. Valproic acid pharmacokinetics in children. IV. Effects of age and antiepileptic drugs on protein binding and intrinsic clearance. *Clin Pharmacol Ther*. 1993; 53:22–9.
28. Herngren L, Negardh A. Pharmacokinetics of free and total sodium valproate in adolescents and young adults during maintenance therapy. *J Neurol*. 1988; 235:491–5.
29. Bauer LA, Davis R, Wilensky A, et al. Valproic acid clearance: unbound fraction and diurnal variation in young and elderly adults. *Clin Pharmacol Ther*. 1985; 37:697–700.
30. Perucca E, Grimaldi R, Gatti G, et al. Pharmacokinetics of valproic acid in the elderly. *Br J Clin Pharmacol*. 1984; 17:665–9.
31. Cloyd JC, Kriel RL, Fischer JH, et al. Pharmacokinetics of valproic acid in children: I. Multiple antiepileptic drug therapy. *Neurology*. 1983; 33:185–91.
32. Beydoun A, Sackellares JC, Shu V. Safety and efficacy of divalproex sodium monotherapy in partial epilepsy: A double-blind, concentration-response design clinical trial. Depakote monotherapy for partial seizures study group. *Neurology*. 1997; 48:182–8.
33. Gidal BE, Spencer NW, Collins DM, et al. Valproate mediated disturbances of hemostasis: relationship to concentration and dose. *Neurology*. 1994; 44:1418–22.
34. May CA, Garnett WR, Small RE, et al. Effect of three antacids on the bioavailability of valproic acid *Clin Pharm*. 1982; 1:244–7.
35. Webster LK, Mihlay GW, Jones DB, et al. Effect of cimitidine and ranitidine on carbamazepine and sodium valproate pharmacokinetics. *Eur J Clin Pharmacol*. 1984; 27:341–3.

36. Goulden KJ, Dooley JM, Camfield PR, et al. Clinical valproate toxicity induced by acetylsalicylic acid. *Neurology.* 1987; 37:1392–4.
37. Orr JM, Abbott FS, Farrell K, et al. Interaction between valproic acid and aspirin in epileptic children: serum protein binding and metabolic effects. *Clin Pharmacol Ther.* 1982; 31:642–9.
38. Bowdle TA, Levy RH, Cutler RE. Effects of carbamazepine on valproic acid kinetics in normal subjects. *Clin Pharmacol Ther.* 1979; 26:629–34.
39. McKauge L, Tyrer JH, Eadie MJ. Factors influencing simultaneous concentrations of carbamazepine and its epoxide in plasma. *Ther Drug Monit.* 1981; 3:63–70.
40. Brodie MJ, Forrest G, Rapeport WG. Carbamazepine 10, 11 epoxide concentrations in epileptics on carbamazepine alone and in combination with other anticonvulsants. *Br J Clin Pharmacol.* 1983; 16:747–50.
41. Levy RH, Moreland TA, Moreselli PL, et al. Carbamazepine/valproic acid interaction in man and rhesus monkey. *Epilepsia.* 1984; 25:338–45.
42. Patel IH, Levy RH, Cutler RE. Phenobarbital–valproic acid interaction. *Clin Pharmacol Ther.* 1980; 27:515–21.
43. Suganuma T, Ishizaki T, Chiba K, et al. The effect of concurrent administration of valproate sodium on phenobarbital plasma concentration/dosage ratio in pediatric patients. *J. Pediatr.* 1981; 99:314–7.
44. Pisani F, Narbone MC, Trunfio C, et al. Valproic acid–ethosuximide interaction: a pharmacokinetic study. *Epilepsia.* 1984; 25:229–33.
45. Anderson GD, Yau MK, Gidal BE, et al. Bidirectional interaction of valproate and lamotrigine in healthy subjects. *Clin Pharmacol Ther.* 1996; 60:145–56.
46. Anderson GD, Gidal BE, Kantor ED, et al. Lorazepam-valproate interaction: Studies in normal subjects and isolated perfused rat liver. *Epilepsia.* 1994; 34:221–5.
47. Mihaly GW, Wajda FJ, Miler JL, et al. Single and chronic dose pharmacokinetic studies of sodium valproate in epileptic patients. *Eur J Pharmacol.* 1979; 15:23–9.
48. Cramer JA, Mattson RH, Bennett DM, et al. Variable free and total valproic acid concentrations in sole and multi drug therapy. *Ther Drug Monit.* 1986; 8:411–6.
49. Orr JM, Abbott FS, Farrell K, et al. Interaction between valproic acid and aspirin in epileptic patients: serum protein binding and metabolic effects. *Clin Pharmacol Ther.* 1982; 31:642–9.
50. Levy RH, Shen D. Valproic acid. Absorption, distribution and excretion. In: Antiepileptic drugs, 4th ed. Levy RH, Mattson RH, Meldrum BS, eds. New York, NY: Raven Press; 1995:605–19.
51. Riva R, Albani F, Contin M, et al. Mechanism of altered drug binding to serum proteins in pregnant women: studies with valproic acid. *Ther Drug Monit.* 1984; 6:25–30.
52. Anderson GD, Gidal BE, Hendryx RJ, et al. Decreased plasma protein binding of valproate in patients with acute head trauma. *Br J Clin Pharmacol.* 1994; 37:559–62.

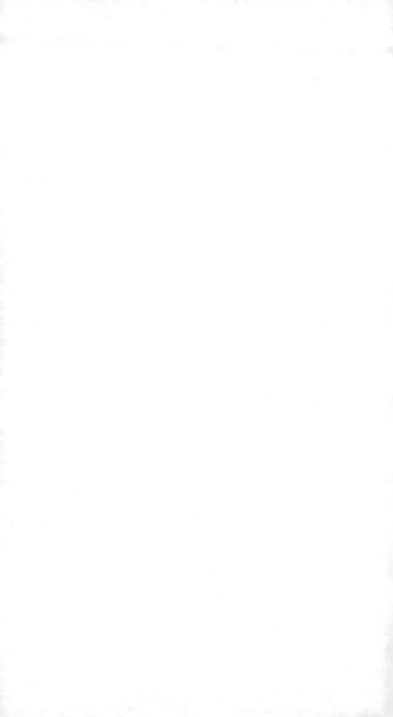

Chapter 20
Reginald F. Frye & Gary R. Matzke

Vancomycin (AHFS 8:12.28)

Usual Dosage Range in Absence of Clearance-Altering Factors

Vancomycin is a tricyclic glycopeptide antibiotic that is active against many gram-positive organisms. Vancomycin is used principally for the treatment of severe and/or resistant staphylococcal and enterococcal infections but may also be used for moderate infections in patients who may be allergic to first-line antibiotics (e.g., cephalosporins).

Dosage Form	Initial Dosage
Intravenous	
Premature neonates[1,2]	
<30 weeks PCA[a]	10 mg/kg/12–24 hr
30–34 weeks PCA[a], <1.2 kg	10 mg/kg/12 hr
30–42 weeks PCA[a], ≥1.2 kg	10 mg/kg/8 hr
>42 weeks PCA[a], >2 kg	10 mg/kg/6 hr
Full-term neonates[3-5]	
<1 week	10–15 mg/kg/12 hr
≥1 week–<1 month	10–15 mg/kg/8 hr
Infants and children[4] (≥1 month–<16 years)	10–15 mg/kg/6 hr
Adults[4] (≥16–<65 years)	15 mg/kg/12 hr
Geriatrics[4] (≥65 years)	10–15 mg/kg/12–24 hr

Oral[4] (for treatment of pseudomembranous
colitis only)
  Children (<20 kg and ≥1–<16 years)   12.5 mg/kg/6 hr
  Adults (≥16–<65 years)   125–250 mg/6 hr

Intrathecal[4]
  Neonates, infants, and children   5–10 mg/day
    (<16 years)
  Adults (≥16–<65 years)   10–20 mg/day

[a] *PCA = Postconceptional age: the sum of the gestational age at birth and chronological age.*

Dosage Form Availability[6]

Dosage Form	Product
Powder for intravenous injection: 500 mg and 1, 5, and 10 g per vial	Vancocin Vancoled Vancomycin HCl
Oral capsules: 125 and 250 mg	Vancocin HCl
Powder for oral solution: 1 and 10 g	Vancocin HCl

Bioavailability (F) of Dosage Forms

Dosage Form	Bioavailability Comments
Intravenous	100%. Not recommended for intramuscular use
Oral capsules and powder	<5% but significant oral absorption was demonstrated in patients with pseudomembranous colitis or severe renal failure.[7] Serum concentrations in the therapeutic range were observed in these patients, so periodic monitoring should be considered, especially for patients receiving >2 g/day for ≥10 days.

General Pharmacokinetic Information

Disposition

The disposition of vancomycin is best characterized by a two- or three-compartment pharmacokinetic model. In the three-compartment model, the half-life of the initial phase is approximately 7 min and that of the second phase is approximately 0.5–1 hr; the terminal elimination half-life ranges from 3 to 9 hr in adults with normal renal function. Approximately 80–90% of the intravenously administered dose is recovered unchanged in the urine of adult patients with normal to moderately impaired renal function.[7]

Elimination
Since elimination is primarily via glomerular filtration, dosage adjustment is necessary for disease- and age-related alterations in renal function. Although some nonrenal clearance of vancomycin may occur, it does not warrant any alteration of vancomycin dosage in patients with hepatic impairment (having normal renal function).

Fraction excreted unchanged	80–90%
Fraction nonrenally excreted	<5%
Active and inactive metabolites	None
Protein binding	30–55%

Protein binding
The proportion of vancomycin bound to plasma proteins averages between 30 and 55% and is dependent on the patient's albumin concentration. In patients with reduced albumin concentrations, the protein binding is lower. For example, in end-stage renal disease and burn patients, the mean protein binding is 19 and 29%, respectively.[8,9]

Clearance (CL)

Age	Clearance (mean ± SD)
Premature neonates[1]	
<30 weeks PCA[a]	Not available
30–34 weeks PCA[a], <1.2 kg	0.043 ± 0.014 L/hr/kg
30–42 weeks PCA[a], ≥1.2 kg	0.095 ± 0.039 L/hr/kg
>42 weeks PCA[a], >2 kg	0.169 ± 0.051 L/hr/kg
Full-term neonates[3]	1.80 L/hr/1.73 m²

Infants[3] (≥1 month–<1 year)	3.47 ± 0.83 L/hr/1.73 m²
Children[3] (≥1–<16 years)	8.45 ± 0.85 L/hr/1.73 m²
Adults[10–16] (≥16–<65 years)	0.073 ± 0.025 L/hr/kg
Geriatrics[10] (≥65 years)	0.053 ± 0.0034 L/hr/kg

[a]*PCA = Postconceptional age: the sum of the gestational age at birth and chronological age.*

In neonates and infants, several equations have been developed that relate vancomycin clearance to patient-specific variables including postconceptional age, body weight, and CrCl.[17] One such equation is

$$CL_{Vanc} \text{ (L/hr/kg)} = [(0.411 \times CrCl) + 0.541] \times 0.06$$

where CrCl is in milliliters per minute.

Numerous investigators have evaluated the relationship between vancomycin clearance and CrCl in adult patients, and several regression equations are available for predictive purposes.[10,13,14,18] The following equation was determined using a one-compartment pharmacokinetic model:[18]

$$CL_{Vanc} \text{ (L/hr)} = [0.711(CrCl) + 18.9] \times 0.06$$

where CrCl is in milliliters per minute.

Such equations should be used with caution in patients with significantly impaired renal function due to the unpredictable nonrenal clearance component (intercept term).

Volume of Distribution (*V*)

Age	Volume[a] (mean ± SD)
Premature neonates[1]	
<30 weeks PCA[b]	Not available
30–34 weeks PCA[b], <1.2 kg	0.47 ± 0.21 L/kg
30–42 weeks PCA[b], ≥1.2 kg	0.48 ± 0.13 L/kg
>42 weeks PCA[b], >2 kg	0.47 ± 0.06 L/kg
Full-term neonates[3]	0.69 L/kg
Infants[3] (≥1 month–<1 year)	0.69 ± 0.17 L/kg

Children[3] (≥1–<16 years)	0.70 ± 0.12 L/kg
Adults[10-16] (≥16–<65 years)	0.62 ± 0.15 L/kg
Obese adults (>30% over IBW)[c]	0.56 ± 0.18 L/kg
Geriatrics[10] (≥65 years)	0.76 ± 0.06 L/kg

[a]Total body weight.
[b]PCA = Postconceptional age: the sum of the gestational age at birth and chronological age.
[c]IBW = Ideal body weight.

Half-Life and Time to Steady State

Age	Half-Life (mean ± SD)	Time to Steady State
Premature neonates[1]		
<30 weeks PCA[a]	Not available	Not available
30–34 weeks PCA[a], <1.2 kg	7.8 ± 3.0 hr	23–39 hr
30–42 weeks PCA[a], ≥1.2 kg	3.8 ± 1.4 hr	11–19 hr
>42 weeks PCA[a], >2 kg	2.1 ± 0.8 hr	6–11 hr
Full-term neonates[3]	6.7 hr	20–34 hr
Infants[3] (≥1 month–<1 year)	4.1 hr	12–21 hr
Children[3] (≥1–<16 years)	2.6 ± 0.4 hr	8–13 hr
Adults[10-16] (≥16–<65 years)	7.0 ± 1.5 hr	21–35 hr
Geriatrics[10] (≥65 years)	12.1 ± 0.8 hr	36–61 hr

[a]PCA = Postconceptional age: the sum of the gestational age at birth and chronological age.

The elimination rate constant (K) of vancomycin can be predicted from the observed relationship with CrCl in adult patients with reduced renal function (CrCl <50 ml/min), as determined by numerous investigators. The following regression equation approximates the mean of the reported values and was determined using a one-compartment pharmacokinetic model:[13]

$$K = 0.00083 \, (CrCl) + 0.0044$$

where CrCl is in milliliters per minute.

Therapeutic Range

Sampling Time	Therapeutic Range
Peak	Not applicable
Trough (≤1 hr before next dose)	5–15 mg/L[a] or 5–20 mg/L[b]

[a] *Conventional treatment*
[b] *Alternative range when no other nephrotoxins are present.*

Suggested Sampling Times and Effect on Therapeutic Range

Because no clear relationship between serum concentrations and therapeutic response is evident, vancomycin concentration monitoring remains controversial. Peak concentrations reported in the literature are often confounded by the timing of the blood sample relative to the end of the infusion and vancomycin's two-compartment pharmacokinetics. Conventional vancomycin therapy based on achieving peak concentrations of 30–40 mg/L and trough concentrations of less than 10 mg/L was based on empirical rather than scientific evidence.

Vancomycin exhibits concentration-independent killing. Time above the minimum inhibitory concentration (MIC) (≤4 mg/L) is a critical determinant of therapeutic efficacy. For patients with stable renal function, obtaining a "trough" concentration after 5 or more days of therapy is adequate monitoring, if therapy is to be continued.[19] If the measured trough concentration is within 20% of the desired trough concentration, the patient may remain on the same regimen. If the concentration is not within the desired range, the dosing regimen should be adjusted accordingly.

Vancomycin concentration monitoring may be necessary for certain patient groups, including patients with fluctuating renal function, patients receiving concurrent treatment with known nephrotoxins (e.g., aminoglycosides or furosemide), patients requiring higher than usual doses (>4 g/day), obese patients, patients receiving dialysis, and pediatric patients (especially premature neonates).[19,20] Vancomycin pharmacokinetics are unpredictable in these patient groups, so obtaining concentrations early in therapy is needed to ensure that vancomycin concentrations are therapeutic (above MIC). A "peak" concentration obtained 1.5–2.5 hr after a 1-hr infusion and a "trough" drawn within 1 hr of the next scheduled dose are adequate. Due to variability in vancomycin removal by dialysis with biocompatible membranes (noncellulose-based filters such as polysulfone and polymethylmethacrylate), an additional sample should be obtained at least 1 hr after the end of dialysis, which allows for vancomycin redistribution from tissues. The concentration values should be used to re-estimate the patient's pharmacokinetic parameter values, which can then be used to modify the dosage regimen to achieve desired concentrations.[7]

Vancomycin concentration sampling should be repeated if there is a change in renal function (increase or decrease in serum creatinine) or a lack of therapeutic response (despite sensitive organism).

Pharmacodynamic Monitoring—Concentration-Related Efficacy

Since no specific monitoring of pharmacodynamics is possible with vancomycin, the signs and symptoms of infection should be used to assess its efficacy. The patient's temperature and white blood cell count should be monitored daily for return to normal, and blood cultures should be repeated every 3 days until negative. The ratio of the minimal bacteriocidal concentration (MBC) to the MIC can be used to monitor or predict the response to therapy; an MBC:MIC ratio of greater than 32 is associated with poor therapeutic response.[21] The MBC should not be determined routinely. However, in patients who are not responding to therapy or who have a serious infection (e.g., endocarditis and osteomyelitis), its determination may be warranted.

Pharmacodynamic Monitoring—Concentration-Related Toxicity

Concentration-related toxicities

Although ototoxicity and nephrotoxicity are associated with vancomycin therapy, the incidence is generally less than 2% and less than 5%, respectively. A causal relationship between attainment of peak concentrations of 25–50 mg/L and/or trough concentrations of 13–32 mg/L and ototoxicity has been reported. Nephrotoxicity is associated with trough concentrations of greater than or equal to 10 mg/L.[22,23] Relating ototoxicity and nephrotoxicity to specific concentration values or a range of values is difficult, however, because most reports do not specify when the samples were taken after a dose.

Early adjustment of vancomycin dosage to produce concentrations in the recommended therapeutic range should minimize these toxicities.[7,12] Serum creatinine should be monitored every 3 days for patients with stable renal function or daily if the patient is renally unstable or is receiving other nephrotoxic agents (e.g., aminoglycosides, loop diuretics, and amphotericin B).

Nonconcentration-related toxicities

Intravenous administration of vancomycin may result in a histamine-like reaction characterized by flushing, tingling, pruritus, tachycardia, and an erythematous macular rash involving the face, neck, upper trunk, back, and arms. This adverse effect is often referred to as "red neck syndrome." Systemic arterial hypotension or shock also may occur. This syndrome usually can be avoided by infusion of vancomycin at 15 mg/min or less or by pretreatment with an antihistamine.

Eosinophilia, neutropenia, urticarial rashes, and drug fever also have been reported.[6,7]

Drug–Drug Interactions

No pharmacokinetic drug interactions have been reported with vancomycin. However, its concomitant use with other ototoxic and nephrotoxic drugs may increase the incidence of these toxicities. Data from several investigations suggest that vancomycin has some potential for causing nephrotoxicity, with the incidence ranging from 5 to 15%. When vancomycin was administered concomitantly with an *aminoglycoside* to adults, the incidence of nephrotoxicity increased in some—but not all—studies (range of 22–35%).[7,24]

Concurrent use of a *loop diuretic* (e.g., furosemide) was associated with a fivefold increase in the risk of developing nephrotoxicity; the risk may be greatest in individuals over 60 years of age.[25] In addition, *amphotericin B* was shown to increase the risk of nephrotoxicity by 6.7-fold.[25]

There is evidence to suggest that the elimination half-life of vancomycin is prolonged in neonates receiving *indomethacin* (for patent ductus arteriosus). Thus, an empiric increase in the vancomycin dosing interval and concentration monitoring may be warranted.[17]

Drug–Disease State Interactions

Patients with *thermal injuries* require higher doses of vancomycin to achieve similar target concentrations.[16,27] The total body clearance and renal clearance in these patients are highly correlated with CrCl,[26,27] and the increase in clearance appears to be due to a significant nonrenal component, as well as enhanced net tubular secretion.[27] The volume of distribution is unaltered.

Hepatic insufficiency and *critical illness* have not been associated with any alteration in the elimination of vancomycin. The degree of protein binding, however, is reduced (to approximately 20%) and the unbound V increases by approximately 8%.[28] Vancomycin therapy should be guided in these patients on the basis of their residual renal function (CrCl) and volume status.

The impact of *acute renal failure* on the disposition of vancomycin is dependent on the severity and acuity of the insult. Since the nonrenal clearance of 0.96–1.2 L/hr is preserved for up to 7–10 days after injury,[29] the standard relationship between CrCl and CL_{Vanc} can be used to project the degree of dosage adjustment if the patient is not receiving dialysis. Patients who are receiving intermittent hemodialysis with a biocompatible dialyzer or continuous renal replacement therapy[30,31] require higher dosage regimens since vancomycin clearance is significantly enhanced. Furthermore, if the drug is given during hemodialysis the dosage may need to be increased further due to the enhanced rate of removal.[32,33]

Vancomycin use in *chronic hemodialysis* patients is complicated by the near absence of nonrenal clearance (residual of 0–0.24 L/hr) and the impact of the hemodialysis procedure. The dialytic clearance is dependent on the dialyzer membrane and the rate of blood flow through it.[33–39] The intradialytic clearance and $t½$ of vancomycin observed in chronic hemodialysis patients for commonly utilized dialyzers are

Dialyzer	CL (L/hr)	$t½$
Cuprophane[35]	0.3–1	35.1
Polysulfone F-40[35]	2.7	11.8
Polysulfone F-60[35]	4.4	6.7
Polysulfone F-80[33,35,37]	5.1–8.8	3.3–4.5
CT-190, Baxter[38]	6	4.5
PMMA, Toray, BK-2.1U[39]	3.6–7.9	3.7–8.0
AN69, Hospal Filteral 16[34]	3.2–4.3	6.1–7
PMMA, Toray B3-2.0A[39]	4.3–6.4	4.5–7

References

1. Lisby-Sutch SM, Nahata MC. Dosage guidelines for the use of vancomycin based on its pharmacokinetics in infants. *Eur J Clin Pharmacol*. 1988; 35(6):637–42.
2. Gabriel MH, Kildoo GC, Gennrich JL, et al. Prospective evaluation of a vancomycin dosage guideline for neonates. *Clin Pharm*. 1991; 10(2):129–32.
3. Schaad UB, McCracken GH, Nelson JD. Clinical pharmacology and efficacy of vancomycin in pediatric patients. *J Pediatr*. 1980; 96(1):119–26.
4. Miscellaneous antibacterial drugs. In: Bennett DR, ed. Drug evaluations. Chicago, IL: American Medical Association; 1992:4.
5. Sanford JP. Guide to antimicrobial therapy 1992. Dallas, TX: Antimicrobial Therapy Inc.; 1992:103.
6. Vancomycin. In: Facts and comparisons. St. Louis, MO: J.B. Lippincott Co.; 1999:2372.
7. Matzke GR. Vancomycin. In: Applied pharmacokinetics: principles of therapeutic drug monitoring. Spokane, WA: Applied Therapeutics; 1992:15-1–31.
8. Tan CC, Lee HS, Ty TL, et al. Pharmacokinetics of intravenous vancomycin in patients with end-stage renal failure. *Ther Drug Monit*. 1990; 12:29.
9. Zokufa HZ, Solem LD, Rodvold KA, et al. The influence of serum albumin and alpha1-acid glycoprotein on vancomycin protein binding in patients with burn injuries. *J Burn Care Rehabil*. 1989; 10:425–8.
10. Cutler NR, Narang PK, Lesko LJ, et al. Vancomycin disposition: the importance of age. *Clin Pharmacol Ther*. 1984; 36:803–10.
11. Golper TA, Noonan HM, Elzinga L, et al. Vancomycin pharmacokinetics, renal handling, and nonrenal clearances in normal human subjects. *Clin Pharmacol Ther*. 1988; 43:565–70.
12. Healy DP, Polk RE, Garson ML, et al. Comparison of steady-state pharmacokinetics of two dosage regimens of vancomycin in normal volunteers. *Antimicrob Agents Chemother*. 1987; 31:393–7.
13. Matzke GR, McGory RW, Halstenson CE, et al. Pharmacokinetics of vancomycin in patients with various degrees of renal function. *Antimicrob Agents Chemother*. 1984; 25:433–7.
14. Rodvold KA, Blum RA, Fischer JH, et al. Vancomycin pharmacokinetics in patients with various degrees of renal function. *Antimicrob Agents Chemother*. 1988; 32:848–52.
15. Hurst KA, Yoshinaga MA, Mitani GH, et al. Application of a Bayesian method to monitor and adjust vancomycin dosage regimens. *Antimicrob Agents Chemother*. 1990; 34:1165–71.
16. Garrelts JC, Peterie JD. Altered vancomycin dose vs. serum concentration relationship in burn patients. *Clin Pharmacol Ther*. 1988; 44:9–13.
17. Rodvold KA, Everett JA, Pryka RD, et al. Pharmacokinetics and administration regimens of vancomycin in neonates, infants and children. *Clin Pharmacokinet*. 1997; 33(1):32–51.
18. Ducharme MP, Slaughter RL, Edwards DJ. Vancomycin pharmacokinetics in a patient population: effect of age, gender, and body weight. *Ther Drug Monit*. 1994; 16(5):513–8.

19. Karam CM, McKinnon PS, Neuhauser MM, et al. Outcome assessment of minimizing vancomycin monitoring and dosing adjustments. *Pharmacother*. 1999; 19(3):257–66.
20. Miles MV, Li L, Lakkis H, et al. Special considerations for monitoring vancomycin concentrations in pediatric patients. *Ther Drug Monitor*. 1997; 19(3):265–70.
21. Sorrell TC, Packham DR, Shanker S, et al. Vancomycin therapy for methicillin-resistant *Staphylococcus aureus*. *Ann Intern Med*. 1982; 97:344–50.
22. Cimino MA, Rotstein C, Slaughter RL, et al. Relationship of serum antibiotic concentrations to nephrotoxicity in cancer patients receiving concurrent aminoglycoside and vancomycin therapy. *Am J Med*. 1987; 83:1091–7.
23. Rybak MJ, Albrecht LM, Boike SC, et al. Nephrotoxicity of vancomycin, alone and with an aminoglycoside. *J Antimicrob Chemother*. 1990; 25:679–87.
24. Farber BF, Moellering RC. Retrospective study of the toxicity of preparations of vancomycin from 1974 to 1981. *Antimicrob Agents Chemother*. 1983; 23:138–41.
25. Vance-Bryan K, Rotschafer JC, Gilliland SS, et al. A comparative assessment of vancomycin-associated nephrotoxicity in the young versus the elderly hospitalized patient. *J Antimicrob Chemother*. 1994; 33(4):811–21.
26. Brater DC, Bawdon RE, Anderson SA, et al. Vancomycin elimination in patients with burn injury. *Clin Pharmacol Ther*. 1986; 39(6):631–4.
27. Rybak MJ, Albrecht LM, Berman JR, et al. Vancomycin pharmacokinetics in burn patients and intravenous drug abusers. *Antimicrob Agents Chemother*. 1990; 34(5):792–5.
28. Li L, Miles MV, Lakkis H, et al. Vancomycin-binding characteristics in patients with serious infections. *Pharmacother*. 1996; 16(6):1024–9.
29. Macias WL, Mueller BA, Scarim SK. Vancomycin pharmacokinetics in acute renal failure: preservation of non-renal clearance. *Clin Pharmacol Ther*. 1991; 50:688–94.
30. Joy MS, Matzke GR, Frye RF, et al. Determinants of vancomycin clearance by continuous venovenous hemofiltration and continuous venovenous hemodialysis. *Am J Kidney Dis*. 1998; 31(6):1019–27.
31. Joy MS, Matzke GR, Armstrong DA, et al. A primer on continuous renal replacement therapy for critically ill patients. *Ann Pharmacother*. 1998; 32:362–75.
32. Scott MK, Macias WL, Kraus MA, et al. Effects of dialysis membrane on intradialytic vancomycin administration. *Pharmacother*. 1997; 17(2):256–62.
33. Foote EF, Dreitlein WB, Steward CA, et al. Pharmacokinetics of vancomycin when administered during high flux hemodialysis. *Clin Nephrol*. 1998; 50(1):51–5.
34. Barth RH, DeVincenzo N. Use of vancomycin in high-flux hemodialysis: Experience with 130 courses of therapy. *Kidney Int*. 1996; 50:929–36.
35. Lanese DM, Alfrey PS, Molitoris BA. Markedly increased clearance of vancomycin during hemodialysis using polysulfone dialyzers. *Kidney Int*. 1989; 35:1409–12.

36. Schaedeli F, Uehlinger DE. Urea kinetics and dialysis treatment time predict vancomycin elimination during high-flux hemodialysis. *Clin Pharmacol Ther*. 1998; 63:26–38.

37. Pollard TA, Lampasona V, Akkerman S, et al. Vancomycin redistribution: dosing recommendations following high-flux hemodialysis. *Kidney Int*. 1994; 45(1):232–7.

38. Welage LS, Mason N, Hoffman EJ, et al. Influence of cellulose triacetate hemodialyzers on vancomycin pharmacokinetics. *J Am Soc Nephrol*. 1995; 6(4):1284–90.

39. Matzke GR, Frye RF, Nolin TD, et al. Vancomycin removal by low and high flux hemodialysis with polymethylmethacrylate dialyzers. *J Am Soc Nephrol*. 1999; 10:193A.

Chapter 21
Douglas F. Covey

Warfarin (AHFS 20:12.04)

Clinical trials have established warfarin sodium as the oral anticoagulant of choice since its discovery at the University of Wisconsin in 1948. Unfortunately, safe prescribing of warfarin is complicated by a narrow therapeutic range and a vast array of drug, disease, and dietary interactions. If not properly and respectfully utilized, this medication can lead to severe complications. Therefore, to minimize the morbidity and mortality associated with warfarin, a thorough working knowledge of this medication is essential.

Warfarin sodium and its derivatives are indirect-acting anticoagulants, active only in vivo. They inhibit the synthesis of blood coagulation factors II (prothrombin), VII (proconvertin), IX (Christmas factor), and X (Stuart factor) in the liver by interfering with the action of vitamin K-mediated gamma-carboxylation of precursor proteins.[1] The full anticoagulant effect does not occur for 2–7 days, and not until the remaining circulating coagulation factors are removed by normal catabolism. This effect is dependent on the half-lives of these clotting factors in circulation, which are 6, 24, 40, and 60 hr for factors VII, IX, X, and II, respectively. When warfarin sodium therapy is discontinued, blood concentrations of the four clotting fac-

The contributions made by Terrence A. Killilea to this chapter are gratefully acknowledged.

tors return to pretreatment levels. Warfarin has no direct thrombolytic effects on established intraluminal thrombi. Clotting factors will inhibit thrombus formation when venous stasis is present and may prevent extension of existing thrombi.

One difficulty found in monitoring warfarin and making dose adjustments is that serum assays do not actually measure the concentration of warfarin, but rather the consequence of that concentration. Optimal dosing of warfarin is monitored by a pharmacodynamic coagulation assay (prothrombin time or PT) that does not necessarily reflect the patient's thrombotic status, particularly during initial stages of treatment.[2] An understanding of several pharmacodynamic and pharmacokinetic components contributes to educated warfarin dosing. These components (reviewed in the following sections) provide the rationale for interpatient variability in regard to susceptibility, magnitude, duration of action, and onset of anticoagulant effect.

Usual Dosage Range in Absence of Clearance-Altering Factors

The dosages listed here are for reference only—they should not be used to establish actual dosage strategies. The initiation dose given for children is derived from the only prospective trial in children and should be utilized cautiously. (For complete guidelines on planning warfarin therapy, see the warfarin dosing strategies section.)

Age	Initiation Dose	Maintenance Dosage
Children (1–<18 years)	0.2 mg/kg/day × 2 days[3]	Based on response
Adults (18–70 years)	7.5–15 mg/day × 2 days	2.5–7.5 mg/day, determined individually
Geriatrics (>70 years)	5–10 mg/day × 2 days	May be lower than for adults[4]

The initiation dose is designed to place a patient's PT in the therapeutic range and allow for maintenance dose estimation. Monitoring of PTs should begin with *the first dose* to detect "hyper-responders."

Maintenance doses greater than 15 mg/day are rarely required in the absence of genetic[5] or external factors.[6] Although some patients have required up to 2.6 mg/kg/day,[7] maintenance dose requirements exceeding 0.25 mg/kg/day are extremely rare.

Dosage Form Availability

Warfarin is currently available in both oral tablet and injectable form. Generic warfarin is available from many sources, but an individual patient should probably not change brands unless the patient is closely monitored.[8,9] Coumadin is the prominent proprietary form of warfarin. Each strength of Coumadin is readily recognizable by its color, and all Coumadin tablets are scored.

Coumadin Dosage Size	Color
1 mg	Pink
2 mg	Lavender
2.5 mg	Green
3 mg	Tan
4 mg	Blue
5 mg	Peach
6 mg	Teal
7.5 mg	Yellow
10 mg	White

General Pharmacokinetic Information[3,10]

Warfarin has excellent bioavailability when taken orally. The drug is rapidly and completely absorbed from the stomach and proximal small intestine with peak blood concentrations in 2–6 hr. Food decreases the rate but not the extent of absorption. The onset of the antithrombogenic effects are similar with oral, intramuscular, or intravenous administration. Larger doses will not hasten the onset but may prolong the duration of action after the drug is discontinued. The half-life of warfarin can be up to 4 days, depending on the individual. Warfarin is highly bound to albumin and is virtually 100% catabolized in the liver through hydroxylation by hepatic microsomal enzymes to inactive metabolites and eliminated via the intestines.

Pharmacokinetics Summary Table

F	95–100%
t_{peak}	1–6 hr
V	0.1–0.2 L/kg
protein binding	97–99% (primarily to albumin)
$t\frac{1}{2}$	40 hr (25–60 hr)
CL	0.09–0.3 L/hr/70 kg
therapeutic serum concentration	0.7–2.6 mg/L

Warfarin distributes to breast milk (inactive form) and crosses the placenta.

Warfarin contains an asymmetric carbon atom (chiral) and, therefore, can exist as two enantiomers: (R)- and (S)-warfarin, which differ with respect to both pharmacodynamic and pharmacokinetic properties.[11] Current products contain equal quantities of the two enantiomers (a racemic mixture). Anticoagulant activity of (S)-warfarin in humans is two to five times that of (R)-warfarin, and (R)-warfarin has the longer half-life.[12,13] Since only the unbound fraction is available for inhibiting the clotting factor conversions, displacement of even 1% may double the activity. Furthermore, if the (S)-enantiomer is selectively displaced, the activity would be proportionately greater (see the drug—drug interactions section for further discussion regarding clinical relevance).

The enantiomers of warfarin are also cleared in a highly stereoselective manner by two different metabolic pathways.[14] The major metabolic pathway for the less active anticoagulant, (R)-warfarin, involves reduction of the ketone function of the acetenyl side chain to secondary alcohols, which are excreted in urine.[15] In contrast, the more active (S)-warfarin is primarily oxidized via ring hydroxylation of the coumarin nucleus to 7-hydroxywarfarin, which is excreted via the bile.[16] The main site of warfarin metabolism is within the microsomal fraction of the endoplasmic reticulum of the liver, but alcohols may be formed by soluble enzymes in the hepatic and renal parenchyma. Enterohepatic recirculation also occurs with this drug.

The stereoselective, regioselective oxidative metabolism of warfarin is as follows:[16]

(R)-Warfarin
    P450-1A2   (R)-6-hydroxywarfarin
                                  (R)-7-hydroxywarfarin
                                  (R)-8-hydroxywarfarin
    P450-3A4   (R)-10-hydroxywarfarin

(S)-Warfarin
    P450-2C9   (S)-6-hydroxywarfarin
                                    (S)-7-hydroxywarfarin
    P450-3A4   (S)-4'-hydroxywarfarin

Clotting factors II, VII, IX, and X, as well as proteins C and S, are synthesized by hepatocytes but must undergo vitamin K dependent carboxylation to become biologically active.

The *average normal clotting factor half-lives* are[11]

- Factor II (prothrombin), 48–120 hr.
- Factor VII, 2–6 hr.
- Factor IX, 18–40 hr.
- Factor X, 30–70 hr.
- Protein C, 8 hr.

Pharmacodynamic Basis of Action

Warfarin, which is structurally similar to vitamin K, competitively inhibits the enzyme required for active vitamin K regeneration. Without regeneration of active (reduced) vitamin K, clotting factor carboxylation fails to occur. The unmodified clotting factors are released and circulate in the blood functionally inactive. Because warfarin acts to prevent the activation and not the synthesis of vitamin K dependent clotting factors, its biologic effects are not apparent until the previously activated clotting factors become depleted. This depletion takes place according to the biologic half-life of each clotting factor. The resultant reduced serum concentrations of factors II, IX, and X provide true antithrombosis.[17,18] PT is sensitive to factor VII depletion and virtually insensitive to factor IX depletion.[10,19]

Thus the initial PT increase (first 2–3 days) due to diminished factor VII (extrinsic pathway) does *not* reflect an antithrombotic state.[18,20] The patient may actually be in a "procoagulant" state due to the diminished protein C concentration and normal factor II and X concentrations.[21]

The reductions of clotting factor concentrations during steady-state warfarin dosing are not equal. Factor II and X (the factors most indicative of antithrombosis) concentrations in plasma are diminished more than are factor VII and IX concentrations.[22]

Prothrombin complex activity and half-life

The ability of the combined coagulation factors to form a clot has been termed the prothrombin complex activity (PCA). Generally, the therapeutic PCA goal in warfarin therapy is 30–50% of normal.[2] PCA has been mathematically linked to the prothrombin ratio (PR) by the equation[23]

$$\text{PCA (\%)} = \frac{100\%}{(3.636)(PR) - 2.636}$$

This relationship appears to vary according to the sensitivity of thromboplastin used (see the therapeutic range section). The synthesis of the prothrombin complex has been estimated to be 5%/hr/70 kg. The elimination half-life of prothrombin is approximately 17 hr.[2] The administration of warfarin decreases the synthesis rate of the prothrombin complex, while its elimination rate remains unchanged. Thus, PCA decreases as the pharmacodynamic effects of warfarin commence. Eventually, the patient reaches a pharmacodynamic steady state where the diminished synthesis of the prothrombin complex is in balance with new clotting factor concentrations and the preexisting elimination rate. Ideally, this maintenance dose equilibrium occurs with PT in the therapeutic range.

Time course of PT elevation

Administration of a large "loading dose" (1.5 mg/kg) elevates PT to above 20 sec (35% PCA) within 1 day. While this method was popular prior to the mid-1960s, its advantage has not been demonstrated. The early rise in PT is primarily due to factor VII depletion, but the intrinsic path of thrombogenesis is independent of factor VII activity.[20,24]

An "initiation" dose (10 mg daily) elevates PT to the therapeutic range in 2–5 days in most patients. This elevation of PT (and apparent decrease in PCA) more accurately reflects a patient's decreased factor II and X concentrations and antithrombotic state (although it may take 7 or more days for these factors to achieve steady state).[25] The rate of PT elevation is dependent on patient-specific factors such as hepatic status, nutrition, and concomitant drug therapy.

The maximum effect of a single warfarin dose typically occurs approximately 36 hr after that dose.[24] This finding cannot necessarily be extrapolated to the change in PCA suppression occurring when a warfarin maintenance dose is changed. The time needed for a fixed warfarin dose to establish a new steady-state elevation of PT is highly variable and may be best estimated at 7–10 days (five times the half-life of the longest clotting factor).

Therapeutic Range

Prothrombin time

The primary method for determining anticoagulation in the United States is the measurement of PT. PT is often interpreted in terms of the prothrombin ratio (PT ratio or PR):

$$\text{PT ratio} = \frac{\text{PT (patient)}}{\text{PT (control)}}$$

PT (control) is often either (a) a standard (such as 12 sec), which is reevaluated periodically by the laboratory, or (b) established daily using pooled unanticoagulated blood.

It is imperative to know the International Sensitivity Index (ISI) of thromboplastin utilized by a specific laboratory for determining PT. This index determines the therapeutic range for patients monitored with a specific lot of thromboplastin. A specific thromboplastin's ISI can be found on the insert distributed with the reagent. The variations in thromboplastin sensitivity are due to differences in manufacturing, source, an d method of preparation. A more responsive thromboplastin, such as that used in the United Kingdom and early clinical trials, produces less rapid stimulation of factor X, resulting in greater prolongation of the PT time for a given reduction in clotting factors.[26–30] A less responsive thromboplastin activates residual factor X more rapidly and results in a less prolonged PT, despite a comparable decrement in clotting factors. ISI values range from 0.95 to 2.9. The higher the number, the less sensitive is the reagent.

International Normalized Ratio (INR)[19]

The INR is a mathematical "correction" for differences in the sensitivity of thromboplastin reagents (see previous section). In 1977, the World Health Organization designated a batch of human brain thromboplastin as the first International Reference Preparation (IRP). A calibration system was developed to describe the linear relationship between the logarithm of the PT ratios of the reference and test thromboplastins. This system allows the conversion of the PT ratio observed with a local thromboplastin into an INR. The INR is the value obtained if the "reference" preparation had been used in the test. In this way, results obtained at different laboratories can be compared, and results from lot-to-lot of thromboplastin used at the same laboratory can be compared.[31]

Various methods of standardizing the PT ratio have been described.[19] The most common and useful method to determine an INR is

$$INR = (PT\ ratio)^{ISI}$$

With this equation, one can readily calculate the variability in PT ratios utilizing reagents with different ISIs, setting the INR constant. Table 1 shows this relationship. Theoretically, these values could represent the same patient going to five different laboratories.

For example, $(2.2)^{1.2} = 2.6$ INR.

TABLE 1. Comparison of PT Ratio (PTR) and International Normalized Ratio (INR) Utilizing Thromboplastin with Different International Sensitivity Indexes (ISI).

Thromboplastin	Patient's PT	Mean Normal	PTR	ISI	INR
A	16 sec	12 sec	1.3	3.2	2.6
B	18 sec	12 sec	1.5	2.4	2.6
C	21 sec	13 sec	1.6	2.0	2.6
D	24 sec	11 sec	2.2	1.2	2.6
E	38 sec	14.5 sec	2.6	1.0	2.6

The INRs considered therapeutic for most indications (prophylaxis/treatment of venous thrombosis and pulmonary embolism, prevention of systemic embolism, atrial fibrillation) are 2–3. For patients with mechanical prosthetic heart valves or recurrent systemic emboli, an INR of 2.5–3.5 is recommended. Specific conditions (such as antiphospholipid antibody syndrome) may require even higher targets.[32]

One final note on INRs, the calibration of the INR for each thromboplastin is carried out using normal plasma samples and plasma samples from persons receiving anticoagulant therapy for at least 6 weeks. This process means that the INR system is designed for monitoring long-term anticoagulation therapy; it is less valuable for patients during the induction phase of oral anticoagulant therapy. It is also less reliable for patients with significant liver dysfunction or for preoperative screening for bleeding disorders. In these cases, the PT and PT ratio will still be the most accurate assessment of therapy.

Warfarin Dosing Strategies and Suggested Sampling Times

Overlap with heparin therapy

A patient receiving warfarin will have an elevated partial thromboplastin time (PTT).[33] The extent of this effect becomes apparent as the serum concentration of factor X diminishes (after 3–5 days of warfarin therapy). Patients may demonstrate a heightened response (increase in PTT to over 80 sec) to a previously established maintenance dose of heparin when warfarin is added. The practitioner faced with this situation can either

- Decrease the heparin administration rate.
- Maintain the same heparin administration rate that provided PTTs in the therapeutic range (in spite of PTTs above the therapeutic window).

The optimal course of action has yet to be determined, but alteration of the heparin infusion rate to assure a PTT of under 100 sec would be prudent.

Heparin, in therapeutic concentrations, can elevate the PT of patients who are receiving[34,35] or not receiving[36] warfarin. The extent of PT elevation is generally 1–3 sec (but can be more). This phenomenon is not always observed in patients receiving concomitant heparin and warfarin. It has not been determined whether this elevation of PT correlates to PTT elevation. It appears to be more related to heparin concentration. The effect of a set heparin infusion rate on PT can vary day to day (or even hour to hour), probably due to different concentrations of heparin in the blood sample.

"Heparin neutralization" has been discussed as a method of negating heparin's effect on PT.[37,38] However, methods of heparin neutralization are unreliable and may lead to underestimation of heparin's effect on PT.[39]

A drop in PT when heparin therapy is ceased can be expected in some patients. This situation often occurs when maintenance dosing of warfarin is being established. Focusing on data obtained after heparin has been stopped can improve accuracy and precision of warfarin maintenance dose estimation.[40,41]

Heparin therapy should not be stopped until the practitioner is confident that factors II and X have been therapeutically reduced—generally in 4–6 days. Another indication that therapeutic antithrombosis has been achieved is when PT has been elevated to the therapeutic range for longer than 2 days. From these considerations arise the recommendation to overlap heparin and warfarin therapy for a minimum of 4 days and, more optimally, 7 days.[21,42–44] Low molecular weight heparin and intermittent subcutaneous heparin have also been shown effective in overlapping therapy for patients with venous thromboembolism.[32] Such use enables the patient to be discharged from the hospital quicker but does not eliminate the need for close monitoring.

Commencement of warfarin therapy
Warfarin therapy should commence as soon as the practitioner is positive that the patient requires long-term anticoagulation, the patient can take oral medications, and the patient apparently does not possess definitive contraindications to anticoagulation. Warfarin therapy should be delayed until after all invasive procedures are completed during the hospitalization and until after heparin therapy is in the therapeutic range.

Warfarin may be started on the first day of hospital admission. This approach can minimize length of stay and allow for full overlap of heparin and warfarin therapy.[45,46]

Phase one: initiation dose—The purpose of this phase is to elevate the patient's PT safely to a value in or near the determined therapeutic range. Necessary baseline information and laboratory values should be obtained including age, height, weight, potentially interacting diseases or drugs, PT, PTT, and hematocrit and hemoglobin (H/H). Further analysis should be performed if hematologic laboratory values appear abnormal. Both PT and H/H should be monitored daily during inpatient warfarin therapy. The patient should be evaluated for relative or absolute contraindications toward warfarin therapy. Any risk of hemorrhaging should be identified, and a monitoring strategy should be established.

A target therapeutic range should be defined. The practitioner must know the target PT ratio for thromboplastin used by the laboratory. Identification of heparin as a potential source of PT elevation should be monitored.

In adults, a warfarin dose of 10 mg is usually given on the first day. If the patient is elderly or expected to respond robustly (due to concomitant drug therapy or disease state), the initial warfarin dose should be only 7.5 or 5 mg.

The dose for the second day is based on the initial response. A patient's PT may remain near baseline after the first dose. If PT rises less than 2 sec, a dose equivalent to the first day's dose is warranted. If PT is within 2 sec of the therapeutic range, a reduction to half of the first day's dose should further elevate PT while avoiding overanticoagulation. If PT is in the therapeutic range after one dose of warfarin, withholding of the second day's dose should be considered.

If there is no reason to achieve therapeutic anticoagulation promptly (i.e., long-term prophylactic therapy can be established for outpatient), the patient can be commenced on an expected maintenance dose (e.g., 5 mg daily for 3 days). Elevation of PT will be slow.[1]

Phase two: maintenance dose determination—The purposes of this phase are to evaluate the patient's PT response to phase one and to initiate a maintenance dose that will place the patient's PT in the therapeutic range at steady state.

If the patient's PT ratio remains below the therapeutic range after two doses, the initial daily dose should be continued. The initial daily dose may have to be increased by 2.5 or 5 mg/day if PT rises less than 1 sec from baseline after 3 days.

Many methods of maintenance dosage estimation have been evaluated. While several methods commence with 10 mg daily for 3 days,[47] these methods have serious limitations. Many patients are overanticoagulated with this regimen,[48] thereby placing these patients at unnecessary risk of an adverse event and confounding subsequent dose stabilization. Trials of these methods have utilized inappropriately high and broad therapeutic ranges. Utilization of one of these methods in a young, healthy patient may be acceptable.

Another method utilizes factor VII concentrations found after a single warfarin dose to determine the maintenance dose.[49] This method is not presented here because few institutions routinely determine factor VII concentrations.

For the most part, there have been few methods of determining maintenance doses that have shown predictability surpassing that of an experienced provider and close monitoring. In predicting the maintenance dose and determining dosage adjustments with each INR, the practitioner should always remember the following concepts:[17]

- PTs often do not elevate after the first 1–2 days of warfarin therapy, even when dosing is initiated at 10 mg daily for 2 days.
- The intensity of the initial response observed generally correlates to the eventual maintenance dose requirement (a robust response to a low dose probably indicates a low maintenance requirement).
- Elderly patients with multiple comorbidities generally require smaller doses than a younger relatively healthy person.
- Concomitant drug therapy and diet influence the warfarin effect.

Phase three: initial maintenance response evaluation—The purpose of this phase is to determine whether the patient's response to the maintenance dose will maintain the patient's PT in the therapeutic range at steady state without heparin. With the expected discontinuance of heparin, PTs 1–2 sec above the therapeutic range are acceptable if heparin therapy is ceased promptly (see overlap with heparin therapy section). If PT drops below the therapeutic range when heparin is stopped, heparin therapy can be reinstituted.

The practitioner should evaluate a patient's PT after 2 days of the anticipated maintenance dose. Minor (1–2 mg/day) modifications of therapy may be necessary if the patient's PT remains sub- or supratherapeutic. Large modifications should be avoided.

Phase four: definitive maintenance response evaluation—If a patient's PT has varied less than 1.5 sec (while remaining therapeutic) with the same daily dose for 5 days, the practitioner can be confident that this amount is the long-term maintenance dose. The patient may be discharged early in this period of analysis as confidence in the selected maintenance dose grows. An algorithm for management of long-term warfarin therapy has been published.[21]

Maintenance dose adjustment

Any method evaluating nontherapeutic response to warfarin therapy (and subsequent dosing adjustments) must take into account confounding patient factors such as noncompliance, diet, and concomitant pharmacotherapy (see pharmacodynamic monitoring—concentration-related toxicity section).

Steady-state dose response to warfarin is not linear throughout the dosing range.[50] Since it takes 7–10 days to reach steady state at any dosage level, adjustments may be made dependent on the total weekly quantity of warfarin the patient is ingesting. An acceptable starting point for altering a dose in a supra- or subtherapeutic patient is 10%. For instance, a patient taking 5 mg qd is taking 35 mg/week. An adjustment may be made by lowering or raising the weekly dose by 3.5 mg. A slightly higher or lower dose may be made to enable use of current tablet size (e.g., 2.5 mg is ½ of the 5 mg tablet and is 7% of the weekly dose). So the resultant schedule for a patient with a slightly supratherapeutic INR would be: "5 mg qd, except take 2.5 mg on Mondays." When maintenance therapy is adjusted, changes greater than 15% of previous therapy should usually be avoided unless the patient is dramatically sub or supratherapeutic.

One to two held doses and/or vitamin K_1 may be necessary in patients with high INRs, with or without bleeding complications. (See section on pharmacodynamic monitoring for further discussion.)

Outpatient monitoring

Longitudinal management of the anticoagulant effect generally relies on the calculated INR (based on the patient's PT) and predetermined target ranges as a basis for dosage adjustment (see therapeutic range section). An optimal sampling strategy for outpatient INR monitoring has not been developed. General considerations include the patient specific history of dose to INR relationship, number and significance of changes recently made to drug therapy, stability of disease, and risk of new clot formation (e.g., high with recent DVT, lower with chronic atrial fibrillation). At a minimum, the following should be performed.

1. *Two weeks postdischarge*—Monitoring during this period depends on the practitioner's confidence in the stability of postdischarge dosing (as assessed by predischarge INR stability). For most patients, initial monitoring of INR every 3–5 days should allow for safe modification of therapy. The frequency can be reduced if the first two or three INRs appear to be therapeutic and relatively consistent. The initial postdischarge INR may be lower than desired because of an improved outpatient diet as compared to the inpatient diet or improved or different overall health.

    An INR more than 0.5 below the therapeutic range may require a single "booster dose" of 1.5 times the new maintenance dose. This booster may transiently elevate INR above the therapeutic range (if the initial observed low INR response is actual), but the net effect is to minimize the time that the patient has a subtherapeutic INR. If a near return to baseline INR is observed, temporary reinstitution of heparin or low molecular weight heparin should be considered to protect against thrombosis while a therapeutic warfarin dose is sought.

    If INR is near the therapeutic range, dosing modifications of greater than 15% may lead to wide fluctuations in INR ratios.

2. *Two weeks to 2 months postdischarge*—INR should be monitored weekly or biweekly, depending on stability and convenience. Potential noncompliance problems should become evident during this period.

3. *Two months postdischarge and later*—Monthly INR determinations are warranted early in this period. If patient compliance, dietary stability, and safety are assured, INR determinations every 6 weeks may suffice.[51]

Pharmacodynamic Monitoring

During the early dosing phase of warfarin therapy, an abnormally low response can indicate

- Drug interactions.
- Diet high in vitamin K.
- Edema.
- Hypothyroidism.
- Patient is nonadherent.
- Patient unable to absorb warfarin.
- Hereditary warfarin resistance.[5]
- Primary and secondary hypercoagulable states.[52]
- Inappropriate dosing.
- Laboratory value obtained from wrong patient.

During this same period, an abnormally high response may be caused by

- Concomitant heparin therapy.
- Cancer.
- Diarrhea.
- Malabsorption.
- Hyperthyroidism.
- Liver disease.
- Specimen was drawn from a heparinized line.
- Specimen was not obtained or handled properly.
- Drug interactions.
- Hereditary warfarin sensitivity.
- Very low vitamin K intake.
- Inappropriate dosing.
- Laboratory value obtained from wrong patient.

Additionally, a classic way to tell if the INR is in error is to observe the trend of the PTT. If the INR is higher than expected, and the PTT is very high (>120 sec when the PTT was in range before), the practitioner should redraw the sample.

During the *maintenance dosing phase* of warfarin therapy, an abnormal PT should be evaluated for the following causes:

- Laboratory inaccuracy or change in thromboplastin.
- Poor patient compliance (excessive or insufficient).
- Initiation, adjustment, or cessation of interacting drug.
- Major alteration in vitamin K intake.
- Recent alcohol ingestion.
- Recent onset of illness affecting response (i.e., severe CHF or liver disease).
- Change in warfarin brand.
- Recent onset of thromboembolic disease.
- PT drawn from wrong patient.

Dosage adjustments based on INR values

Multiple elaborate schemes have been developed for adjusting warfarin doses based on INR values. These are helpful, particularly to the relatively inexperienced practitioner. However, no table or flow chart can account for the multitude of variables found within a single patient. Therefore, any use of these methods must be coupled with appropriate patient assessment and practitioner knowledge and experience. One example of a basic method of dosage adjustment in patients with a target treatment INR of 2–3 is outlined in Table 2. Follow-up is also patient specific but should be every 1–2 weeks when making dosage adjustments or expecting an external influence and 4–6 weeks when the patient stabilizes.

Safe practice recommendations for using vitamin K_1 to reverse excessive warfarin anticoagulation

The Fifth Consensus Conference on Antithrombotic Therapy statement on use of phytonadione (vitamin K_1) is

TABLE 2. Sample Protocol for Dosage Adjustments and Monitoring Frequency Based on INR Values and Target Treatment INR of 2–3.

Patient INR Value	Dosage Adjustment Guidelines
<1.5	Increase maintenance dose by 10–20%
1.5–1.8	Increase maintenance dose by 5–15%
1.8–2.0	No dosage adjustment necessary unless two consecutive INR values in this range; if dosage adjustment needed, increase maintenance dose by 5–15%
2.0–3.0	No dosage adjustment necessary
3.0–3.5	No dosage adjustment necessary unless two consecutive INR values in this range; if dosage adjustment needed, decrease maintenance dose by 5–15%
3.5–4.0	Decrease maintenance dose by 5–15%
4.0–5.0	Hold one dose; decrease maintenance dose by 10–20% if increase not accounted for by contributing factors
5.0–6.0	Hold two doses; decrease maintenance dose by 15–20%
>6.0	Hold dose indefinitely (recheck in 24–72 hr); administer vitamin K_1 (see Table 3)

summarized in Table 3. The route for administering vitamin K_1 for excessive warfarin anticoagulation is controversial. Subcutaneous use was not studied and has sometimes been found to be ineffective. The intravenous route is likely to give the most predictable response, but it can be complicated by anaphylactoid reactions, can more easily overcorrect, and may induce warfarin resistance for up 14 days. The oral dose is effective in most cases if the INR <10, and

TABLE 3. Vitamin K_1 Administration Based on INR Value.[32]

Patient INR Value	Vitamin K_1 Use Guidelines
<5.0	Hold one dose, resume at lower dose
5.0–9.0	• If no bleeding and no risk of bleeding, hold one or two doses • If no bleeding but a risk of bleeding, hold one dose, then 2.5 mg of vitamin K_1 orally • If rapid reversal needed (surgery) then 2–4 mg of vitamin K_1 orally
>9.0	• If no bleeding, then 3–5 mg of vitamin K_1 • If rapid reversal needed (surgery, INR >20), then 10 mg q12 hr prn of vitamin K_1 intravenously, plus fresh frozen plasma if urgency dictates

it has the advantages of being safer and more convenient than parenteral administration.

Currently, there are two formulations available in the United States: an oral 5-mg tablet (Mephyton) and an injectable preparation available as a 2-mg/ml or 10-mg/ml aqueous dispersion (Aquamephyton). With oral vitamin K_1, blood coagulation factors increase in 6–12 hr and INR values return to normal within 24–48 hr. With intravenous vitamin K_1, coagulation factors increase in 1–2 hr, bleeding is controlled within 3–8 hr, and INR values return to normal after 12–14 hr. The intravenous route produces the most rapid effect with progressively reduced effects seen in the following order: subcutaneous, intramuscular, and oral.

Ideally, vitamin K_1 should be administered in a dosage that rapidly reduces the INR into a safe range without (1) overshooting the lower limit of the targeted range, (2) rendering the patient resistant to warfarin when therapy with it is restarted, and (3) exposing the patient to a risk of an anaphylactoid reaction. There is a strong relationship between the level of the INR and the risk of bleeding.

The risk of bleeding rises sharply when the INR exceeds 5.0, but bleeding is increased, particularly in high-risk patients, when the INR exceeds 3.0.[32]

Drug–Drug Interactions

Many frequently prescribed drugs affect a patient's response to warfarin. Modification of response—increased or decreased—can lead to serious clinical sequelae. The actual pharmacokinetic and pharmacodynamic elements of a particular warfarin–drug interaction, as well as the time course and extent of response alteration, must be understood.

Warfarin has often been labeled a textbook example of drug interactions, since it exhibits virtually every interaction possible for a drug. The pharmacokinetic drug interactions may occur by several mechanisms, including interference with absorption (e.g., cholestyramine), displacement from plasma protein binding sites (e.g., sulfamethoxazole), inhibition of metabolism (e.g., amiodarone) and increased metabolism (e.g., rifampin). Pharmacodynamic reactions result primarily from the influence of concomitant drug therapy on clotting factor metabolism (e.g., levothyroxine) or platelet function (e.g., NSAIDs). When starting, stopping, or changing the dose of drugs suspected to interact with oral anticoagulants, it may be necessary to monitor for changes in anticoagulant activity. This approach is also advisable with new products for which clinical data regarding drug interactions are lacking. Patients should be advised of the potential drug interactions of oral anticoagulants with oral contraceptives and over-the-counter products (e.g., aspirin, cimetidine, NSAIDs) and be encouraged to consult their pharmacist or physician before taking these products.[53-55]

In addition, another reason why warfarin drug interactions are interesting is that the R- and S-isomers are metabolized via different CYP pathways. The R-isomer is metabolized through CYP450-1A2, and the S-isomer is metabolized via CYP450-2C9. That is why CYP450-2C9 inhibitors seem to affect warfarin more so than CYP450-1A2 inhibitors.

Time course of drug interaction

The clinical effects of an interaction may be seen within a few days (for most drugs) or several months (e.g., amiodarone). Most drug interactions with warfarin have a delayed pharmacodynamic onset, particularly interactions that alter the serum warfarin concentration. The effect is the equivalent of altering the warfarin dosage. Therefore, the time to observe the full effect of a warfarin-drug interaction (at initiation or discontinuation of the affecting drug) is often the same as the time to observe the full effects of a dosage change (5–7 days).

If an interacting drug increases the INR response to warfarin, its discontinuance leads to a decrease in INR. The opposite is true when a drug that decreases the INR response is discontinued. Furthermore, just as the time for observation of a drug interaction (as INR response) may be up to 7 days, the return to a noninteracted state after the drug is discontinued may require the same length of time.

Specific drug interactions

Since there are well over 400 drugs that influence the therapeutic effect of warfarin, it is impossible for any practitioner to learn each one in detail. Recognizing drugs within a category, learning the nature of the interaction within these categories, and applying this knowledge to other similar agents may not be as cumbersome. This approach is particularly true for newer agents. It is helpful that FDA now requires new medications to list the isoenzyme involved in their P450 metabolism, thus allowing better prediction of interference with warfarin and other drugs. The following lists indicate drug interactions that may lead to life-threatening sequelae. These lists are not complete; many warfarin–drug interactions have been cited in case reports but not subsequently investigated. Several excellent publications elaborate on the mechanism and management of drug interactions with warfarin. If there is a question, the clinician should refer to more in-depth drug interaction texts.

Agents that pharmacokinetically increase response to warfarin include

- Alcohol (acute)
- Allopurinol
- Amiodarone
- Azole antifungals (fluconazole unlikely in doses <400 mg/day)
- Cefoperazone
- Cephalosporins
- Chloramphenicol
- Cimetidine
- Ciprofloxacin
- Clarithromycin
- Clofibrate
- Danazol
- Disulfiram
- Erythromycin
- Gemfibrozil
- Lovastatin
- Metronidazole
- Nalidixic acid
- NSAIDs
- Omeprazole
- Phenylbutazone
- Quinidine
- Salicylates
- Simvastatin
- SSRIs (fluvoxamine has the greatest effect)
- Thyroid hormones
- Trimethoprim–sulfamethoxazole
- Vitamin E >800 IU/day

Agents that pharmacokinetically *decrease response to warfarin* include

> Alcohol (chronic)
> Barbiturates
> Carbamazepine
> Cholestyramine
> Griseofulvin
> Rifampin

Agents that increase the synthesis of clotting factors include

> Estrogens
> Oral contraceptives
> Propylthiouracil
> Vitamin K

Agents that increase catabolism of clotting factors include

> Androgens
> Thyroid hormones

Agents that affect hemostasis include

Aspirin
Clopidegrel
Dipyridamole
NSAIDs
Pentoxifylline
Ticlopidine

Most drug interactions with warfarin, like drug interactions in general, are highly variable from patient to patient. Appropriate laboratory and clinical monitoring of the anticoagulant response to warfarin can help evaluate possible drug interactions and substantially reduce the consequences of these events.[56] Avoidance is not always possible or necessary, but close monitoring is!

Drug–Disease State or Condition Interactions

Several disease states may make the patient abnormally sensitive to warfarin.[17] This problem should be considered for a chronic disease state as well as when a patient develops a disease or is restored to normal health.

- *Liver disease*—Severe liver disease impairs a patient's ability to eliminate warfarin and decreases the synthesis rate of prothrombin complex factors.[57]
- *Congestive heart failure*—Severe heart failure possibly may cause a patient to be more sensitive to warfarin.[58]
- *Cardiac valve replacement*—Patients commencing warfarin therapy after cardiac valve replacement appear to have increased response to warfarin.[59] This phenomenon usually vanishes several weeks after surgery, and outpatient warfarin dosage requirements appear to be higher. Close postdischarge monitoring of cardiac valve patients is warranted.
- *Nephrotic syndrome*—Nephrotic syndrome patients with low serum albumin appear to have a higher free fraction of warfarin. This status leads to an increase in plasma clearance. The net effect is unlikely to affect maintenance dose requirements, although response to a single warfarin dose may increase or the maintenance dose response may fluctuate.[60]
- *Malignancy*—While the direct effect of malignancy on warfarin dose determination has not been investigated, the coagulopathies observed often involve clotting proteins related to warfarin therapy.[61–63]
- *Diet*—Variations in dietary vitamin K content can alter response to warfarin.[6,64] However, a single intake of food high in vitamin K may not significantly affect a patient's anticoagulation status.[65] Variations of daily dietary vitamin K intake of less than 250–500 mcg do not appear to disturb anticoagulation.[66]

Chronic consumption (or cessation of consumption) of various vitamin K-rich foods should be considered when a patient's response to maintenance warfarin appears abnormal.[67] The vitamin K content in enteral feeding products also should be considered for patients receiving these products.[68]

- *Smoking*—Cigarette smoking does not appear to affect warfarin dosing requirements.[69,70]
- *Pregnancy*—Oral anticoagulants are contraindicated at any time during pregnancy and should not be used in women planning pregnancy. Long-term heparin therapy is a therapeutic alternative.[71]

Summary

Warfarin is a valuable agent for the prevention and treatment of thrombosis. Several therapeutic suggestions should be kept in mind:

1. When possible, warfarin should be initiated as soon as heparin therapy is commenced.
2. The specific therapeutic PT ratio range (using ISI) for the thromboplastin used by the laboratory should be known or patient response should be reported as INR.
3. Initial response should be monitored closely for accurate estimation of maintenance requirements and to avoid unnecessary risk.
4. A drop in INR should be expected when heparin therapy is discontinued.
5. The extent and time course of the addition or deletion of interacting medications or disease states must be understood.

References

1. Hirsh J. Oral anticoagulant drugs. *New Engl J Med*. 1991; 324:1865–75.
2. Holford NHG. Clinical pharmacokinetics and pharmacodynamics of warfarin. *Clin Pharmacokinet*. 1986; 11:483–504.
3. Doyle JJ, Koren G, Cheng MY, et al. Anticoagulation with sodium warfarin in children: effect of a loading regimen. *J Pediatr*. 1988; 113:1095–7.

4. Wickramasinghe LSP, Basu SK, Bansal SK. Long-term anticoagulant therapy in elderly patients. *Age Ageing*. 1988; 17:388–96.
5. Alving BM, Strickler MP, Knight RD, et al. Hereditary warfarin resistance. *Arch Intern Med*. 1985; 145:499–501.
6. Walker FB. Myocardial infarction after diet-induced warfarin resistance. *Arch Intern Med*. 1984; 144:2089–90.
7. O'Reilly RA, Aggeler PM, Hoag MS. Hereditary transmission of exceptional resistance to coumarin anticoagulant drugs. *N Engl J Med*. 1964; 271:809–15.
8. Neutel JM, Smith MD. A randomized crossover study to compare the efficacy and tolerability of Barr warfarin sodium to the currently available Coumadin. *CVR&R* 1998; Feb:49–59.
9. Scheidt S. Generic warfarin: a difficult decision. *CVR&R* 1998; Feb:46–8.
10. Porter RS, Sawyer WT. Warfarin. In Evans WE, ed. Applied pharmacokinetics: Principles of therapeutic drug monitoring, 3rd Ed. Vancouver, WA: Applied Therapeutics, Inc.; 1992: 31.1–31.46.
11. Park BK. Warfarin: metabolism and mode of action. *Biochem Pharmacol*. 1988; 37:19–27.
12. Yacobi A, Levy G. Protein binding of warfarin enantiomers in serum of humans and rats. *J Pharmacokinet Biopharm*. 1977; 5:123–31.
13. Breckenridge AM, Orme M, Wesselling H, et al. Pharmacokinetics and pharmacodynamics of the enantiomers of warfarin in man. *Clin Pharmacol Ther*. 1974; 15:424–30.
14. Lewis RL, Trager WF, Chan KK, et al. Warfarin: stereochemical aspects of its metabolism and the interaction with phenylbutazone. *J Clin Invest*. 1974; 53:1607–17.
15. Chan KK, Lewis RJ, Trager WF. Absolute configurations of the four warfarin alcohols. *J Med Chem*. 1972; 15:1265–70.
16. Rettie AE, Korzekwa KR, Kunze KL, et al. Hydroxylation of warfarin by human cDNA expressed cytochrome p450: a role for P450-2C9 in the etiology of S-warfarin drug interactions. *Chem Res Toxicol*. 1992; 5:54–9.
17. Stults BM, Dere WH, Caine TH. Long-term anticoagulation. *West J Med*. 1989; 151:414–29.
18. Wessler S, Gitel SN. Pharmacology of heparin and warfarin. *J Am Coll Cardiol*. 1986; 8:10B–20B.
19. Hirsh J, Dalen JE, Anderson DR, et al. Oral anticoagulants: mechanism of action, clinical effectiveness, and optimal therapeutic range. *Chest* 1998; 114(5):445S–69S.
20. O'Reilly RA, Aggeler PM. Studies on coumarin anticoagulant drugs: initiation of warfarin therapy without a loading dose. *Circulation*. 1968; 38:169–77.
21. Carter BL. Therapy of acute thromboembolism with heparin and warfarin. *Clin Pharm*. 1991; 10:503–18.
22. Kumar S, Haigh JR, Tate G, et al. Effect of warfarin on plasma concentrations of vitamin K dependent coagulation factors in patients with stable control and monitored compliance. *Br J Haematol*. 1990; 74:82–5.

23. Sheiner LB. Computer-aided long-term anticoagulation therapy. *Comput Biomed Res.* 1969; 2:507–18.
24. Nagashima R, O'Reilly RA, Levy G. Kinetics of pharmacologic effects in man: the anticoagulant action of warfarin. *Clin Pharmacol Ther.* 1968; 10:22–35.
25. Breckinridge AM. Interindividual differences in the response to oral anticoagulants. *Drugs.* 1977; 14:367–75.
26. Hirsh J, Levine MN. The optimal intensity of oral anticoagulant therapy. *J Am Med Assoc.* 1987; 258:2723–6.
27. Hirsh J, Deykin D, Poller L. Therapeutic range for oral anticoagulant therapy. *Arch Intern Med.* 1986; 146:466.
28. Hirsh J, Poller L, Deykin D, et al. Optimal therapeutic range for oral anticoagulants. *Chest.* 1989; 95:5S–11S.
29. Vanscoy GJ, Krause JR. Warfarin and the international normalized ratio: reducing interlaboratory effects. *DICP Ann Pharmacother.* 1991; 25:1190–2.
30. Boston Area Anticoagulation Trial for Atrial Fibrillation Investigators. The effect of low-dose warfarin on the risk of stroke in patients with nonrheumatic atrial fibrillation. *N Engl J Med.* 1990; 323:1505–11.
31. WHO Expert Committee on Biological Standardization 33rd Report. WHO Tech Rep Ser. #687; 1983.
32. Fifth ACCP consensus conference on antithrombotic therapy. *Chest* 1998; 114(5):439S–769S.
33. Hauser VM, Rozek SL. Effect of warfarin on the activated partial thromboplastin time. *Drug Intell Clin Pharm.* 1986; 20:964–7.
34. Sawyer WT, Raasch RH. Effect of heparin on prothrombin time. *Clin Pharm.* 1984; 3:192–4.
35. Lutomski DM, Djuric PE, Draeger RW. Warfarin therapy: the effect of heparin on prothrombin time. *Arch Intern Med.* 1987; 147:432–3.
36. Bark CJ. Coagulation nondisease. *N Engl J Med.* 1970; 282:1214.
37. Hutt ED, Kingdon HS. Use of heparinase to eliminate heparin inhibition in routine coagulation assays. *J Lab Clin Med.* 1972; 79:1027–34.
38. Thompson AR, Counts RB. Removal of heparin and protamine from plasma. *J Lab Clin Med.* 1976; 88:922–9.
39. Wenz B, Burns ER. Rapid removal of heparin from plasma by affinity filtration. *Am J Clin Pathol.* 1991; 96:385–90.
40. Thomas P, Fennerty A, Blackhouse G, et al. Monitoring effects of oral anticoagulants during treatment with heparin. *Br Med J.* 1984; 288:191.
41. Killilea T, Aebi M, Asbury M. Evaluation of the effect of heparin therapy on warfarin dose estimation. *Pharmacotherapy.* 1990; 10:244.
42. Shetty HGM, Fennerty AG, Routledge PA. Clinical pharmacokinetics consideration in the control of oral anticoagulant therapy. *Clin Pharmacokinet.* 1989; 16:238–53.
43. Hull RD, Raskob GE, Rosenbloom D, et al. Heparin for 5 days as compared with 10 days in the initial treatment of proximal venous thrombosis. *New Engl J Med.* 1990; 322:1260–4.
44. Schulman S, Lockner D, Bergstrom K, et al. Intensive initial oral anticoagulation and shorter heparin treatment in deep vein thrombosis. *Thromb Haemost.* 1984; 52:276–80.

45. Gallus A, Jackaman J, Tillett J, et al. Safety and efficacy of warfarin started early after submassive venous thrombosis or pulmonary embolism. *Lancet*. 1986; 2:1293–6.
46. Westblom TU, Marienfeld RD. Prolonged hospitalization because of inappropriate delay of warfarin therapy in deep venous thrombosis. *South Med J*. 1985; 78:1164–7.
47. Sawyer WT, Poe TE, Canaday BR, et al. Predictability of warfarin maintenance dose, comparison of six methods. *Clin Pharm*. 1985; 4:440–6.
48. Fennerty A, Dolben J, Thomas P, et al. Flexible induction dose regimen for warfarin and prediction of maintenance dose. *Br Med J*. 1984; 288:1268–70.
49. Jupe DML, Peterson GM, Coleman RL, et al. Warfarin dosage requirements: prospective clinical trial of a method for prediction from the response to a single dose. *Br J Clin Pharmacol*. 1988; 25:607–10.
50. Murray B, Coleman R, McWaters D, et al. Pharmacodynamics of warfarin at steady state. *Ther Drug Monit*. 1987; 9:1–5.
51. Bussey HI, Rospond RM, Quandt CM, et al. The safety and effectiveness of long-term warfarin therapy in an anticoagulation clinic. *Pharmacotherapy*. 1989; 9:214–9.
52. Thomas JH. Pathogenesis, diagnosis, and treatment of thrombosis. *Am J Surg*. 1990; 160:547–51.
53. Tatro DS, ed. Drug Interaction Facts. St. Louis, MO: Wolters Kluwer; 1999 (Quarterly Updates).
54. Hansten PD, Horn JR. Drug Interactions and Updates Quarterly. Vancouver, WA: Applied Therapeutics; 1999.
55. Harder S, Thurmann P. Clinically important drug interactions with anticoagulants. *Clin Pharmacokinet*. 1996; 30:416–44.
56. Hansten PD, Horn JR, Koka-Kimble MA, et al. Drug Interactions and Updates Quarterly. Vancouver, WA: Applied Therapeutics; 1995.
57. Blanchard RA, Furie BC, Jorgensen M, et al. Acquired vitamin k-dependent carboxylation deficiency in liver disease. *New Engl J Med*. 1981; 305:242–8.
58. Ristola P, Kaleui P. Determinants of the response to coumarin anticoagulants in patients with acute myocardial infarction. *Acta Med Scand*. 1972; 192:183–8.
59. Killilea TA, White R, Coleman RW. Increased response to warfarin in valve-replacement patients compares to PE/DVT patients. *Clin Pharmacol Ther*. 1988; 43:161.
60. Ganeval D, Fischer AM, Barre J, et al. Pharmacokinetics of warfarin in the nephrotic syndrome and effect on vitamin k-dependent clotting factors. *Clin Nephrol*. 1986; 25:75–80.
61. Lindahl AK, Sandset PM, Abildgaard U, et al. High plasma levels of extrinsic pathway inhibitor and low levels of other coagulation inhibitors in advanced cancer. *Acta Chir Scand*. 1989; 155:389–93.
62. Blaisdell WF. Acquired and congenital clotting syndromes. *World J Surg*. 1990; 14:664–9.
63. Fengler SA, Berenberg JL, Lee YTM. Disseminated coagulopathies and advanced malignancies. *Am Surg*. 1990; 56:335–8.
64. Fletcher DC. Do clotting factors in vitamin k-rich vegetables hinder anticoagulant therapy? *J Am Med Assoc*. 1977; 237:1871.

65. Karlson B, Leijd B, Hellstrom K. On the influence of vitamin k-rich vegetables and wine on the effectiveness of warfarin treatment. *Acta Med Scand*. 1986; 220:347–50.

66. Ott P, Hamberg O, Ovesen LF. Optimizing warfarin treatment. *Ugeskr Laeger*. 1991; 153:263–7.

67. Ensminger A. Food and nutrition encyclopedia, vol 2. Clovis, CA: Pegus Press; 1983:2208, 2270–4.

68. Rombeau J, Caldwell M. Clinical nutrition: enteral and tube feeding, 2nd ed. Philadelphia, PA: W. B. Saunders; 1990:503.

69. Bachmann K, Shapiro R, Fulton R, et al. Smoking and warfarin disposition. *Clin Pharmacol Ther*. 1979; 25:309–15.

70. Weiner B, Faraci PA, Fayad R, et al. Warfarin dosage following prosthetic valve replacement: effect of smoking history. *Drug Intell Clin Pharm*. 1984; 18:904–6.

71. Ginsberg JS, Hirsh J. Optimum use of anticoagulants in pregnancy. *Drugs*. 1988; 36:505–12.

Chapter 22
Ana M. Lopez-Samblas, Philip R. Diaz &
Kim H. Binion

Drug Dosing in the Neonate

Neonates are a unique patient population with regard to drug disposition and therapeutic responsiveness. Within this population, marked differences are found when premature neonates are compared to full-term newborns. Extreme caution should be employed when extrapolating data and clinical experience from adults and other pediatric patients to the treatment of neonates. Furthermore, some of the information in this chapter differs from that found in previous chapters because of differences in interpretation of study results or in the patient populations cited.

For the dosage recommendations in Table 1, the following classifications and terminology are used:[18,19]

- Premature neonate—gestational age of 37 weeks or less.
- Full-term neonate—gestational age of 38–41 weeks.
- Post-term neonate—gestational age of 42 weeks or more.
- Gestational age—number of weeks from the first day of the last menstrual period to birth.
- Postnatal age (PNA)—number of weeks since birth.
- Postconceptional age (PCA)—gestational age plus postnatal age in weeks.

The contributions made by Kamal Behbahani, Jorge Chivite, and Helena Wang to this chapter are gratefully acknowledged.

TABLE 1. Neonatal Dosing Guidelines

Drug	Empiric Dosage[a]	Comments
Amikacin[1]	PCA ≤30 weeks: 9 mg/kg/18 hr PCA >30 weeks: 9 mg/kg/12 hr Term, PNA >1 week: 7.5 mg/kg/8 hr	Infusion should be over 30 min, preferably with syringe pump
Aminophylline[2]	LD = 6 mg/kg Premature MD = 2.5 mg/kg/12 hr Term MD = 2.5 mg/kg/6–8 hr	Neonates asphyxiated at birth may require MD reductions due to a decrease in CL of 20–50%; aminophylline contains 80–85% theophylline
Caffeine[3]	LD = 10 mg/kg (20 mg/kg salt form) MD = 2.5 mg/kg/day (5 mg/kg salt form)	Caffeine citrate salt forms contain 50% caffeine base (S = 0.5); higher MD may be needed with increasing PNA
Carbamazepine[4]	MD = 5 mg/kg/12 hr	Limited data are available
Digoxin[5,6]	Premature TDD = 15–25 µg/kg Premature MD = 4–6 µg/kg/day Term TDD = 20–30 µg/kg Term MD = 5–8 µg/kg/day	TDD is divided by one-half, one-fourth, and one-fourth and given at 8-hr intervals; doses are for intravenous route; oral dose is 20% higher
Gentamicin or tobramycin[7,8]	3.5 mg/kg/day	Infusion should be over approximately 30 min, preferably with syringe pump
Indomethacin[9,10]	LD = 0.25 mg/kg MD = 0.2 mg/kg/12 hr × 2 (0.2 mg/kg/day may be continued for 5 additional days)	Furosemide 2 mg/kg should be given within 20 min to minimize renal toxicity; indomethacin 0.1 mg/kg may be used for intraventricular hemorrhage prophylaxis

TABLE 1. (*continued*)

Drug	Empiric Dosage[a]	Comments
Pentobarbital[11]	LD = 10 mg/kg over 20 min MD = 1 mg/kg/hr	Continuous infusions induce barbiturate coma for intractable seizures
Phenobarbital[12,13]	LD = 20 mg/kg MD = 3–5 mg/kg/day (every 12–24 hr)	Neonates asphyxiated at birth only require 3 mg/kg/day; need for 12-hr dosing is questionable due to long half-life
Phenytoin[14]	LD = 15–20 mg/kg MD = 4–8 mg/kg/day (every 8–12 hr)	Intravenous LD rate is 0.5–1 mg/kg/min; oral absorption is erratic, and administration with feedings should be avoided
Fosphenytoin[15]	Same dose as Phenytoin, express as PE (Phenytoin equivalents)	Can be given intramuscularly; intravenous LD rate up to 3 mg/kg/min
Valproic acid[16]	LD = 20 mg/kg MD = 4–8 mg/kg/day (every 8–12 hr)	Sodium syrup (commercially available) should be diluted 1:1 with formula to minimize GI irritation
Vancomycin[17]	PCA <27 weeks 18 mg/kg/36 hr PCA 27–30 weeks 16 mg/kg/24 hr PCA 31–36 weeks 18 mg/kg/18 hr PCA >36 weeks 15 mg/kg/12 hr	Infusion should be over ≥1 hr, preferably with syringe pump

[a]*LD = loading dose, MD = maintenance dose, and TDD = total digitalizing dose.*

The information should be used only as a guide; as with any patient population, the clinical status of the neonate should be the primary consideration when choosing a dosage regimen.

General Pharmacokinetic Information[20-23]

Absorption

GI absorption in the newborn is variable because of irregular and prolonged gastric-emptying time, erratic peristalsis, and extreme fluctuations in gastric pH. Due to study design limitations inherent with this patient population, few bioavailability studies are available.

Serum concentrations of *caffeine, phenobarbital,* and *theophylline* after oral administration are comparable to those produced by corresponding intravenous doses. Absorption of *phenytoin*, however, may be erratic and incomplete.

Rectal absorption can be an adequate alternative with a proper formulation. Suppositories are often impractical for drugs with narrow therapeutic windows since dosing requirements in neonates depend on body weight. In addition, cutting suppositories may result in an unpredictable dose because the drug is not uniformly dispersed throughout the preparation. Rectally administered liquid preparations, such as *valproic acid* and *diazepam,* have been used effectively to treat seizures in neonates. However, they may be impractical if neonates cannot retain the volume required.

Intramuscular absorption is variable because a premature newborn has a small percentage of body weight that is skeletal muscle and subcutaneous fat compared to older infants, children, and adults. In addition, circulatory insufficiency, hypoxia, and exposure to a cold environment may decrease intramuscular absorption. For example, the intramuscular administration of *aminoglycosides* in premature neonates is discouraged due to inconsistent serum concentrations, but it is routinely employed in full-term, otherwise healthy, infants. Furthermore, the stress resulting from intramuscular injections in low birth weight neonates should always be considered.

Percutaneous absorption is pronounced in the premature neonate because the epidermal barrier is thin and often poorly developed. The use of adhesive tape on a newborn's skin further increases that area's permeability. Topical drugs with limited safety experience in neonates should be employed cautiously. Toxic effects have been reported with agents such as *hexachlorophene solution* and *boric acid powder.*

Distribution
The volume of distribution for water-soluble drugs is generally increased in neonates, especially premature infants, due to their large total body water composition (87% water for premature neonates and 77% for full-term neonates versus 55% for adults) and their higher percentage of extracellular to intracellular water (45% for neonates versus 20% for adults). In neonates, the volume of distribution for *theophylline* and the *aminoglycosides* can be more than double the mean adult value.

Although adipose tissue and skeletal muscle mass are limited, high volumes of distribution have been reported for some lipophilic drugs. This result is possibly due to the size of lipid-rich organs (e.g., brain and liver) in neonates relative to their total body weight. Decreased plasma protein binding may further increase the volume of distribution for highly protein-bound drugs.

In view of the distribution factors typical of neonates, larger milligram per kilogram doses than those required in adults are often necessary to produce equivalent serum drug concentrations.

Metabolism
Since the neonate's enzyme systems are not fully developed, the rate of metabolic degradation is delayed, especially in the first 2 weeks of life. The various metabolic pathways mature at different rates.

Phase I reduction and hydroxylation reactions, which occur in the cytochrome P450 enzyme systems, are in general terms low in occurrence (50–70% of adult values). Cytochrome P450 isoenzymes do not exhibit the same degree of activity during the neonatal period. Preliminary research suggest that CYP2A6, 2C9, 2D6, 2E1, and 3A are present during the prenatal and infant period; CYP1A2, 2B6, and 2C8 are highly active in children over 1 year of age; and the activity of CYP3A7 disappears after infancy. Pharmacokinetic studies performed during the neonatal period support a prolonged half-life for the xanthines, phenobarbital, and phenytoin. Ongoing research will afford a better understanding of the effect of specific isoenzyme activity on drug disposition during the neonatal period.

Of the phase II reactions, sulfate conjugation is present while glucuronidation and acetylation are minimal. As a result, neonates cannot conjugate *chloramphenicol* as well as adults; if used, chloramphenicol doses should be adjusted accordingly.

Neonates can exhibit alternative metabolic pathways such as the conversion of *theophylline* to *caffeine* and the excretion of higher percentages of unchanged theophylline.

Exposure to an enzyme-inducing agent before or after birth may increase or stimulate oxidative pathways.

Elimination

In the neonate, kidneys are anatomically and functionally immature. Filtration, secretion, and reabsorption evolve at different rates. At 34–36 weeks gestational age, the renal system develops rapidly due to changes in the glomeruli.

Glomerular filtration exceeds tubular function at birth and persists for the first 6 months. Inulin clearance is 30–50% of adult values in full-term newborns (per body surface area). Although the glomerular filtration rate is related to gestational age, this relationship is not linear.

In the premature neonate, renal function is impaired compared to full-term infants; renal development relates linearly with postconceptional age. Since the half-lives of drugs excreted renally (e.g., vancomycin) are prolonged, dosing intervals should be extended. Dosing guidelines based on postconceptional age have been used effectively to initiate therapy because they approximate the degree of renal function maturity.

Protein binding

The plasma protein binding of various drugs is less in the neonate compared to other patient populations because

1. The total plasma protein concentration is smaller.
2. Fetal albumin is present, which has a decreased affinity for drugs.
3. Endogenous substances such as free fatty acids and unconjugated bilirubin may compete with drugs for binding sites.

A decrease in protein binding results in increased free unbound drugs in these patients. Therefore, the therapeutic ranges of certain highly bound drugs are lower for neonates (e.g., 6–14 versus 10–20 mg/L in adults for *phenytoin*).

Therapeutic Range

Suggested therapeutic ranges and monitoring parameters for drugs frequently used in the neonate are listed in Table 2. Note that some of these therapeutic ranges have been extrapolated from the adult population and that others are based on limited neonatal literature.

Factors Interfering with Therapeutic Monitoring[31-34]

Methods of intravenous drug administration

Since the volumes of drugs administered to neonates are small, the method of drug infusion can considerably

TABLE 2. Suggested Therapeutic Ranges and Monitoring Parameters for Selected Drugs Used in the Neonate[24–26]

Therapeutic Range	Pharmacodynamic Monitoring		Comments
	Efficacy	Toxicity	
Amikacin[1] Peak = 20–30 mg/L Trough = 5–10 mg/L	• Resolution of laboratory[a] and clinical[b] markers of sepsis	• Nephrotoxicity: BUN and serum creatinine (S_{Cr}) • Urine output: <1 ml/kg/hr • Ototoxicity: brain stem auditory-evoked responses	• Peak should be drawn 0.5 hr after end of infusion • Trough should be drawn within 0.5 hr prior to subsequent dose
Caffeine:[3,25,26] 4–25 mg/L	• Resolution or acceptable decrease in apnea and bradycardia	• Tachycardia: mean baseline heart rate calculated prior to initiation of caffeine or theophylline therapy; when heart rate is >180/min, other causes of tachycardia (e.g., fluid overload) should be ruled out before dose is reduced or discontinued • Other signs: feeding intolerance, aspiration, vomiting, excessive agitation, and hyperglycemia	• Toxicity rarely occurs at concentrations of <50 mg/L • *Caution* is required in patients who cannot mount tachycardic response (e.g., patients receiving digoxin)

Drug	Clinical/Therapeutic Monitoring	Toxicity Monitoring	Comments
Carbamazepine:[4,20] 4–12 mg/L	• Resolution of seizure activity documented on EEG • Improvement in clinical manifestation of seizure	• GI irritation • Sedation • Leukopenia documented by CBC • Hepatotoxicity documented by liver function tests (LFTs) • Serious skin reactions	• Limited data exist for use in neonates • Protein binding may be diminished
Digoxin:[5,6] 0.5–2 µg/L	• Resolution of CHF documented by chest X-ray and echocardiogram • Clinical improvement in weight, urine output, dependent edema, delayed capillary refill time, and hypotension • Resolution or control of supraventricular tachycardia, atrial fibrillation, or flutter documented by ECG	• Feeding intolerance • Bradycardia • Diarrhea • Lethargy • Cardiac dysrhythmias on ECG	• Endogenous digoxin-like substances cross-react with some reagents commonly used to detect digoxin in serum, therefore by *falsely elevating apparent digoxin levels*; therefore, specificity of the assay in neonates needs to be considered. • Clinical monitoring is critical; concentrations should be interpreted only in light of clinical findings
Gentamicin or tobramycin: Peak = 5–10 mg/L Trough = <2 mg/L	• Resolution of laboratory[a] and clinical[b] markers of sepsis	• Nephrotoxicity: BUN and S_{Cr} • Urine output: <1 ml/kg/hr	• Peak concentrations correlate with therapeutic effect but not with toxicity

TABLE 2. (continued)

Therapeutic Range	Pharmacodynamic Monitoring		Comments
	Efficacy	Toxicity	
		• Ototoxicity: brain stem auditory-evoked responses	• Peak should be drawn 0.5 hr after end of infusion • Trough should be drawn within 0.5 hr prior to subsequent dose
Indomethacin:[9,10] 0.4–3.6 mg/L[c]	• Closure of patent ductus arteriosus (PDA) on ECG with resolution of clinical signs • Resolution of clinical signs, including increased precordial activity, bounding peripheral pulses, murmur, widened pulse pressures, and high or fluctuating ventilatory requirements	• Nephrotoxicity: S_{Cr} (baseline and before each dose throughout therapy; drug might need to be held if S_{Cr} increases >0.5 mg/dl) • Urine output: <1 ml/kg/hr • Hyponatremia • Decreased platelet function • GI bleeding • Necrotizing enterocolitis • Decreased myocardial contractility • Decreased cerebral blood flow • Hypoglycemia at higher drug levels	• Aminoglycosides, digoxin, and vancomycin may accumulate during indomethacin therapy; patient should be observed for toxicity • In all cases, pharmacodynamic monitoring is necessary

Drug and therapeutic range	Efficacy monitoring	Toxicity monitoring	Comments
Pentobarbital:[11] 10–40 mg/L	• Inducement of coma in patients with intractable seizures • Resolution of seizure activity documented on EEG	• Respiratory depression • Hypotension	• Patient should receive artificial ventilation prior to coma induction
Phenobarbital:[12] 10–40 mg/L	• Degree of sedation[28]	• Lethargy • Excessive sedation • Respiratory depression • Hypotonia • Urinary retention • Systemic hypotension	
Phenytoin:[14] 6–15 mg/L (unbound 1–3 mg/L)	• Resolution of seizure activity documented on EEG • Improvement in clinical manifestation of seizure	• Rash • Fever • Lethargy • Hypotension during infusion • Hypotension in patients receiving dopamine • Excessive sedation • Hypotonia • Seizures at high concentrations	• Peak concentrations of patients on *fosphenytoin* should be obtained at least 4 hr after intramuscular dosing and 2 hr after intravenous dosing to ensure complete conversion to phenytoin

TABLE 2. (*continued*)

Therapeutic Range	Pharmacodynamic Monitoring		Comments
	Efficacy	Toxicity	
Theophylline:[25] 4–20 mg/L	• Resolution or acceptable decrease in apnea and bradycardia • Ventilator weaning of patients on low settings (i.e., FiO_2 <40, PIP <25, and rate <30) • Prevention of intubation in patients with $pO_2:FiO_2$ >130[27]	• See caffeine	• Theophylline converts to caffeine
Valproic acid:[16] 25–100 mg/L	• Resolution of seizure activity documented on EEG • Improvement in clinical manifestation of seizure	• Hepatotoxicity documented by LFTs • Hyperammonemia documented by plasma ammonium • GI irritation and bleeding • Potentiated bleeding secondary to platelet inhibition	

Drug	Therapeutic Goal	Adverse Effects	Comments
Vancomycin:[17] Peak = 30–40 mg/L Trough = 5–15 mg/L	Resolution of laboratory[a] and clinical[b] markers of sepsis	Red baby syndrome (histamine reaction): hypotension, flushing (rate related), and tachycardia	• Drug concentration may not correlate with toxic response • Peak should be drawn 1 hr after end of infusion • Trough should be drawn within 0.5 hr prior to subsequent dose

[a]*Laboratory markers of sepsis include CBC with differential, increased immature to total (I:T) neutrophil ratio,[25] absolute neutrophil count,[26] decreased platelet count, increased bilirubin, serial cultures/sensitivities, cerebral spinal fluid information, and C-reactive protein.[30]*
[b]*Clinical markers of sepsis include abnormal chest X-rays, apnea and bradycardia, respiratory distress, lethargy, glucose intolerance, feeding intolerance, temperature instability, abdominal distension, cholestasis, and hypotension.*
[c]*Concentrations outside this range may be therapeutic.*

influence the time to attain peak drug concentrations and, thus, the reliability of "timed" peak and trough concentration levels. Three administration methods are commonly used: antegrade, retrograde, and syringe pump.

In antegrade infusion, drug delivery can be substantially delayed based on the intravenous flow rate (slow rates are less accurate) and injection site (distal sites are less accurate). When flow rates are less than 25 ml/hr, antegrade infusion should not be used if the accuracy of infusion time is important for therapeutic drug monitoring.

Syringe pumps are the preferred method for drug administration in most neonatal intensive care units. Although superior to the antegrade method, their accuracy is influenced by a variety of factors. Studies have demonstrated that elevating syringe pumps during infusion can result in a rapid bolus injection followed by a period of no flow. Lowering the devices may result in aspiration into the syringe system. To improve consistency of drug delivery, the following measures are recommended: (1) position the syringe pump above the infusion port, (2) ensure that the pump remains stationary during infusions, (3) use microbore tubing, (4) attach the microbore tubing to the injection site closest to the patient, and (5) utilize the highest volume/rate tolerated by the patient.

Because of the small drug volumes typical of neonates, trapping in the dead space of stopcocks and other administration ports should be considered, regardless of the method of drug administration. All administration sites should be flushed with just enough volume to clear the dead space without causing a bolus effect.

Concentration measurements drawn from intravenous lines[22]

When drug concentrations appear to be inconsistent with the dose and clinical picture, the blood collection site should be considered. Sample collections from an intravascular line (e.g., umbilical artery catheter or other central line) may result in artificially elevated serum drug concentrations due to contamination with the drug administered via that line.

This problem might be greater in neonates than in other patients because dosage volumes are small and significant amounts of drug may be "trapped" in dead spaces of stopcocks. To prevent this situation, drug administration sites should be flushed prior to sample collection or separate drug administration and blood collection sites should be employed.

Medication errors

Errors in medication dose calculations for neonates occur with alarming frequency and, therefore, should be considered if serum drug concentrations appear to be inconsistent with the prescribed dose. The following items should be verified: dose calculation per kilogram, patient's weight and gestational and postconceptional ages, dosage units, and specially calculated drug dilutions if needed for accurate dose measurement.

Digoxin-like substances[35,36]

An endogenous digoxin-like substance (DLS) can cause falsely elevated serum digoxin concentrations in neonates and infants. Commercially available digoxin assays differ significantly in their degree of specificity. Therefore, validity of the specific assay used for digoxin should be determined prior to monitoring or making pharmacokinetic calculations. Emphasis should be placed on clinical monitoring of response and signs of toxicity when dosing digoxin in neonates.

Factors Influencing Drug Disposition

Asphyxia[37-39]

The elimination of aminoglycosides, phenobarbital, and theophylline in neonates asphyxiated at birth is markedly reduced due to decreased renal and liver perfusion during severe hypoxia. In neonates with Apgar scores of less than 3 at 1 or 5 min or with cardiac and respiratory arrest requiring resuscitation, concentrations of drugs with narrow therapeutic windows should be closely monitored; dosage requirements might need to be decreased by approximately 50%. Since the duration of this effect is not well established, followup is warranted.

Asphyxiated neonates receiving *phenobarbital* or *theophylline* can be empirically dosed with half the usual maintenance dose, followed by drug concentration monitoring for dosage adjustment (no adjustment is needed for loading doses). For neonates receiving *aminoglycosides* or *vancomycin,* urine output should be evaluated to assess the need for dosing interval adjustments. Urine output can serve as an immediate indicator of decreased renal clearance due to hypoxia.

Exchange transfusion[40–42]

Information regarding the effect of exchange transfusions on serum concentrations of drugs commonly administered to neonates is limited and often controversial. Drug loss has varied from 1 to 55%, depending on the medications, study design, and timing and frequency of procedures. The magnitude of the decline in drug concentrations is greatest when the procedure is performed shortly after dose administration (since concentrations are higher) and can be considered clinically inconsequential at the end of the dosing interval. The effect is augmented by the number of blood volumes exchanged (on the same dose) and the rate utilized.

When exchange transfusions are at the beginning of the dosing interval and a drop in concentration might be clinically consequential, drug concentrations should be obtained to assess drug loss and to calculate a "replacement" dose. Concentrations obtained following exchange transfusions should not be employed for routine pharmacokinetic calculations since they do not reflect steady-state conditions.

Extracorporeal membrane oxygenation (ECMO)[43–48]

The pharmacokinetics of gentamicin and vancomycin have been studied in neonates undergoing ECMO. Some studies found little difference between pharmacokinetic parameters in infants undergoing ECMO compared to literature values. In contrast, other studies found significantly larger volumes of distribution and lower clearances when compared to literature values and patients were utilized as their own controls. The increased V may be explained by the administration of fluids and blood required to perform ECMO. Decreased organ perfusion and ischemia prior to ECMO as well as the nonpulsative blood flow of the ECMO circuit are potential explanations for the decrease in clearance. In addition, studies have shown that when medications are administered into the ECMO circuit there may be delayed or reduced drug delivery. One hypothesis is that drug pooling may occur with low flow rates. Other investigations suggest binding of drug to the ECMO circuit, which occurs to a greater extent with a new circuit and declines when the circuit has been used over several days. Therefore, dosing during ECMO should take into account the patient's response and be individualized based on drug concentrations.

Patent ductus arteriosus (PDA)[49–51]

Significant differences in the volume of distribution (depending on whether the ductus arteriosus is open or closed) have been shown for several drugs including *gentamicin, indomethacin,* and *vancomycin*. In addition, the calculated volume of distribution significantly decreases after PDA closure, potentially changing dosing requirements that were therapeutic beforehand. When utilizing indomethacin for the pharmacological closure of the PDA, its nephrotoxic effects may decrease renal clearance of *aminoglycosides, digoxin,* and *vancomycin*.

References

1. Kenyon CF, Knoppert DC, Lee SK, et al. Amikacin pharmacokinetics and suggested dosage modifications for the preterm infant. *Antimicrob Agents Chemother.* 1990; 34(2):265–8.
2. Gilman JT, Gal P, Levine RS, et al. Factors influencing theophylline disposition in 179 neonates. *Ther Drug Monit.* 1986; 8:4–10.
3. Thomson AH, Kerr S, Wright S. Population pharmacokinetics of caffeine in neonates and young infants. *Ther Drug Monit.* 1996; 18:245–53.
4. MacKintosh DA, Biard-Lampert J, Buchanan N. Is carbamazepine an alternative maintenance therapy for neonatal seizures? *Dev Pharmacol Ther.* 1987; 10:100–6.
5. Park MK. Use of digoxin in infants and children with specific emphasis on dosage. *J Pediatr.* 1986; 108(6):871–7.
6. Bendayan R, McKenzie MW. Digoxin pharmacokinetics and dosage requirements in pediatric patients. *Clin Pharm.* 1983; 2(3):224–35.
7. Murphy JE, Austin ML, Frye RF. Evaluation of gentamicin pharmacokinetics and dosing protocols in 195 neonates. *Am J Health-Syst Pharm.* 1998; 55:2280–8.
8. Skopin H, Heiman G. Once daily aminoglycosides in full-term neonates. *Pediatr Infect Dis.* 1995; 14(1):71–2.
9. Gal P, Ransom JL, Schall S, et al. Indomethacin for patent ductus arteriosus closure: application of serum concentrations and pharmacodynamics to improve response. *J Perinatol.* 1990; 1:20–6.
10. Hammerman C, Aramburo MJ. Prolonged indomethacin therapy for the prevention of recurrences of patent ductus arteriosus. *J Pediatr.* 1990; 117:771–6.
11. Weity TE, Kriel RL. Pentobarbital coma for treating intractable seizures in a neonate. *Clin Pharm.* 1985; 4:330–2.
12. Gal P, Toback J, Boer H, et al. Efficacy of phenobarbital monotherapy in the treatment of neonatal seizures; relationship to blood levels. *Neurology.* 1982; 32:1401–4.
13. Fisher JH, Lockman LA, Zaske D, et al. Phenobarbital maintenance dose requirements in treating neonatal seizures. *Neurology.* 1981; 31:1042–4.
14. Loughnan PM, Greenwald A, Purton WW, et al. Pharmacokinetic observations of phenytoin disposition in the newbornland young infant. *Arch Dis Child.* 1977; 52:303–9.
15. Pellock JM. Fosphenytoin use in children. *Neurology.* 1996; 46(*Suppl 1*):S14–S16.
16. Gal P, Oles KS, Gilman JT, et al. Valproic acid efficacy, toxicity, and pharmacokinetics in neonates with intractable seizures. *Neurology.* 1988; 38:467–71.
17. McDougal A, Ling EW, Levine M. Vancomycin pharmacokinetics and dosing in premature neonates. *Ther Drug Monit.* 1995; 17(4):319–26.
18. Fanaroff AA, Martin RJ, eds. Neonatal–perinatal medicine, diseases of the fetus and infant, 4th ed. St. Louis, MO: C. V. Mosby; 1987.
19. Fanaroff AA, Klaus MH. Care of the high-risk neonate, 3rd ed. Philadelphia, PA: W. B. Saunders; 1986.

20. Morselli PL, Franco-Morselli R, Bossi L. Clinical pharmacokinetics in newborns and infants; age-related differences and therapeutic implications. *Clin Pharmacokinet.* 1980; 5:485–527.
21. Stewart CF, Hampton EM. Effect of maturation on drug disposition in pediatric patients. *Clin Pharm.* 1987; 6:548–64.
22. Walson PD, Edwards R, Cox S. Neonatal therapeutic drug monitoring: its clinical relevance. *Ther Drug Monit.* 1989; 11:425–30.
23. Tateishi T, Nakura H, Asoh M, et. al. A comparison of hepatic cytochrome P450 protein expression between infancy and postinfancy. *Life Sci.* 1997; 61(26):2567–74.
24. Bonati MM, Marchetti F, Zullini MT, et al. Adverse drug reactions in neonatal intensive care units. *Acute Poisoning Rev.* 1990; 9:103–18.
25. Roberts RJ. Drug therapy in infants: pharmacologic principles and clinical experience. Philadelphia, PA: W. B. Saunders; 1984:94–118.
26. Monroe BL, Weinberg AG, Rosenfeld CR, et al. The neonatal blood count in health and disease: I. Reference ranks for neutrophil cells. *J Pediatr.* 1979; 95:89–98.
27. Farkas VA, Gal P, Ranson JL, et al. Predictors of pharmacodynamic effect of theophylline for the prevention of intubation in premature neonates with respiratory distress syndrome. *Pharmacotherapy.* 1990; 10:237.
28. Mimaki T, Walson PD, Suzuki Y. Anticonvulsants. In: Yaffe SJ, Aranda JV, eds. Pediatric pharmacology, 2nd ed. Philadelphia, PA: W. B. Saunders; 1992:299.
29. Maloley PA, Gal P, Mize R, et al. Lorazepam dosing in neonates: application of objective sedation scores. *DICP.* 1990; 24:326–7.
30. Gerdes JS. Clinicopathologic approach to the diagnosis of neonatal sepsis. *Clin Perinatol.* 1991; 18:361–81.
31. Roberts RJ. Intravenous administration of medication in pediatric patients; problem and solutions. *Pediatr Clin North Am.* 1981; 28: 23–34.
32. Nahata MC. Influence of infusion methods on therapeutic drug monitoring in pediatric patients. *DICP.* 1986; 20:367–9.
33. Morgan ED, Bergadale S, Ziegler EE. Effect of syringe-pump position on infusion of fat emulsion with a primary solution. *Am J Hosp Pharm.* 1985; 42:1110–1.
34. Lönnquist PA. Design flaw can convert commercially available continuous syringe pumps to intermittent bolus injections. *Intensive Care Medicine.* 1997; 23:998–1001.
35. Valdes R Jr, Geaves SW, Brown BA, et al. Endogenous substance in newborn infants causing false positive digoxin measurements. *J Pediatr.* 1983; 102:947.
36. Pudek MR, Secombe DW, Jacobson BE, et al. Seven different digoxin immunoassay kits compared with respect to immunoreactive substance in serum from premature and full-term infants. *Clin Chem.* 1983; 29:1972.
37. Friedman CA, Parks BR, Rawson JE. Gentamicin disposition in asphyxiated newborns: relationship to mean arterial blood pressure and urine output. *Pediatr Pharmacol.* 1982; 2:189–97.

38. Gal P, Toback J, Erkan NV, et al. The influence of asphyxia on phenobarbital dosing requirements in neonates. *Dev Pharmacol Ther.* 1984; 7:145–52.
39. Gal P, Boer HR, Toback J. Effect of asphyxia on theophylline clearance in newborns. *South Med J.* 1982; 75:836–8.
40. Assael BM, Caccamo ML, Gerna M, et al. Effect of exchange transfusion on elimination of theophylline in premature neonates. *J Pediatr.* 1977; 91:331–2.
41. Kliegman RM, Bertino JS, Fanaroff AA, et al. Pharmacokinetics of gentamicin during exchange transfusions in neonates. *J Pediatr.* 1980; 96:927–30.
42. Roberts RJ. Drug therapy in infants: pharmacologic principles and clinical experience. Philadelphia, PA: W. B. Saunders; 1984.
43. Southgate WM, DiPiro JT, Robertson AF. Pharmacokinetics of gentamicin in neonates on extracorporeal membrane oxygenation. *Antimicrob Agents Chemother.* 1989; 33:817–9.
44. Hoie EB, Swigart SA, Leushen MP. Vancomycin pharmacokinetics in infants undergoing extracorporeal membrane oxygenation. *Clin Pharm.* 1990; 9:711–5.
45. Bhatt-Mehta V, Johnson CE, Schumacher RE. Gentamicin pharmacokinetics in term neonates receiving extracorporeal membrane oxygenation. *Pharmacotherapy.* 1992; 12:28–32.
46. Amaker RD, Dipiro JT, Bhatia J. Pharmacokinetics of vancomycin in critically ill infants undergoing extracorporeal membrane oxygenation. *Antimicrob Agents Chemother.* 1996; 40(5):1139–42.
47. Cohen P, Collart L, Prober CG, et al. Pharmacokinetics of gentamicin in neonatal patients undergoing extracorporeal membrane oxygenation. *Pediatr Infect Dis.* 1990; 9(8):562–6.
48. Buck ML. Administration of medications to neonates receiving extracorporeal membrane oxygenation. *J Pediatr Pharm Pract.* 1996; 1:155–62.
49. Watterberg KL, Kelly WH, Johnson JD, et al. Effect of patent ductus arteriosus on gentamicin pharmacokinetics on very low birth weight (< 1500 g) babies. *Dev Pharmacol Ther.* 1987; 10:107–17.
50. Spivey J, Gal P. Vancomycin pharmacokinetics in neonates. *Am J Dis Child.* 1986; 140:859.
51. Zarfin Y, Koren G, Maresky D, et al. Possible indomethacin–aminoglycoside interaction in preterm infants. *J Pediatr.* 1985;106: 511–3.

Chapter 23
Vinita B. Pai & Milap C. Nahata

Drug Dosing in Pediatric Patients

Pediatric patients have been labeled "therapeutic orphans" because of the lack of pharmacokinetic, pharmacodynamic, efficacy, and safety data necessary to provide safe and effective drug therapy to this population. Efficacy and safety trials of new drugs are initially conducted in adult patients, most often excluding children and pregnant women. Safety and efficacy data in the pediatric population may come from a trial and error method after use of these drugs. Numerous drugs, routinely used in pediatric patients, do not have pediatric labeling. Children should not be considered miniature adults; adult doses, scaled down based on body weight, may not be as safe and effective in the pediatric population as in adults. As neonates develop into toddlers and young adolescents, several physiologic events occur that change the body composition (e.g., changes in body water, body fat, plasma proteins, and hormonal composition) and influence drug disposition. The pediatric population, based on age, can be classified into five distinct groups as follows:

Premature (preemie)	born at gestational age <38 weeks
Neonate (newborn)	0–4 weeks postnatal age
Infant	1–<12 months of age
Child	1–12 years of age
Adolescent	13–18 years of age

Physiological changes resulting in growth and development of a human body may not strictly remain in these age-related boundaries and may not be linearly related to age. Drug disposition in pediatric patients may change due to certain intrinsic factors such as gender, race, heredity, and inherited diseases and certain extrinsic factors such as acquired diseases, diet, and prior exposure to drug therapy. To provide safe and effective drug therapy to pediatric patients, it is important to gain knowledge of the pharmacokinetic and pharmacodynamic properties of each drug and the effect of development on its disposition. This chapter focuses on the influence of growth and maturation on drug disposition and pharmacodynamic response to drugs in the pediatric population, ranging from infants to adolescents. Drug dosing in the neonate is addressed in chapter 22.

Absorption

Intravenous

Factors such as site of injection, intravenous flow rate, the infusion system, and the dosage volume influence the delivery of an intravenously administered drug into the systemic circulation.[1-5] A site of injection distant from the patient, a slow intravenous flow rate, and a large dose volume result in lower and delayed peak concentrations of the drug. This reduction may potentially influence therapeutic efficacy and/or safety of some drugs. A timed drug concentration measurement, especially one different from what was predicted, should be evaluated only after giving careful consideration to these factors. Accurate drug delivery can be achieved by using syringe pumps and low-volume microbore tubings, by choosing as close a site as possible to the patient, and by flushing or priming the pump and the intravenous tubing with sufficient volume of the drug solution to be administered.

Oral

Most drugs administered by the oral route are absorbed by passive diffusion. Gastric pH, gastric and intestinal motility, pancreatic enzyme activity, bacterial colonization of the intestines, bile salt production, blood flow to the GI tract, and the surface area of absorption affect the rate and extent of GI absorption.[6-9] These factors undergo considerable maturational changes as an infant grows into an adult. The volume and acid concentration of the gastric juice are dependent on age and approach the lower limit of adult values by 3 months of age; they reach adult values only after 2 years of age.[10-14] The rate and extent of absorption for drugs that are weak acids or bases may depend on their partition coefficients.[15-17] Gastric pH may change with ingestion of certain foods. For example, orange juice, cranberry juice, and carbonated beverages decrease the gastric pH causing acidic drugs to be absorbed more readily. An acidic gastric pH is necessary for complete absorption of itraconazole, which may be altered in patients receiving H_2-antagonists such as ranitidine. In pediatric patients administering itraconazole with carbonated beverages or orange juice increases its absorption. Absorption of acidic drugs decreases when given with milk or infant formula due to increases in gastric pH.[18]

Gastric emptying rate appears to be a function of gestational age, postnatal age, and the nature of feedings. It is considerably delayed in infants, reaching adult values by 6–8 months of age.[19-21] Most orally administered drugs are absorbed in the small intestine; therefore, a shorter gastric emptying time leads to a faster rate of absorption. The rate and extent of drug absorption may be significantly altered in patients with acute changes in the GI tract. Decreased and delayed absorption of ampicillin and nalidixic acid was observed in infants and children treated with these drugs for acute shigellosis.[22] In another study involving use of ampicillin in the treatment of gastroenteritis in children, the mean concentrations of ampicillin were lower in the children with gastroenteritis than in children without the malady, possibly due to malabsorption.[23] Beyond the neonatal age group, differences in GI maturation and absorption between the different age groups may not be significant enough to impact oral dosing recommendations for most drugs.

Pancreatic enzymes increase bioavailability of certain drugs whose oral dosage forms require intraluminal (GI) hydrolysis prior to absorption (e.g., oral liquid ester formulations of clindamycin and chloramphenicol palmitate).[24] Pancreatic enzyme activity is low at birth.[25] Amylase activity remains low (approximately 10% of adult values) even after the first month of life.[24] Lipase activity increases 20-fold during the first 9 months after birth.[19,25] Trypsin secretion in response to pancreozymin and secretin develops during the first year of life.[26]

Bile salts may influence the absorption of certain fat-soluble drugs and nutrients. Bile salt metabolism matures postnatally within the first few months of life and continues during the first year of life.[27]

Composition and rate of GI colonization by bacterial flora depend more on diet than on age;[28] however, the effect of bacteria on intestinal motility and drug metabolism is not completely known. For example, intestinal colonization by oral digoxin-reducing anaerobic bacteria approaches adult values by 2 years of age;[29] however, the reduction of digoxin by these bacteria that is observed in adults may not be achieved until adolescence. Therefore, when compared to adults, higher digoxin bioavailability can be anticipated in infants.

Intramuscular

The surface area over which the injected solution can be distributed, the blood flow to the site of injection, the ease of penetration through the endothelial capillary walls, and muscle activity may all influence the absorption of drugs after intramuscular administration. This route is more commonly used for administration of vaccines. However, drugs administered by this route are generally well absorbed in infants and children. Obviously, it can be a painful route of administration and should be used only when oral administration is not indicated or intravenous access is unavailable.

Percutaneous

Greater skin hydration, thinner and/or immature stratum corneum, and greater body surface area to weight ratio increase percutaneous drug absorption in pediatric patients.[30] However, the skin of a full-term neonate has barrier properties to drug absorption similar to adult skin.[31] Increased absorption of topically applied compounds may be observed in infants as compared to children and adults with equal dose applications (Table 1).[32] Since percutaneous absorption is increased through damaged skin, application of high potency corticosteroids to diaper rashes with severe perianal inflammation should be avoided.[33]

Rectal

The rectal route of administration is a useful alternative when oral administration is precluded by nausea, vomiting, seizures, preparation for surgery, or when the intravenous route is precluded by lack of intravenous dosage form or lack of intravenous access. The rate and extent of absorption of certain drugs may be much improved when rectal solutions are used rather than suppositories.[34] However, factors such as delay in onset of action and failure to reach minimal effective concentrations in the plasma for some drugs make the rectal route of drug administration inferior to oral and intravenous routes for most drugs.

TABLE 1. Age-Dependent Differences in Physiologic Functions and Drug Disposition

Physiologic Variability	Neonate	Infant	Child	Pharmacokinetic Consequences
Absorption				
Gastric pH	Increased (>5)	Increased (2–4)	Normal (2–3)	Increase in bioavailability of acid-labile drugs, e.g., penicillin G, ampicillin, and nafcillin in neonates and infants compared to children and adults; decreased bioavailability of weak organic acids, e.g., phenobarbital[1,5–17,100]
Gastric and intestinal emptying time	Reduced and irregular	Increased	Increased	Possible elimination of a significant portion of theophylline dose from certain sustained-release products (Theo-Dur, Slo-bid Gyrocaps) in the stool before being absorbed due to slower rates of absorption compared to the GI transit time in the young (8 months to 4 years of age)[101]
Biliary function	Immature	Near adult pattern	Adult pattern	Increased absorption of fat and fat-soluble vitamins D and E in infants and children compared to neonates[27]

Pancreatic function	Immature	Near adult pattern	Adult pattern	Increased hydrolysis and bioavailability of oral liquid ester formulations of clindamycin and chloramphenicol in infants and children compared to neonates[24]
Gut microbial colonization	Reduced	Near adult pattern	Adult pattern	Increased bioavailability of digoxin in neonates compared to adults due to lack of microbial gut colonization with an oral digoxin-reducing anaerobic bacteria[29]
Intramuscular absorption	Variable	Increased	Increased or near adult pattern	Benzathine penicillin G more rapidly absorbed in children compared to adults since no measurable activity was detected in children 18 days after the injection[102]
Skin permeability and percutaneous absorption	Increased	Increased	Near adult pattern	EMLA (eutectic mixture of local anesthetics lidocaine and prilocaine) contraindicated in patients less than 3 months of age due to risk of methemoglobinemia due to increased percutaneous absorption of prilocaine and decreased methemoglobin reductase[32]
Rectal absorption	Increased	Increased	Near adult pattern	Specific example not available

TABLE 1. (*continued*)

Physiologic Variability	Neonate	Infant	Child	Pharmacokinetic Consequences
Distribution				
Total body water and extracellular water	Increased	Increased	Near adult pattern	Increase in mean apparent volume of distribution (V) for hydrophilic drugs, e.g., gentamicin[36,37]: $V_{<34\,wk} = 0.67 \pm 0.13$ L/kg; $V_{34-48\,wk} = 0.52 \pm 0.10$ L/kg; $V_{1-4.9\,yr} = 0.38 \pm 0.16$ L/kg; $V_{5-9.9\,yr} = 0.33 \pm 0.14$ L/kg; $V_{10-16\,yr} = 0.31 \pm 0.12$ L/kg; $V_{adult} = 0.30$ L/kg
Total body fat	Reduced	Reduced	Increasing by ages 5–10 yr	Increase in mean apparent V for lipophilic drugs, e.g., diazepam[39] 1.3–2.6 L/kg in infants vs 1.6–3.2 L/kg in adults
Total plasma proteins	Reduced	Reduced or near adult pattern	Adult pattern	Increase in V and free phenytoin concentration in neonates and infants[45]

Renal Elimination			
Glomerular filtration	Reduced	Adult pattern	Adult pattern	Famotidine–80% excreted unchanged in the urine in older children and adults; renal clearance equivalent to adults by 1 year of age[103]
Tubular secretion	Reduced	Near adult pattern	Adult pattern	Penicillins–increased elimination half-life due to decreased excretion both by glomerular filtration and tubular secretion, therefore lengthening the dosing interval in neonates and perhaps infants compared to children and adolescents[24]
Tubular reabsorption	Reduced	Near adult pattern	Adult pattern	Specific example not available

Distribution

The volume of distribution is greater for drugs highly distributed in the tissues. Factors such as the relative proportion of body water and body fat and differences in protein binding determine the differences in drug distribution between children and adults. The total body water decreases from approximately 71% in a full-term neonate to 60% (25% is extracellular water and 35% is intracellular) by one year of age.[35] Total body water approaches adult values of 50–60% (20% extracellular and 40% intracellular) by 12–13 years of age.

Hydrophilic drugs such as aminoglycoside antibiotics largely distribute into the extracellular fluid and thus have larger volumes of distribution in neonates compared to older infants and children (Table 1).[36,37] Larger volumes of distribution require larger milligram-per-kilogram doses of aminoglycosides to achieve recommended peak concentrations. Caution should be exercised in using actual body weight in calculating aminoglycoside doses in obese children due to the relatively lower percentage of extracellular water in obesity.

Total body fat increases from 12–16% of body weight at full-term to 20–25% at one year of age. It then increases between 5 and 10 years of age, followed by a decrease in boys around age 17. At puberty, there is a rapid increase in percent body fat in females, approaching twice the value compared to males.[35,38] Lipophilic drugs will have a larger volume of distribution in adults and children than neonates and infants due to higher percentage of body fat (Table 1).[39]

The binding of drugs to circulating plasma proteins depends on multiple factors such as total amount of proteins, the number of binding sites, the binding affinity, and the presence of pathophysiologic conditions (e.g., change in blood pH) and/or endogenous compounds (e.g., bilirubin, free fatty acids) that may alter the drug–protein interaction. Albumin, alpha-1-acid glycoprotein, and lipoproteins are the important drug-binding proteins; albumin comprises 58% of all plasma proteins.[40] Total protein concentration including serum albumin and alpha-1-acid glycoprotein as well as their function and binding capacity approach adult values by the first year of age and remain consistently stable in healthy children between 2 and 18 years of age.[39,41,42]

Acidic and neutral drugs such as beta-lactam antibiotics, warfarin, and digoxin exhibit great binding affinity for albumin; basic compounds such as propranolol and alprenolol bind to alpha-1-acid glycoprotein, lipoproteins, and beta-globulins.[43] Several endogenous substances such as bilirubin and free fatty acid compete for the albumin binding sites and influence the drug–protein binding capacity. For example, bilirubin is often increased in neonates and infants with increased red cell destruction and limited liver capacity to conjugate it. The binding capacity of bilirubin to plasma albumin is decreased in newborn infants but approaches adult values by 5 months of age. Drugs highly bound to the plasma proteins, e.g., sulfonamides, may displace bilirubin and contribute to kernicterus in neonates and infants.[44] The pharmacological action of a drug moiety is usually attributed to the free (unbound) form of the drug. Conditions that decrease serum plasma proteins may increase the free, active fraction of highly protein-bound drugs.

Metabolism

Drug metabolism primarily occurs in the liver; however, kidneys, intestines, lungs, and skin may also be involved.[46] Most drugs that are metabolized are converted to more water-soluble compounds for easy excretion from the body by the kidneys. Active parent compounds may be transformed into inactive or active (e.g., theophylline to caffeine or procainamide to N-acetylprocainamide) metabolites. Pharmacologically inactive compounds or prodrugs may also be converted to their active moiety (e.g., cyclophosphamide is hydroxylated to 4-hydroxycyclophosphamide and aldophosphamide).

Hepatic blood flow, extraction efficacy, binding affinity, and enzyme activity may affect hepatic drug metabolism. Of these factors, enzyme activity is greatly dependent on patient age. Two primary enzymatic processes, phase I (nonsynthetic) reactions and phase II (synthetic) reactions are involved in drug biotransformation. Phase I reactions include oxidation, reduction, hydrolysis, and hydroxylation that introduce or reveal a functional group within the substrate that will serve as a site for a phase II conjugation reaction. In phase II reactions, the substrate may be conjugated with endogenous agents such as sulfate, acetate, glucuronic acid, glutathione, and glycine, resulting in a more polar, water-soluble compound that can be eliminated easily by the renal and/or the biliary system.

The activity of the oxidizing enzymes is greatly reduced at birth, resulting in prolonged elimination of drugs such as phenytoin and diazepam.[47-50] The hepatic mono-oxygenase system approaches and exceeds adult capacities by approximately 6 months of age.[47,48,51,52] Alcohol dehydrogenase activity, detectable at ≤3–4% of adult activity at 2 months of age, approaches adult capacity after 5 years of age.[53] Demethylation activity may not be seen until 14–15 months of age and may increase thereafter. Hydrolytic activity reaches adult values within the first few months of life. Quantitatively, cytochromes P450 are the most important phase I enzymes with CYP1, CYP2, and CYP3 genes being important in human drug metabolism (Table 2).[54-56]

The phase II enzymes consist of glucuronosyltransferases, sulfotransferases, arylamine N-acetyltransferases, glutathione S-transferases, and methyltransferases, all of which play an important role in biotransformation of drugs (Table 3).[57-59] Important differences exist between

TABLE 2. Age-Dependent Differences in Activity of Important Drug-Metabolizing Phase I Enzymes and Drug Metabolism

Enzyme	Neonate	Infant	Child	Adolescent	Pharmacokinetic Consequences
CYP2D6	Reduced (20% of adult activity)	Reduced	Adult pattern (by age 3–5 years)	Adult pattern	O-Demethylation of codeine to morphine decreases in neonates and infants, resulting in reduced efficacy and poor pain control[55]
CYP2C19	Reduced	Adult pattern (reached by age 6 months)	Increased (peak activity at ages 3–4 years)	Adult pattern (decreases to adult value at puberty)	Diazepam half-life increases in neonates and infants (25–100 hr) compared to children (7–37 hr) and adults (20–50 hr) due to decreased oxidative activity[50]
CYP2C9	Reduced	Adult pattern (reached by age 1–6 months)	Increased (peak activity at ages 3–10 years)	Adult pattern (decreases to adult value at puberty)	Phenytoin half-life decreases from 80 hr at 0–2 days, to 15 hr at 3–14 days, to 6 hr at 14–150 days after birth[47,48]
CYP3A4	Reduced (30–40% of adult activity)	Adult pattern (by age 6 months)	Increased (between ages 1 and 4 years, then progressively decreases)	Adult pattern (at puberty)	Increased metabolism of carbamazepine to its 10,11-epoxide in infants and children with increased CYP3A4 activity compared to neonates and adults[56]

TABLE 3. Age-Dependent Differences in Activity of Important Drug-Metabolizing Phase II Enzymes and Drug Metabolism

Enzyme	Neonate	Infant	Child	Adolescent	Pharmacokinetic Consequences
N-Acetyltransferase-2	Reduced	Reduced	Adult pattern (present by ages 1–3 yr)	Adult pattern	Decreased acetylation of sulfapyridine (sulfasalazine metabolite) results in increased side effects of nausea, headache, and abdominal pain[57]
Methyltransferase	Increased (50% higher than adults)	Adult pattern	Adult pattern	Adult pattern	Specific example not available
Glucuronosyl-transferase	Reduced	Adult pattern (by ages 6–18 months)	Adult pattern	Adult pattern	The ratio of glucuronide conjugate to sulfate conjugate of acetaminophen increases with age as the glucuronosyl enzyme system matures[59]; newborn 0.34; child (3–10 yr) 0.8; adolescent 1.61, and adult 1.8–2.3
Sulfotransferase	Reduced (10–20% of adult activity)	Increased (for specific substrates)	Increased (for specific substrates)	Adult pattern	Specific example not available

children and adults, and phase II enzymes do not all follow the same developmental patterns.

Elimination

Most drugs or their water-soluble metabolites are excreted through the kidneys. The functional capacity of the kidney increases with age up to early adulthood. Glomerular filtration, tubular secretion, and reabsorption all impact on the renal elimination of drugs. Glomerular filtration of drugs depends on the functional capacity of the glomerulus, the integrity of renal blood flow, and the extent of drug–protein binding. The amount of drug filtered through the glomerulus is inversely proportional to the degree of protein binding. The glomerular filtration rate (GFR) increases with an increase in renal blood flow. In utero, high renal vascular resistance decreases the renal blood flow, which approaches adult values by approximately 5–12 months of age.[47,48,60] The GFR dramatically increases from birth and approaches adult values by approximately 3–5 months of age.[61,62] The increase in GFR is related to changes in renal blood flow; at birth, clamping of the umbilical cord increases the cardiac output and perfusion, decreases the renal vascular resistance, and thus increases renal blood flow.

The tubular secretory function does not mature at the same rate as the GFR because the proximal convoluted tubules are small relative to their corresponding glomeruli at birth.[63] Tubular function approaches adult values by approximately 30 weeks of life, thus affecting drugs eliminated by tubular secretion in addition to glomerular filtration (Table 1).[60,64]

Dosing recommendations for renally excreted drugs, especially those with a narrow therapeutic range, should be based on the patient's renal function to avoid toxicity due to decreased elimination and increased accumulation. Monitoring parameters such as urine output, creatinine clearance, and serum creatinine can assess renal function clinically. A urine output of approximately 1 mL/kg/hr in neonates may be considered normal.[65] However, urine output varies with fluid intake, hydration status, renal solute load, and urine concentration capabilities and may not accurately reflect renal clearance of drugs primarily excreted through the kidneys, especially drugs eliminated by tubular secretion rather than glomerular filtration.

The GFR can be estimated by assessing creatinine clearance. This estimation requires a 24-hr urine collection that is difficult to obtain in infants and children. Incomplete collections will lead to inaccurate results; complete collection may require catheterization of the patient, making the process more invasive. Creatinine clearance can be estimated from single serum creatinine values by using nomograms or mathematical formulas which are most convenient but less accurate.[65-67] In patients receiving aminoglycosides, renal clearance of the aminoglycoside approximates creatinine clearance, since >90% of the dose is filtered through the glomeruli without being secreted or absorbed and can be used to estimate the GFR.[68]

Drug Disposition in Cystic Fibrosis

Drug disposition may be altered by different disease states. A pathological disorder of the organs involved in absorption, distribution, metabolism, or excretion of drugs may alter the rate and/or the extent of absorption, the apparent volume of distribution, plasma protein binding, and elimination half-life and clearance. Recommendations for changes in drug dosing should be made based on the type of alteration in drug disposition. For drugs with a narrow therapeutic range and accurate methods available for measuring drug concentrations, dosing recommendations should be made based on these concentrations.

Cystic fibrosis (CF) is an autosomal recessive disease, predominantly seen in the Caucasian population, affecting approximately 30,000 children and young adults in the United States.[69] Mutation of a single gene on chromosome 7 encoding the CF transmembrane conductance regulator leads to abnormalities affecting multiple organs; this mutation then impacts all aspects of drug disposition.[70] Factors such as lower rate of absorption, larger apparent volume of distribution, and greater metabolic and renal clearances may alter drug disposition and lower plasma concentrations after administration of age-appropriate doses of many drugs in patients with CF when compared to normal patients.

Drug absorption in patients with CF may be decreased due to altered GI physiology such as gastric acid hypersecretion, bile acid malabsorption, and proximal small intestinal mucosal injury.[71,72] Bioavailability studies of oral and intravenous cloxacillin in patients with CF and healthy individuals exhibited no significant difference between the two groups, only greater variability in the CF patients.[73] Fluoroquinolone bioavailability data in patients with CF have been conflicting, with some studies suggesting no change while others showing an increase in the bioavailability compared to the normal population.[74–77] The rate of absorption was significantly slower and the time (t_{max}) to achieve maximum plasma concentration (C_{max}) was significantly greater in patients with CF for cloxacillin and ciprofloxacin.

Alteration in protein binding of drugs due to hypoalbuminemia and hypogammaglobulinemia in patients with CF[78,79] could alter their distribution volume. The choice of units using body surface area (L/m^2) and body weight (L/kg) may affect the apparent volume of distribution because body weight is affected much earlier than linear growth during the course of CF. A higher volume of distribution has been reported for cloxacillin, theophylline, and ceftazidime in patients with CF compared to healthy individuals when expressed by units of body weight. For drugs such as methicillin and ticarcillin, the distribution volume was not significantly different when expressed per unit of body surface area (BSA). It has been recommended that volume of distribution should be normalized by lean body mass (LBM) rather than BSA.[80] However, the appropriateness of one approach over another is still unknown.[81]

Hepatobiliary dysfunction, increase in hepatic enzymes, and reduced synthesis of proteins are reported in approximately 30–40% of patients with CF.[82,83] Hepatic clearance of drugs is largely influenced by the hepatic blood flow and activity of liver enzymes. Evidence of an increase in portal venous blood flow in CF patients is conflicting; therefore, increased hepatic blood flow may be unrelated to the CF gene defect. Age, severity of CF disease, and extent of hepatic dysfunction may influence the hepatic blood flow.

Hepatic biotransformation of drugs by phase I and II reactions may either be increased or remain unchanged in patients with CF compared to healthy individuals. The formation clearance values for 3-hydroxymethylantipyrine were significantly higher in the patients with CF compared to healthy adults, after intravenous administration of antipyrine. Antipyrine is metabolized to 3-hydroxymethylantipyrine via the CYP2C8 and CYP1A2 pathways, suggesting that activity mediated through these two pathways may be enhanced. However, data on the CYP1A2 pathway are conflicting.[83–86] CYP2C9 activity was found to be similar in patients with CF and the control group for S-warfarin.[87] CYP3A4-dependent metabolic activity was not found to be induced or activated in patients with CF for conversion of R-warfarin to 1-hydroxywarfarin.[88]

Disease-specific alterations in hepatic biotransformation in patients with CF are not limited to the monooxygenase system. Ibuprofen is mainly metabolized by glucuronosyltransferase to a glucuronide conjugate.[89] A significant increase in the apparent total clearance of ibuprofen was observed after oral administration in children with CF compared with healthy children,[90] suggesting that glucuronidation is enhanced in this population. Both in vitro and in vivo data showed increased metabolic clearance of unbound sulfamethoxazole to N4-acetylsulfamethoxazole and thus confirmed that the intrinsic activity of N-acetyltransferase (NAT1) was significantly increased in patients with CF.[91,92] However, activity of N-acetyltransferase (NAT2) is not significantly different in the patients with CF compared to healthy individuals.

Results from studies measuring renal function, i.e., GFR and tubular clearance, are conflicting with both parameters either increased or unchanged in patients with CF. These results are attributed to differences in age and severity of the CF disease, e.g., glomerulomegaly and hyperfiltration.

The renal clearance of ceftazidime was significantly increased in patients with CF compared to healthy adults due to increased glomerular filtration.[93,94] Aminoglycosides are primarily eliminated by glomerular filtration; however, they are also reabsorbed by the proximal tubule. Studies comparing renal clearance of amikacin to inulin and tobramycin to iodothalamate indicated that the glomerular filtration of aminoglycosides is not altered in patients with CF.[95,96] Therefore, the decrease in tubular reabsorption and/or clearance into the respiratory tract was speculated to be the cause of increased plasma clearance of aminoglycosides.

Tubular secretion of penicillin derivatives such as cloxacillin, methicillin, and ticarcillin, primarily eliminated renally by tubular secretion, was significantly higher in patients with CF compared to healthy individuals.[97-99]

Altered drug disposition in patients with CF impacts drugs with a narrow therapeutic index and their plasma concentrations and drugs with large pharmacokinetic variabilities. Therefore, the normal age-appropriate drug doses should be altered in CF patients based on plasma concentrations.

TABLE 4. Recommended Ranges for Selected Drugs

Drug and Empiric Doses[104] (Infants and Children)	Therapeutic Range	Comments
Ethosuximide Children: <6 yr Initial: 15 mg/kg/day in two divided doses (max. = 250 mg/dose); increase every 4–7 days Maintenance: 15–40 mg/kg/day in two divided doses (max. = 1.5 g/day) Children >6 yr: use adult dose	40–100 mg/L	A concentration as high as 150 mg/L may be needed to achieve seizure control; a trough or predose concentration measurement is most appropriate to recommend dosing changes
Lidocaine Loading dose: 1 mg/kg, repeat in 10–15 minutes if needed for two doses Continuous infusion: 20–50 mcg/kg/min to be titrated to therapeutic range	1.5–5.0 mg/L	Evaluate serum concentration 1–2 hr into infusion if no response; within 12–24 hr after initiation to estimate steady state; every 24–48 hr to monitor for adequate clearance

Drug	Therapeutic range	Comments
Caffeine Apnea of prematurity Loading dose: 10–20 mg/kg as caffeine citrate (5–10 mg/kg as caffeine base) Maintenance dose: 5–10 mg/kg/day as caffeine citrate (2.5–5 mg/kg/day as caffeine base) once daily starting 24 hr after the loading dose.	8–20 mg/L	If patient already on theophylline, doses of caffeine need to be adjusted; adjust maintenance doses based on patient response and caffeine concentrations
Flucytosine Infants, children, and adults: 100–150 mg/kg/day in divided doses every 6 hr	25–100 mg/L	Determine a peak concentration to monitor for adequate absorption; determine peak 2 hr postdose at least 4 days after start of therapy (A concentration between 40 and 60 mg/L is necessary for treatment of invasive candidiasis.)

Therapeutic Drug Monitoring (TDM)

Table 4 lists several drugs and their therapeutic ranges used in the pediatric population that require TDM. The ultimate goal of TDM is to document positive therapeutic outcomes, e.g., eradication of infection with absence of nephrotoxicity after aminoglycoside therapy and control of seizures with phenytoin.

References

1. Gould T, Roberts RJ. Therapeutic problems arising from the use of the intravenous route for drug administration. *J Pediatr*. 1979; 95(3):465–71.
2. Nahata MC, Powell DA, Glazer JP, et al. Effect of intravenous flow rate and injection site on in vitro delivery of chloramphenicol succinate and in vivo kinetics. *J Pediatr*. 1981; 99(3):463–6.
3. Nahata MC, Powell DA, Durrell D, et al. Delivery of tobramycin by three infusion systems. *Chemotherapy*. 1984; 30(2):84–7.
4. Nahata MC, Powell DA, Durrell D, et al. Effect of infusion methods on tobramycin serum concentrations in newborn infants. *J Pediatr*. 1984; 104(1):136–8.
5. Leff RD, Roberts RJ. Methods for intravenous drug administration in the pediatric patient. *J Pediatr*. 1981; 98(4):631–5.
6. Parsons RL. Drug absorption in gastrointestinal disease with particular reference to malabsorption syndromes. *Clin Pharmacokinet*. 1977; 2(1):45–60.
7. Radde IC. Mechanisms of drug absorption and their development. In: MacLeod SM, Radde IC, eds. Textbook of pediatric clinical pharmacology. Littletown: PSG Publishing; 1985:17–43.
8. Welling PG. Influence of food and diet on gastrointestinal drug absorption: a review. *J Pharmacokinet Biopharm*. 1977; 5(4):291–334.
9. Welling PG. Interactions affecting drug absorption. *Clin Pharmacokinet*. 1984; 9(5):404–34.
10. Agunod M, Yomaguchi N, Lopez R, et al. Correlative study of hydrochloric acid, pepsin and intrinsic factor secretion in newborns and infants. *Am J Dig Dis*. 1969; 14(6):400–14.
11. Harada T, Hyman PE, Everett S, et al. Meal–stimulated gastric acid secretion in infants. *J Pediatr*. 1984; 104(4):534–8.
12. Hyman PE, Clark DD, Everett SL, et al. Gastric acid secretory function in preterm infants. *J Pediatr*. 1985; 106(3):467–71.
13. Lebenthal E, Lee PC, Heitlinger LA. Impact of development of the gastrointestinal tract on infant feeding. *J Pediatr*. 1983; 102(1):1–9.
14. Morselli PL. Clinical pharmacokinetics in neonates. *Clin Pharmacokinet*. 1976; 1(2):81–98.
15. Huang NN, High RH. Comparison of serum levels following the

administration of oral and parenteral preparations of penicillin to infants and children of various age groups. *J Pediatr*. 1953; 42:657–68.
16. O'Connor WJ, Warren GH, Edrada LS, et al. Serum concentrations of sodium nafcillin in infants during the perinatal period. *Antimicrob Age Chemother*. 1965; 5:220–2.
17. Sliverio J, Poole JW. Serum concentrations of ampicillin in newborn infants after oral administration. *Pediatrics*. 1973; 51(3):578–80.
18. Pinkerton CR, Welshman SG, Glasgow JF, et al. Can food influence the absorption of methotrexate in children with acute lymphoblastic leukaemia? *Lancet*. 1980; 2(8201):944–6.
19. Cavell B. Gastric emptying in preterm infants. *Acta Paediatr Scand*. 1979; 68(5):725–30.
20. Grand RJ, Watkins JB, Torti FM. Development of human gastrointestinal tract: A review. *Gastroenterol*. 1976; 70(5PT1):790–810.
21. Gupta M, Brans YW. Gastric retention in neonates. *Pediatrics*. 1978; 62(1):26–9.
22. Nelson JD, Shelton S, Kusmiesz HT, et al. Absorption of ampicillin and nalidixic acid by infants and children with acute shigellosis. *Clin Pharmacol Ther*. 1972; 13(6):879–86.
23. Elliot RB, Stokes EJ, Maxwell GM. Ampicillin in paediatrics. *Arch Dis Child*. 1964; 39:101–5.
24. Reed MD, Besunder JB. Developmental pharmacology: ontogenic basis of drug disposition. *Pediatr Clin N Am*. 1989; 36:1053–74.
25. Kearns GL, Reed MD. Clinical pharmacokinetics in infants and children: a reappraisal. *Clin Pharmacokinet*. 1989; 17(Suppl. 1):29–67.
26. Hadron B, Zoppi G, Shmerling DH, et al. Quantitative assessment of exocrine pancreatic function in infants and children. *J Pediatr*. 1968; 73(1):39–50.
27. Heubi JE, Balistreri WF, Suchy FJ. Bile salt metabolism in the first year of life. *J Lab Clin Med*. 1982; 100(1):127–36.
28. Yoshioka H, Iseki K, Fujita K. Development and differences of intestinal flora in the neonatal period in breast-fed and bottle-fed infants. *Pediatrics*. 1983; 72(3):317–21.
29. Linday L, Dobkin JF, Wang TC, et al. Digoxin inactivation by the gut flora in infancy and childhood. *Pediatrics*. 1987; 79(4):544–8.
30. Shear NH, Radde IC. Percutaneous drug absorption. In: Radde IC, MacLeod SM, eds. Pediatric pharmacology and therapeutics. St. Louis: Mosby; 1993:377–83.
31. Harpin VA, Rutter N. Barrier properties of the newborn infant's skin. *J Pediatr*. 1983; 102(3):419–25.
32. Nilsson A, Engberg G, Henneberg S, et al. Inverse relationship between age-dependent erythrocyte activity of methaemoglobin reductase and prilocaine-induced methaemoglobinaemia during infancy. *Br J Anaesth*. 1990; 64(1):72–6.
33. Feinblatt BI, Aceto T Jr, Beckhom G, et al. Percutaneous absorption of hydrocortisone in children. *Am J Dis Child*. 1966; 112(3):218–24.
34. Dhillon S, Ngwane E, Richens A. Rectal absorption of diazepam in epileptic children. *Arch Dis Child*. 1982; 57(4):264–7.
35. Friis-Hansen B. Body water compartments in children: changes

during growth and related changes in body composition. *Pediatrics.* 1961; 28:169–81.

36. Semchok WM, Shevchuk YM, Sankaran K, et al. Prospective randomized controlled evaluation of a gentamicin loading dose in neonates. *Biol Neonate.* 1995; 67(1):13–20.

37. Shevchuk YM, Taylor DM. Aminoglycoside volume of distribution in pediatric patients. *DICP.* 1990; 24(3):273–6.

38. Milsap RL, Hill MR, Szefler SJ. Special pharmacokinetic considerations in children. In: Evans WE, Schentag JJ, Jusko WJ, eds. Applied pharmacokinetics: principles of therapeutic drug monitoring. Vancouver, WA: Applied Therapeutics Inc.; 1992:10-1-32.

39. Divoll M, Greenblatt DJ, Ochs HR, et al. Absolute bioavailability of oral and intramuscular diazepam: effects of age and sex. *Anesth Analg.* 1983; 62:1–8.

40. Wilkinson GR. Plasma and tissue binding considerations in drug disposition. *Drug Metab Rev* 1983; 14(3):427–65.

41. Pacifici GM, Viani A, Taddeucci-Brunelli G, et al. Effects of development, aging, and renal and hepatic insufficiency as well as hemodialysis on the plasma concentration of albumin and alpha 1 acid glycoprotein: implications for binding of drugs. *Ther Drug Monit.* 1986; 8(3):259–63.

42. Radde IC. Drugs and protein binding. In: McLead SM, Radde IC, eds. Textbook of pediatric clinical pharmacology. Littletown: PSG Publishing; 1985:32–43.

43. Piafsky KM. Disease-induced changes in the plasma binding of basic drugs. *Clin Pharmacokinet.* 1980; 5(3):246–62.

44. Walker PC. Neonatal bilirubin toxicity: A review of kernicterus and the implications of drug-induced bilirubin displacement. *Clin Pharmacokinet.* 1987; 13(1):26–50.

45. MacKichan JJ. Influence of protein binding and use of unbound (free) drug concentrations. In: Evans WE, Schentag JJ, Jusko WJ, eds. Applied pharmacokinetics: principles of therapeutic drug monitoring. Vancouver, WA: Applied Therapeutics Inc.; 1992:5-1–48.

46. Litterst CL, Mimnaugh EG, Reagan RL. Comparison of in vitro drug metabolism by lung, liver, and kidney of several common laboratory species. *Drug Metab Dispos.* 1975; 3(4):165–259.

47. Besunder JB, Reed MD, Blumer JL. Principles of drug disposition in the neonate: a critical evaluation of the pharmacokinetic-pharmacodynamic interface. Part I. *Clin Pharmacokinet.* 1988; 14(4):261–86.

48. Besunder JB, Reed MD, Blumer JL. Principles of drug disposition in the neonate: a critical evaluation of the pharmacokinetic-pharmacodynamic interface. Part II. *Clin Pharmacokinet.* 1988; 14(5):189–216.

49. Nitowsky HM, Matz L, Berzofsky JA. Studies on oxidative drug metabolism in the full term newborn infant. *J Pediatr.* 1966; 69(6):1139–49.

50. Morselli PL, Principi N, Tognoni G, et al. Diazepam elimination in premature and full-term infants and children. *J Perinat Med.* 1973; 1(2):133–41.

51. Gladtke E. The importance of pharmacokinetics for paediatrics. *Eur J Pediatr*. 1979; 131(2):85–91.
52. Neims AH, Warner M, Loughman PM, et al. Developmental aspects of the hepatic cytochrome P450 mono-oxygenase system. *Ann Rev Pharmacol Toxicol*. 1976; 16:427–45.
53. Pikkarainen PH, Raiha NCR. Development of alcohol dehydrogenase activity in the human liver. *Pediatr Res*. 1967; 1(3):165–8.
54. Leeder JS, Kearns GL. Pharmacogenetics in pediatrics: implications for practice. *Pediatr Clin N Am*. 1997; 44:55–77.
55. Mortimer O, Persson R, Ladona MG, et al. Polymorphic formation of morphine from codeine in poor and extensive metabolizers of dextromethorphan. Relationship to the presence of immunoidentified cytochrome P 450 IID1. *Clin Pharmacol Ther*. 1990; 47(1):27–35.
56. Korinthenberg R, Haug C, Hannak D. The metabolization of carbamazepine to CBZ–10, 11-epoxide in children from the newborn age to adolescence. *Neuropediatrics*. 1994; 25(4):214–6.
57. Evans DA. N-Acetyltransferase. *Pharmacol Ther*. 1989; 42(2):157–234.
58. Evans WE, Horner M, Chu YQ, et al. Altered mercaptopurine metabolism, toxic effects and dosage requirement in a thiopurine-methyltransferase deficient child with acute lymphoblastic anemia. *J Pediatr*. 1991; 119(6):985–9.
59. Miller RP, Roberts RJ, Fischer LJ. Acetaminophen elimination kinetics in neonates, children and adults. *Clin Pharmacol Ther*. 1976; 19(3):284–94.
60. West JR, Smith HW, Chasis H. Glomerular filtration rate, effective renal blood flow and maximal tubular excretory capacity in infancy. *J Pediatr*. 1948; 32:10–8.
61. Arant BS. Developmental patterns of renal functional maturation compared in the human neonate. *J Pediatr*. 1978; 92(5):705–12.
62. Leake RD, Trygstad CW. Glomerular filtration rate during the period of adaptation to extrauterine life. *Pediatr Res*. 1977; 11(9):959–62.
63. Fitterman GH, Shuplock NA, Phillip FJ. The growth and maturation of human glomeruli and proximal convolutions from term to childhood. *Pediatrics*. 1965; 35:601–19.
64. Trompeter RS, Baratt TM. Clinical evaluation. In: Holliday MA, Baratt TM, Avner ED, eds. Pediatric nephrology. Baltimore: Williams & Wilkins; 1994:366–77.
65. Cockcroft DW, Gault MH. Prediction of creatinine clearance from serum creatinine. *Nephron*. 1976; 16(1):31–41.
66. Jellife RW. Creatinine clearance: bedside estimate. *Ann Intern Med*. 1973; 79:604–5.
67. Schwartz GJ, Brion LP, Apitzer A. The use of plasma creatinine concentration for estimating glomerular filtration rate in infants, children and adolescents. *Pediatr Clin N Am*. 1987; 34 (3):570–90.
68. Koren G, James A, Perlman R. A simple method for the estimation of glomerular filtration rate by gentamicin pharmacokinetics during routine drug monitoring in newborn. *Clin Pharmacol Ther*. 1985; 38(6):680–5.

69. Cystic Fibrosis Foundation. Facts about cystic fibrosis. [Online] Feb. 22, 1999. Available: http://www.cff.org/facts.htm [Feb. 24,1999].
70. Collins FS. Cystic fibrosis: molecular biology and therapeutic implications. *Science*. 1992; 256(5058):774–9.
71. Cox KL, Isenberg JN, Ament ME. Gastric acid hypersecretion in cystic fibrosis. *J Pediatr Gastroenterol Nutr*. 1982; 1(4):559–65.
72. Fondacaro JD, Heubi JE, Kellogg FW. Intestinal bile acid malabsorption in cystic fibrosis: a primary mucosal cell defect. *Pediatr Res*. 1982; 16(6):494–8.
73. Spino M, Chai RP, Isles AF, et al. Cloxacillin absorption and disposition in cystic fibrosis. *J Pediatr*. 1984; 105(5):829–35.
74. Goldfarb J, Wormser GP, Inchiosa MA Jr, et al. Single–dose pharmacokinetics of oral ciprofloxacin in patients with cystic fibrosis. *J Clin Pharmacol*. 1986; 26(3):222–6.
75. Bender SW, Dalhoff A, Shah PM, et al. Ciprofloxacin pharmacokinetics in patients with cystic fibrosis. *Infection*. 1986; 14(1):17–21.
76. LeBel M, Bergeron MG, Vallee F, et al. Pharmacokinetics and pharmacodynamics of ciprofloxacin in cystic fibrosis patients. *Antimicrob Ag Chemother*. 1986; 30(2):260–6.
77. Christensson BA, Nilsson Ehle I, Ljungberg B, et al. Increased oral bioavailability of ciprofloxacin in cystic fibrosis patients. *Antimicrob Ag Chemother*. 1992; 36:2512–7.
78. Strober W, Peter G, Schwartz RH. Albumin metabolism in cystic fibrosis. *Pediatrics*. 1969; 43(3):416–26.
79. Schwartz RH. Serum immunoglobulin levels in cystic fibrosis. *Am J Dis Child*. 1960; 111(4):408–11.
80. Prandota J. Drug disposition in cystic fibrosis: progress in understanding pathophysiology and pharmacokinetics. *Pediatr Infect Dis J*. 1987; 6(12):1111–26.
81. Morgan DJ, Bray KM. Lean body mass as a predictor of drug dosage: implications for drug therapy. *Clin Pharmacokinet*. 1994; 26(4):292–307.
82. Kearns GL. Hepatic drug metabolism in cystic fibrosis: recent developments and future directions. *Ann Pharmacother*. 1993; 27(1):74–9.
83. Isenberg JN. Cystic fibrosis: its influence on the liver, biliary tree and bile salt metabolism. *Semin Liver Dis*. 1982; 2(4):302–13.
84. Kearns GL, Crom WR, Karlson KH, et al. Hepatic drug clearance in patients with mild cystic fibrosis. *Clin Pharmacol Ther*. 1996; 59(15):529–40.
85. Parker AC, Pritchard P, Preston T, et al. Enhanced drug metabolism in young children with cystic fibrosis. *Arch Dis Child*. 1997; 77(3):239–41.
86. Hamelin BA, Xu K, Valle F, et al. Caffeine metabolism in cystic fibrosis: enhanced xanthine oxidase activity. *Clin Pharmacol Ther*. 1994; 56(5):521–9.
87. O'Sullivan TA, Wang JP, Unadkat JD, et al. Disposition of drugs in cystic fibrosis. V. In vivo CYP2C9 activity as probed by (S)-warfarin is not enhanced in cystic fibrosis. *Clin Pharmacol. Ther*. 1993; 54(3):323–8.

88. Wang JP, Unadkat JD, McNamara S, et al. Disposition of drugs in cystic fibrosis. VI. In vivo activity of cytochrome P450 isoform involved in the metabolism of (R)-warfarin (including P450 3A4) is not enhanced in cystic fibrosis. *Clin Pharmacol Ther*. 1994; 55(5):528–34.
89. Albert KS, Gernaat CM. Pharmacokinetics of ibuprofen. *Am J Med*. 1984; 77 (1A):40–6.
90. Konstan MW, Hoppel CL, Chai BL, et al. Ibuprofen in children with cystic fibrosis: pharmacokinetics and adverse effects. *J Pediatr*. 1991; 118(6):956–64.
91. Hutabarat RM, Unadkat JD, Sahajwalla C, et al. Disposition of drugs in cystic fibrosis: I Sulfamethoxazole and trimethoprim. *Clin Pharmacol Ther*. 1991; 49(4):402–9.
92. Hutabarat RM, Smith AL, Unadkat JD, et al. Disposition of drugs in cystic fibrosis. VII. Acetylation of sulfamethoxazole in blood cells: in vitro-in vivo correlation and characterization of its kinetics of acetylation in lymphocytes. *Clin Pharmacol Ther*. 1994; 55(4):427–33.
93. Prandota J. Clinical pharmacology of antibiotics and other drugs in cystic fibrosis. *Drugs*. 1988; 35(5):542–78.
94. Pechere JC, Dugal R. Clinical pharmacokinetics of aminoglycoside antibiotics. *Clin Pharmacokinet*. 1979; 4(3):170–99.
95. Levy J, Smith AL, Koup JR, et al. Disposition of tobramycin in patients with cystic fibrosis: a prospective controlled study. *Pediatrics*. 1984; 105(1):117–24.
96. Finkelstein E, Hall K. Aminoglycoside clearance in patients with cystic fibrosis. *J Pediatr*. 1979; 94(1):163–4.
97. Jusko WJ, Mosovich LL, Gerbracht LM, et al. Enhanced renal excretion of dicloxacillin in patients with cystic fibrosis. *Pediatrics*. 1975; 56(6):1038–44.
98. Yaffe SJ, Gerbracht LM, Mosovich LL, et al. Pharmacokinetics of methicillin in patients with cystic fibrosis. *J Infect Dis*. 1977; 135(5):828–31.
99. de Groot R, Hack BD, Weber A, et al. Pharmacokinetics of ticarcillin in patients with cystic fibrosis: a controlled prospective study. *Clin Pharmacol Ther*. 1990; 47(1):73–8.
100. Wallin A, Jalling B, Boreus LO. Plasma concentrations of phenobarbital in the neonate during prophylaxis for neonatal hyperbilirubinemia. *J Pediatr*. 1974; 85(3):392–8.
101. Hendeles L, Iafrate RP, Weinberger M. A clinical and pharmacokinetic basis for the selection and use of slow release theophylline products. *Clin Pharmacokinet*. 1984; 9:95–135.
102. Ginsburg CM, McCracken GH, Zweighaft TC. Serum penicillin concentrations after intramuscular administration of benzathine penicillin G in children. *Pediatrics*. 1982; 69(4):452–4.
103. James LP, Marshall JD, Heulitt MJ, et al. Famotidine pharmacokinetics and pharmacodynamics in children. *J Clin Pharmacol*. 1996; 36(1):48–54.
104. Pediatric Dosage Handbook. 5th ed. Taketomo CK, Hodding JH, Kraus DM, eds. Hudson, Ohio: Lexicomp Inc.; 1999–2000.

Chapter 24
Susan W. Miller

Therapeutic Drug Monitoring in the Geriatric Patient

While old age is inevitable, much of the disease and disability common in later life is preventable.[1] Researchers have cautioned against a "gerontology of the usual," suggesting that a focus on typical aging as normal ignores the heterogeneity of the population.[2] Although many irreversible changes occur with aging, it is now well recognized that individuals age at different rates (chronological and biological age are not synonomous). Older patients take more medications than younger persons, yet major drug studies are performed on individuals younger than 55 years. It is now recognized that the frailty of a geriatric patient can alter drug metabolism and that this effect appears to vary from drug to drug. The frail elderly have been shown to have reduced drug metabolism.[3]

Studies examining the pharmacokinetics of drugs in the elderly compared with younger patients are beginning to increase in number. This information is sorely needed; current dosing in geriatric patients is often based on broad generalizations ("use one-third to one-half the usual dose") or anecdotal data—not on solid pharmacokinetic or pharmacodynamic studies. Pharmacokinetic/pharmacodynamic differences in older patients may account for either the toxic or subtherapeutic response that often occurs.

Adverse drug reactions (ADRs) and drug–drug interactions (DDIs) occur more frequently in geriatric patients,[4] in part because this population is most likely to be utilizing complex drug therapies. Although considerable evidence suggests that an ADR will not occur simply because a patient is elderly, pharmacokinetic and pharmacodynamic changes in the elderly may significantly alter drug disposition and must be considered.[5,6]

Significant ADRs are most likely with drugs having a narrow therapeutic index or saturable hepatic metabolism (e.g., phenytoin and theophylline) or when elimination is via a single mechanism or pathway. The patients most at risk usually have multiple disease states or compromised organ function, and they receive multiple drug therapy. Complicated drug therapy, poor compliance, and altered pharmacokinetics are among the many possible causes of ADRs and DDIs.

Physiologic Changes

Absorption, distribution, metabolism, and excretion

The processes of absorption, distribution, metabolism, and excretion determine the amount of drug present at any given time within the body's various cellular, tissue, and fluid compartments. The science of pharmacokinetics uses mathematical equations to derive the parameters of bioavailability, half-life, clearance, and volume of distribution from timed measurements of drug concentrations. Comparisons are then possible between different drugs and individuals.

Pharmacokinetic parameters represent a composite of both genetic and environmental effects.[7] The physiologic changes produced by aging that may have important implications for altered pharmacokinetics are summarized in Table 1.

TABLE 1. Physiologic Changes with Aging that May Affect Pharmacokinetics[7]

Process	Physiologic Effect
Absorption	Reduced gastric acid production Reduced gastric-emptying rate Reduced GI motility Reduced GI blood flow Reduced absorptive surface
Distribution	Decreased total body mass Increased percentage of body fat Decreased percentage of body water Decreased plasma albumin Disease-related increase in alpha-1-acid glycoprotein Altered relative tissue perfusion
Metabolism	Reduced liver mass Reduced liver blood flow Reduced hepatic metabolic capacity
Excretion	Reduced glomerular filtration Reduced renal tubular function

Age-related physiologic changes in the GI tract include elevated gastric pH, delayed gastric-emptying time, and decreases in GI motility, intestinal blood flow, and absorptive surface area. Reduced gastric secretion of acid can reduce tablet dissolution and decrease the solubility of basic drugs.

The delay in gastric emptying allows more contact time in the stomach for

- Potentially ulcerogenic drugs such as the nonsteroidal anti-inflammatory drugs (NSAIDs).
- Antacid drug interactions due to an increased chance for binding.
- Increased absorption of poorly soluble drugs.

A higher incidence of diarrhea and a delay in onset action of weakly basic drugs also result from this physiologic effect.

One study reported a threefold decrease in *levodopa* availability in the elderly because delayed gastric emptying allowed the increased degradation by GI dopa-decarboxylase to dopamine.[8] Differences in gastric emptying might explain the unpredictable and inconsistent responses to levodopa in individual patients.[9]

Clorazepate, a benzodiazepine, is converted by acid hydrolysis in the GI tract to an active metabolite, desmethyldiazepam. Desmethyldiazepam concentrations have been reported to be lower in both elderly and gastrectomized patients compared with younger adults. This decrease in active metabolite levels is presumed to be a result of a decreased conversion from the parent drug.[10]

Age influences the active transport mechanisms involved in the absorption of nutrients such as sugars, vitamins (e.g., *thiamine* and *folic acid*), and minerals (e.g., *calcium* and *iron*). In elderly patients, this absorption is often reduced.[11] Age-related physiologic changes alone apparently do not influence the passive transport mechanisms by which most drugs are absorbed; however, some drugs may have reduced bioavailability due to incomplete absorption or first-pass metabolism.

Some drugs with high intrinsic clearance in the liver are metabolized during their passage from the portal vein through the liver to the systemic circulation, thus reducing their bioavailability. Drugs with potentially *increased* bioavailability in the elderly, presumably due to a decrease in first-pass metabolism, include

Amitriptyline	Lidocaine
Chlordiazepoxide	Metoprolol
Clomethiazole	Metronidazole
Cimetidine	Propranolol
Desipramine	Quinidine
Imipramine	Trazodone
Labetalol[12]	Verapamil[13]
Levodopa	

Drugs that undergo first-pass metabolism and may have *decreased* bioavailability in older patients include clorazepate, digoxin, and prazosin.

Although the total amount of absorbed drug reaching the systemic circulation is affected for only a few drugs, age-related physiologic changes can alter the absorption rate, resulting in an erratic and sometimes inconsistent pharmacologic response. Clinical factors such as acute CHF, achlorhydria, and unusual dietary patterns may necessitate the intravenous route of administration because of incomplete absorption via oral and intramuscular routes. The absorption of intramuscularly administered drugs also decreases in bedridden elderly patients, perhaps because of changes in regional blood flow. Considerations involved in using controlled-release dosage formulations include age-related changes in GI transit time, motility, and pH.

Binding proteins

Age can alter the distribution of drugs throughout the body and to target organs. Although total protein generally is unaffected by aging, the plasma albumin portion has been shown to decrease from 4% in young adults to approximately 3.5% in patients over 80.[14] If albumin is decreased, a compensatory increase in unbound (active) drug occurs. In addition to age, disease states such as cirrhosis, renal failure, and malnutrition can lower albumin concentrations. Alpha-1-acid glycoprotein (AAG) binds mostly to lipophilic basic drugs and tends to increase with age. The binding of drugs to AAG increases during acute illness and can return to normal after several weeks or months when the acute stress passes and the acute phase reactant, AAG, decreases.[15]

Increased free (unbound) fraction

Increases in the free fraction of *naproxen, diflunisal,* and *salicylates* have been found in the elderly, presumably as a result of the decrease in albumin protein binding.[16] Increased concentrations of NSAIDs may be responsible for the reported higher incidence of gastric bleeding from peptic ulcers.[17]

Decreased protein binding (as well as the resultant increased free fraction) is also seen with *phenytoin,* which is cleared from the plasma more rapidly because of an increase in free phenytoin.[18] Seizure control should be seen at lower measured total (bound plus unbound) phenytoin concentrations. Although the increase in the free fraction of phenytoin with age is statistically significant, it is unlikely to warrant a compensatory change in dose unless the patient has a total phenytoin concentration that is near the upper limit of the therapeutic range and/or that is sufficient to saturate metabolizing enzymes. With *meperidine,* binding to red blood cells decreases with age,[19] thus increasing the amount of free meperidine available in the elderly patient.

Although higher therapeutic effects of some drugs may be beneficial, the accompanying risks of toxicity are problematic in the geriatric patient. Doses of most highly protein-bound drugs (>90% protein bound) should be reduced initially and increased slowly if there is evidence of decreased albumin. If several highly protein-bound drugs are used together, the chance of a drug interaction increases (Table 2).

Lean body weight to fat ratio

Changes in the ratio of lean body weight to fat also can alter drug distribution and, thus, pharmacologic response. In the average elderly patient, total body water is decreased and total body fat is increased. These changes influence the onset and duration of action of highly tissue-bound drugs (e.g., *digoxin*) and water-soluble drugs (e.g., *alcohol, lithium,* and *morphine*). The dosages of most water-soluble drugs are based on estimates of lean body weight. If a patient's actual weight is less than the estimated lean body weight, the actual weight should be used in most dosage calculations.

TABLE 2. Effects of Age on Plasma Protein Binding of Drugs in Geriatric Population

Drugs with decreased protein binding (increased free fraction)

- Acetazolamide
- Carbenoxolone
- Ceftriaxone
- Clomethiazole
- Desipramine[a]
- Desmethyldiazepam
- Diazepam[a]
- Diflunisal
- Fluphenazine
- Flurazepam
- Lorazepam[a]
- Meperidine[a]
- Naproxen
- Phenylbutazone
- Phenytoin[a]
- Salicylate[a]
- Temazepam
- Theophylline
- Tolbutamide
- Triazolam[a]
- Valproate
- Warfarin[a]

Drugs with increased protein binding (decreased free fraction)

- Amitriptyline[a]
- Chlorpromazine
- Disopyramide[a]
- Haloperidol[a]
- Lidocaine
- Nortriptyline[a]
- Propranolol[a]

Drugs with no change in protein binding

- Alprazolam
- Amitriptyline[a]
- Atropine
- Caffeine
- Canrenone
- Chlordiazepoxide
- Desipramine[a]
- Desmethyldiazepam
- Diazepam[a]
- Disopyramide[a]
- Fentanyl
- Furosemide
- Haloperidol[a]
- Ibuprofen
- Imipramine
- Lorazepam[a]
- Maprotiline
- Meperidine[a]
- Methadone
- Metoprolol
- Midazolam
- Nadolol
- Nitrazepam[a]
- Nortriptyline[a]
- Oxazepam
- Penicillin
- Phenobarbital
- Phenytoin[a]
- Piroxicam
- Propranolol[a]
- Quinidine
- Salicylate[a]
- Sulfadiazine
- Sulfamethoxazole
- Thioridazine
- Triazolam[a]
- Trimethoprim
- Vancomycin
- Warfarin[a]

[a]*Conflicting data have been published.*[16]

Between ages 18 and 85, total body fat increases on average in both females and males; lean body mass eventually decreases in both groups as well. With increasing age, the volume of distribution of lipophilic drugs increases as a result of diminished protein binding and an increased fat to lean muscle ratio. Fat-soluble drugs (e.g., most *tricyclic antidepressants, barbiturates, benzodiazepines, calcium channel blockers,* and *phenothiazines*) may have a delayed onset of action and can accumulate in adipose tissue, prolonging their action sometimes to the point of toxicity.

Drug Elimination

Drugs are primarily cleared from the body by metabolism in the liver, excretion by the kidneys, or some combination of the two processes. A decrease in total body clearance results in higher average drug concentrations and an enhanced pharmacologic response, which can lead to toxicity.

For some drugs, hepatic metabolism is highly dependent on blood flow. Liver blood flow decreases significantly with increasing age and is further compromised in the presence of CHF. With drugs that are highly dependent on hepatic metabolism (e.g., most *beta-blockers, lidocaine,* and *narcotic analgesics*), a decrease in hepatic clearance can increase the drug concentration to toxicity.

In addition to altering hepatic blood flow, age influences the rate of hepatic clearance by causing changes in the intrinsic activity of selected liver enzymes. This process has been found in the Phase I enzymatic pathway. Common drugs utilizing this pathway (and having the potential for metabolism influenced by age) include the longer acting benzodiazepines such as *diazepam, chlordiazepoxide, clorazepate,* and *prazepam*. The enzymatic demethylation of *amitriptyline*,[20] *imipramine*,[21] *thioridazine*,[22] and *theophylline*[23] also decreases in the elderly.

Drugs that undergo Phase II enzymatic biotransformation (e.g., *lorazepam, oxazepam*, and *temazepam)* do not appear to be adversely affected by age; therefore, they are preferred agents for older patients.

At all ages, drug metabolism can also be affected by genetics, smoking, diet, gender, comorbid conditions, and concomitant drugs. The cytochrome P-450 enzyme system, primarily a part of the Phase I hepatic metabolism path, can be affected by many drugs. Of the more than 30 CP450 isoenzymes identified to date, the major ones responsible for drug metabolism include CYP3A4, CYP2D6, CYP1A2, and the CYP2C subfamily. CYPs are increasingly being identified in extrahepatic organs, such as the intestine, kidney, brain, and skin. The full effect of aging on these enzyme systems is yet to be determined.[24] Unlike renal function, no accurate laboratory tests directly measure liver function for drug dosage adjustment. Nonspecific tests to monitor liver function include ALT, plasma albumin, and prothrombin time.

Renal Clearance

Age-related physiologic changes in the kidneys influence drug response and elimination in the geriatric patient more than do hepatic changes. Between ages 20 and 90, the glomerular filtration rate (GFR) may decrease as much as 50% (average decline of 35%). Serum creatinine is frequently utilized to monitor kidney function, but this test is of limited usefulness in monitoring the GFR of the geriatric patient. Serum creatinine does not increase significantly unless kidney function deteriorates greatly. The production of creatinine, which is dependent on muscle mass, decreases in the elderly; therefore, an apparently normal serum creatinine in a geriatric patient may not be a valid predictor of renal function and drug elimination. BUN also is not useful because it can be affected by hydration status, diet, and blood loss.

The most accurate, readily available estimation of GFR in the elderly is CrCl, which correlates well with both GFR and tubular secretion. CrCl can be estimated using a standard equation that considers age, body weight, and serum creatinine in patients with stabilized renal function. Of course, mathematical equations are simply estimates of an individual's actual renal function. Even the best methods for estimating creatinine clearance may result in suboptimal dosing for many elderly patients. For geriatric patients with low serum creatinine (<1.0 mg/dl, 88.4 SI), rounding the serum creatinine to 1.0 mg/dl, 88.4 SI may result in underestimation of creatinine clearance and suboptimal dosing.[25] (See Chapter 1.)

Dosages of *renally excreted drugs* should be adjusted if the patient has lost more than 50% of kidney function. If clearance is less than 30 ml/min, major dosage adjustments may be necessary to avoid drug toxicity. Once the GFR drops below 30 ml/min, drug elimination decreases rapidly and serum drug concentrations increase significantly. Drugs with low therapeutic to toxic ratios that are excreted primarily unchanged by the kidneys are

Acetazolamide	Ethambutol
ACE inhibitors	H_2-antagonists
Amantadine	Lithium
Aminoglycosides	Methotrexate
Cephalosporins	Penicillin
Chlorpropamide	Procainamide
Digoxin	Quinidine
Disopyramide	Tetracycline

Age-Related Pharmacodynamic Changes Influencing Drug Response

With increasing age, the tolerance to drugs decreases as a result of altered pharmacodynamic responses at target organs. Pharmacodynamics govern the type, intensity, and duration of drug action. The clinical manifestation of this altered sensitivity may range from an insignificant response, to an ADR, to therapy failure.

Qualitative differences in drug response also may occur. Pharmacodynamic alterations are often unpredictable and, therefore, frequently lead to toxicity. Altered response may be due to depletion of neurotransmitters, disease, or physiologic changes. With aging, there is evidence of

- Decreased acetylcholine, dopamine, and serotonin.
- Decreased enzymatic degradation of monoamine oxidase.
- Impaired baroreceptor response to blood pressure changes.
- Decreased responsiveness of beta-adrenergic receptors.
- Increased pain tolerance.
- Decreased antibody response to vaccination.
- Decreased insulin sensitivity.
- Decreased cortisol suppression.

Altered end organ sensitivity may result in exaggerated pharmacologic response, as seen with *barbiturates* and *benzodiazepines*, or diminished pharmacologic response, as seen with *beta-blockers, beta-agonists*, and *calcium channel blockers*. Other affected drug classes include the *narcotic analgesics, antihypertensive agents, antiparkinson drugs, phenothiazines*, and *antidepressants*. The incidence and irreversibility of tardive dyskinesia are increased in the elderly and may be due to age-related imbalances in neurotransmitters.[26]

Dosing adjustments are usually necessary since many of these same drugs are also influenced by age-related physiologic changes, especially drug distribution and elimination. The net effect in an individual patient is often difficult to predict. For example, elderly patients have increased bioavailability of *beta-blockers* but decreased responsiveness at the receptor site level (a variable effect is seen with *verapamil*). Another example is that *theophylline's* inotropic effect increases with age but its bronchodilator effect decreases.[27] A decreased pharmacologic response can also be anticipated with *furosemide* in the geriatric patient. Drugs that may exhibit an increased pharmacologic response in the geriatric population include *halothane, hydroxyzine, metoclopramide, warfarin*, and the calcium channel blockers.

More than one in six elderly patients are taking prescription drugs that are not suited for geriatric patients and may lead to physical or mental deterioration and possibly death.[28] Recently strategies have been developed in attempts to foster appropriate prescribing of medications in the geriatric population overall. The explicit criteria for determining potentially inappropriate medication use by elderly patients, labeled the "Beers Criteria" are listed in Table 3.

TABLE 3. Explicit Criteria for Inappropriate Medication Orders

Medications that should be avoided in geriatric patients
Sedative or hypnotic agents
    Long-acting benzodiazepines
    Meprobamate
    Short-acting benzodiazepines

Antidepressants
    Amitriptyline
    Combination antidepressants-antipyschotics

Antihypertensive agents
    Methyldopa
    Propranolol
    Reserpine

Nonsteroidal anti-inflammatory drugs
    Indomethacin
    Phenylbutazone

Oral hypoglycemic agents
    Chlorpropamide

Analgesic agents
    Propoxyphene
    Pentazocine

Dementia treatments
    Cyclandelate
    Isoxsupine

TABLE 3. (*continued*)

Platelet inhibitors
  Dipyridamole

Muscle relaxants or antispasmodic agents
  Cyclobenzaprine
  Orphenidrate
  Methocarbamol
  Carisoprodol

Gastrointestinal antispasmodic agents
  Clidinium
  Hyoscyamine
  Dicyclomine
  Belladonna

Medications with dosage limits
  Antipsychotic agents
    Haloperidol
    Thioridazine

  Digoxin

  Histamine blockers
    Cimetidine
    Ranitidine

  Iron supplements

  Short-acting benzodiazepines
    Oxazepam
    Triazolam

  Antihypertensive agents
    Hydrochlorothiazide

Medications with duration limits
  Decongestants
    Oxymetazoline
    Phenylephrine
    Pseudoephedrine

  Histamine blockers

  Short-acting benzodiazepines
    Oxazepam
    Triazolam
    Alprazolam

These criteria were developed through a consensus panel of experts in geriatric care, geriatric pharmacology, geriatric psychopharmacology, and nursing home care. These experts reached agreement on criteria defining inappropriate drug use in nursing home residents. The criteria relate to certain drugs that should not be used and doses and durations of therapy of some drugs that should not be exceeded in the older patient who is a resident of a nursing facility.[29,30] Practitioners may extrapolate these recommendations to the geriatric patient population at large.

Summary of Changes

Table 4 is a compilation of the pharmacokinetic and pharmacodynamic literature available on the dosing of drugs in the geriatric population. However, dosing of any drug in a specific patient should be based on that patient's response and ability to clear the drug.[31,32]

TABLE 4. Pharmacokinetic Parameters and Average Doses of Drugs Commonly Used in Geriatric Patients[14,25,26,33]

Drug	Volume of Distribution	Clearance	Half-Life	PB (%f)	Time to Peak	Dynamics	Dose (mg/day)	Comment
Acetaminophen	D	D	I		D		1500–3000	Hepatic metabolism not significantly altered; no dosage adjustment necessary unless patient is taking chronic high doses
Alprazolam	D	D	I	NC	D	**	0.75–2	
Amantadine	D		I			200		Dosage reduction in renal failure

Amantadine (continued):

CrCl (ml/min/1.73 m²)	Maintenance Dose
≥80	100 mg twice daily
60–79	200 mg/100 mg on alternate days
40–59	100 mg once daily
30–39	200 mg twice weekly
20–29	100 mg three times weekly
10–19	200 mg/100 mg alternating every 7 days

TABLE 4. (*continued*)

Drug	Volume of Distribution	Clear-ance	Half-Life	PB (%f)	Time to Peak	Dynamics	Dose (mg/day)	Comment
Amikacin	I	D	I				***	Dose conservatively based on CrCl
Aminophylline	I	NC	I	NC			0.4 mg/kg/hr	
Amitriptyline	I	D	I	D*	I		10–150	Prolonged half-life; evaluation of therapeutic effect to be delayed; increased bioavailability
Amoxicillin							750–1500	Dosage reduction in moderate to severe renal impairment
Ampicillin	I	D	I		I		500–2000	Dosage reduction in moderate to severe renal impairment
Aspirin	I	D	I	I*	I		1300–4000	
Atenolol	I	D	I	I			25–150	
Azathioprine	No data	D	I	I	No data		1.5–2.5 mg/kg/day	If CrCl <50 ml/min give 75% of dose; if CrCl <10 ml/min, give 50% of dose

Benazepril	NC	I	NC	NC	Exaggerated	20–40	Preferred class in comorbid CHF, DM, HTN.
Bleomycin	No change	No data*	I	*		10–20 units/m^2	If CrCl <50 ml/min give 75% of dose; if CrCl <10 ml/min, give 50% of dose
Bupropion						150–450	SE profile allows use in patients intolerable to TCAs
Buspirone	NC	D in hepatic failure	I	NC	I	10–60	Slow titration to avoid side effects. Reduced sedation advantageous.
Busulfan	NC	No data	No data	D		4–8	
Captopril					I	12.5–250	Renal impairment monitored for K+; see benazepril
Cefadroxil			I	NC	NC	1–2g/day	Base dose on renal function and severity of infection
Cefaclor	NC	D	I	NC	NC	750–1500	If CrCl <50 ml/min, use 50% of dose BID
Cefamandole	NC	D	I	NC	NC	4–12 g/day	If CrCl <50 ml/min, reduce dose and increase dosage interval

TABLE 4. (continued)

Drug	Volume of Distribution	Clearance	Half-Life	PB (%f)	Time to Peak	Dynamics	Dose (mg/day)	Comment
Cefazolin	NC	D	I					Dosage reduction in renal impairment; all adults receive loading dose of 500 mg <table><tr><th>CrCl (ml/min)</th><th>Dose</th></tr><tr><td>≥55</td><td>Usual adult dose</td></tr><tr><td>35–54</td><td>Usual adult dose at 8-hr intervals</td></tr><tr><td>11–34</td><td>One-half usual adult dose at 12-hr intervals</td></tr><tr><td>≤10</td><td>One-half usual adult dose every 18–24 hr</td></tr></table>
Cefepime	NC	D	I	NC	NC		0.5–4 g/day	Base dose on renal function and severity of infection
Cefixime	NC	D	I	NC	NC		400	If CrCl 21–60 ml/min, give 75% of usual dose
Cefoperazone	NC	D	I	NC	NC		2–12 g/day	Reduce dose in hepatic failure; sodium content is 1 g (1.5 mEq)

Drug					Dose range	Notes
Cefotaxime	I	D	I	NC	NC	2–12 g/day	If CrCl <20 ml/min, reduce dose by 50%
Cefotetan	NC	D	I	NC	NC	1–6 g/day	If CrCl <30 ml/min, increase dosing interval
Cefoxitin	I	I	I	D		3000–8000	Dosage reduction in severe renal impairment (may need to give every 12–48 hr)
Cefpodoxime	NC	D	I	NC	NC	200–800	If CrCl <30 ml/min, admin q 24 hr
Cefprozil	I	D	I	NC	NC	500–1000	Admin for ≥10 days
Ceftazidime	D	D	I	D	NC	*	*Base on renal function; minimum interval = 12 hr
Ceftizoxime	I	D	I	NC	NC	1.5–12 g/day	If CrCl <80, reduce dose
Ceftriaxone	D	D	I	I		500–2000	No dosage reduction with impaired renal or hepatic dysfunction; serum concentration monitoring in severe renal impairment or in both hepatic and substantial renal impairment (maximum dosage of 2 g daily)

TABLE 4. (*continued*)

Drug	Volume of Distribution	Clearance	Half-Life	PB (%f)	Time to Peak	Dynamics	Dose (mg/day)	Comment
Cefuroxime	NC	D	I	NC	NC		O:500–1 g/day P: 3–6 g/day	If CrCl <20 ml/min, reduce dose
Cephalothin	I	D	I		I		3000–6000	Dosage reduction with concurrent renal and hepatic dysfunction CrCl (ml/min) — Dose >50–80 — 2 g every 6 hr >25–50 — 1.5 g every 6 hr >10–25 — 1 g every 6 hr 2–10 — 500 mg every 8 hr
Cephradine								Dose based on degree of renal impairment, severity of infection, and susceptibility of causative organism

THERAPEUTIC DRUG MONITORING IN THE GERIATRIC PATIENT

Drug						CrCl (ml/min)	Dose
						>20	500 mg every 6 hr (intravenous or oral)
						5–20	250 mg every 6 hr (intravenous or oral)
						<5	250 mg every 6 hr (intravenous or oral)
Chlorambucil	NC	No data*	*	*	0.1 mg/kg/day		
Chlordiazepoxide	I	D	I	NC*	10–40		
Chlorpromazine				D	10–800		
Chlorpropamide	I	D	I		100–750		Inactive metabolite excreted via urine
Cholestyramine	Not absorbed*	*	*	*	16–24 g/day		
Cimetidine	D	D	I		300–600		If CrCl <30 ml/min/1.73 m², 300 mg every 12 hr (intravenous or oral); further dosage reduction in concomitant hepatic impairment

TABLE 4. (continued)

Drug	Volume of Distribution	Clearance	Half-Life	PB (%f)	Time to Peak	Dynamics	Dose (mg/day)	Comment
Ciprofloxacin			I					If CrCl = 30–50 ml/min/1.73 m², 250–500 mg every 12 hr (intravenous or oral); if CrCl = 2–25 ml/min/1.73 m², 250–500 mg (oral) every 18 hr or 200–400 mg every 24 hr.
Cisapride	NC	NC	NC	NC	NC		40–80	Css higher, no clinical effect
Cisplatin	No data*	*	*	*	*		2.5–50 mg/m²/day	Hydrate to prevent toxicity. If CrCl <50 ml/min, give 75% of dose; if CrCl <10 ml/min, give 50% of dose
Citalopram	No data*	D	I	*	I			
Clofibrate	I	I	I	NC	NC		1–2 g/day	If CrCl <50 ml/min, dose every 12–18 hr. If CrCl <10 ml/min, avoid use
Colestipol	Not absorbed*	*	*	*	*		13–30 g/day	

Drug							Dose	Comments
Clorazepate	I				I	**	15–30	
Cyclophosphamide	I	D	I	No data	I	No data	1–2 mg/kg/day	If CrCl <10ml/min, give 75% of dose; risk of hemorrhagic cystitis
Daunorubicin	No data*	*	*	*	*		30–45 mg/m²/day	
Desipramine	I	I	I*				20–150	Prolonged half-life; evaluation of therapeutic effect to be delayed
Diazepam	I	D	I	I*		**	2–20	
Diclofenac	NC	NC	NC	NC	NC		50–150	High risk for GI bleed or CNS effects. Reduce dose in CrCl <50 ml/min
Diflunisal	NC	D	I	NC	NC		500–1500	High risk for GI bleed or CNS effects
Digoxin	D	D	I				0.125–0.25	Conservative dosing based on IBW and CrCl
Diltiazem							90–360	Initiation with low dose because of significantly reduced clearance

TABLE 4. (continued)

Drug	Volume of Distribution	Clearance	Half-Life	PB (%f)	Time to Peak	Dynamics	Dose (mg/day)	Comment
Diphenhydramine	NC	D	I				25–50	Elderly more sensitive to anticholinergic and sedative effects
Doxepin			I				25–150	Prolonged half-life; evaluation of therapeutic effect to be delayed
Doxorubicin	NC	NC	NC	NC	NC		50–75 mg/m²	Risk of acute renal failure and nephrotic syndrome
Doxycycline	NC	D	I				50–100	Tetracycline drug of choice in severe renal impairment
Enalapril	D	D	NC				5–40	See benazepril
Erythromycin		I	D				1000–4000	
Ethanol	D							Increased concentrations due to lowered volume of distribution; additive effects with other sedatives
Etodolac	NC	NC	NC	NC	NC		400	High risk for GI bleed or CNS effects

Drug					Dose	
					CrCl (ml/min/1.73 m²)	
Famotidine	NC	NC	NC	NC	30–60 One-half usual adult dose <30 One-fourth usual adult dose or <10 One-tenth usual adult dose	Usual adult dose 40 mg
Fenoprofen	NC	NC	NC	NC	1.2–4 g/day	High risk for GI bleed or CNS effects
Fluorouracil	NC	NC	NC	NC	12 mg/kg/day	
Fluoxetine					20–40	SE profile allows use in patients who can't tolerate TCAs
Flurazepam			I	**	15	Dose-related drowsiness from drug accumulation
Flurbiprofen	NC	NC	NC	NC	200–300	High risk for GI bleed or CNS effects
Flutamide	No data*	*	*	*	450	Gynecomastia; antiandrogenic

TABLE 4. (*continued*)

Drug	Volume of Distribution	Clearance	Half-Life	PB (%f)	Time to Peak	Dynamics	Dose (mg/day)	Comment
Fluvastatin	No data	NC	No data	NC	NC		2–10	No dosage reduction in reduced CrCl
Fosinopril	NC	D	I	NC			10–40	See benazepril
Furosemide	No data*	*	*	*	*		40–2000	
Gatifloxacin	No data	NC	NC	NC				
Gemfibrozil		D	I			**	1200	
Gentamicin							5–40	Conservative dosing based on weight and CrCl; interpatient variation
Glipizide							2.5–20	Inactive metabolite excreted via urine
Glyburide								Reduce dose in CrCl <10 ml/min/ 1.73 m^2
Haloperidol				D*			0.75–50	Elderly more susceptible to side effects; prolonged half-life

Drug					Dose	Comments
Heparin				**	20–200	Increased age may increase risk of major bleeding
Hydralazine			I	**	25–50	
Hydrochlorothiazide						Not effective in CrCl <30 ml/min/1.73 m².
Hydrocodone	I	D	I	NC	NC	I	10–30	Enhanced CNS effects and constipation noted
Hydroxyurea	No data*	*	*	*		20–30 mg/kg/day	If CrCl <50 ml/min, give 50% of dose; if CrCl <10 ml/min, give 20% of dose
Ibuprofen	NC	NC	NC	NC		800–3200	High risk for GI bleed or CNS effects
Imipramine		I	NC			30–150	Prolonged half-life; evaluation of therapeutic effect to be delayed
Indomethacin		I				50–200	Other NSAIDs preferable due to efficacy and lower toxicity
Isoniazid	D	D	I			200–300	Dosage adjustment in slow acetylator patients

TABLE 4. (continued)

Drug	Volume of Distribution	Clearance	Half-Life	PB (%f)	Time to Peak	Dynamics	Dose (mg/day)	Comment
Ketoprofen	I	D	I				150–300	
Ketorolac	NC	D	I	NC	NC		60–120	High risk for GI bleed or CNS effects; reduce dose because of decreased clearance
Labetalol		D					200–2400	Initiation with lower doses because of increased bioavailability with age
Lansoprazole	No data	D	I				15–30	No dosage reduction in reduced CrCl
Levodopa	D	D	D		I			Decreased bioavailability possibly due to slowed gastric emptying
Levofloxacin							250–500	Dosage reduction based on renal impairment. If CrCl = 20–49 ml/min/1.73 m^2, 250 mg every 24 hr (after initial dose of 500 mg). If CrCl 10–19 ml/min/1.73 m^2, 250 mg every 48 hr

(after initial dose of 250 mg for renal infections and 500 mg for others).

Drug						Value	Comments
Lidocaine	I		D	I	D	**	Decreased clearance in presence of CHF or liver disease
Lisinopril						10–40	
Lithium			D		D	150–900	One-half initial dose because of susceptibility to volume depletion; dose based on drug concentrations (0.4–0.7 mEq/L)
Lorazepam	D		D	I	I*	**	1–3	
Lovastatin	No data		NC	NC	NC		20–80	
Meclofenamic Acid	No data		NC	NC	NC	NC	150–400	High risk for GI bleed or CNS effects
Mefenamic Acid	No data		NC	NC	NC	No data	1000	High risk for GI bleed or CNS effects
Melphalan	No data		D	I			6	If CrCl <50 ml/min, give 75% of dose; if CrCl <10 ml/min, give 50% of dose

TABLE 4. (continued)

Drug	Volume of Distribution	Clearance	Half-Life	PB (%f)	Time to Peak	Dynamics	Dose (mg/day)	Comment
Meperidine	I	D	I	I*		**	150–500	Dosage reduction because of increased sensitivity; elderly more susceptible to side effects
Methotrexate	NC	D	I	NC	NC		5–10	Dose for rheumatoid arthritis; if CrCl <50 ml/min, mg/wk give 50% of dose; if CrCl <10 ml/min, avoid; refer to specific disease protocols for neoplastic disease
Methyldopa							250–3000	May be inappropriate due to side effect profile
Metoclopramide	NC	D	I	I	NC	I	O:15–30 P:10–20	Geriatrics more likely to develop dyskinesias
Metoprolol			I	NC	D		25–300	
Morphine	D	D	D				20–100	Dosage reduction because of increased sensitivity; elderly more susceptible to side effects

							Comments
Moxifloxacin	No data*	*	*	*	*	*	1–2 g/day	High risk for GI bleed or CNS effects; reduce dose if CrCl <50 ml/min
Nabumetone	NC	NC	NC	NC	NC	NC		
Nadolol					NC		40–320	
Naproxen	I		D	I	I	I	500–750	
Nefazodone	NC		D	I	NC	NC	200–400	Limited data available
Nifedipine							30–180	
Nizatidine	NC		D	I		Exaggerated	150	
Nortriptyline	I		D	I	D*		10–50	Prolonged half-life; evaluation of therapeutic effect to be delayed
Olanzapine	NC		D	I		NC	5–20	
Omeprazole	no data		D	I			20–40	No dosage reduction in reduced CrCl
Oxaprozin	NC		NC	D*	NC	NC	1200	Dual elimination (renal and hepatic) allows for decreased $t½$ in chronic dosing. High risk for GI bleed or CNS effects

TABLE 4. (*continued*)

Drug	Volume of Distribution	Clearance	Half-Life	PB (%f)	Time to Peak	Dynamics	Dose (mg/day)	Comment
Oxazepam	I	D	I	NC	I	**	10–60	
Oxycodone	I	D	I	I	NC	I	10–20	Enhanced CNS effects and constipation noted
Paroxetine	D		I				10–40	See fluoxetine
Penicillin G		I	I	NC			1000–2000	Dosage reduction in moderate to severe renal impairment
Phenobarbital			I	NC			30–60	Dose administration at bedtime to avoid excessive sedation; tolerance within a few weeks
Phenytoin		D	I*				200–300	Decreased serum albumin concentrations may increase clearance; monitoring of free phenytoin concentrations
Pioglitazone	No data*	*	*	*	*			
Piroxicam	D	D	I	NC	D		10–20	

Drug						Dose	Comments
Pravastatin	NC	NC	NC	NC	NC	10–40	
Prazosin	I	D	I	I		2–10	
Probucol	No data*	*	*	*	*	1000	
Propoxyphene	NC	D	I	I	NC	*65(100)	Not recommended in geriatrics
Propranolol	D	D	I	D*	**	40–480	
Quinidine		D		NC		600–3600	Dosage reduction because of decreased clearance; dose based on side effects, therapeutic response, and concentrations (2–6 mg/L)
Ranitidine	D	D	I		NC	150	Prolonged half-life; if CrCl <50 ml/min, 150 mg every 24 hr orally or 50 mg every 18–24 hr intramuscularly or by intravenous intermittent slow infusion or direct injection (continuous intravenous infusion has not been evaluated in impaired renal function)
Risperidone	NC	D	I	I	NC	0.5–3	Titrate slowly to avoid ADRs

TABLE 4. (*continued*)

Drug	Volume of Distribution	Clearance	Half-Life	PB (%f)	Time to Peak	Dynamics	Dose (mg/day)	Comment
Rosaglitazone	No data*	*	*	*	*			
Sertraline	D						2.5–50	See fluoxetine
Simvastatin	No data*	*	*	NC	*		5–40	
Spironolactone			I		NC		50–100	Dosage reduction in significant renal impairment
Sulindac	No data	NC	NC	NC	NC		400	Hepatic metabolism to active metabolite; high risk for GI bleed or CNS effects
Tamoxifen	NC	No data*	*				20–40	Hot flashes, nausea, vomiting
Temazepam	NC	NC	NC	I	NC	**	15–30	
Tetracycline		I					500–2000	Rarely drug of choice
Theophylline	D	D	I	I		**	0.2–0.4 mg/kg/hr	Elderly more susceptible to side effects; CHF or liver disease

Drug					Comments
Thioridazine		I	NC		decreases clearance; dose based on concentrations (7.5–15 mg/L) Elderly more susceptible to side effects; prolonged half-life
Timolol				10–400	
Tobramycin	NC	D	I	20–80	Dose conservatively based on weight and CrCl
Tolazamide				***	
Tolbutamide	D	D	I	I	100–1000
					500–3000 Inactive metabolite excreted via urine
Tolmetin	NC	NC	NC	NC	1200
Tramadol	NC	D	I	NC	200–300
Trazodone			I	D	50–400 Prolonged half-life; evaluation of therapeutic effect to be delayed
Triamterene			D		50–100 More effective in combination with thiazide diuretic
Triazolam		D	I	I*	I	0.125–0.25

TABLE 4. (*continued*)

Drug	Volume of Distribution	Clearance	Half-Life	PB (%f)	Time to Peak	Dynamics	Dose (mg/day)	Comment
Trimethoprim–Sulfamethoxazole								Dosage reduction based on degree of renal impairment, severity of infection, and susceptibility of causative organism CrCl (ml/min) Dose 15–30 One-half usual adult daily dose <15 Conflicting data (recommendations of reduced dosages or of no use at all)
Verapamil	I with chronic doses	D	I			**	240–480	
Vinblastine		NC	No data				37 mg/m²	

Vincristine	NC	NC	No data		5-8 mg/m²	
Warfarin	I	D	I*	**	***	Increased age and female sex may increase risk of bleeding; 40% dosage reduction

*PB (%f) = protein binding alterations (percent free fraction), dynamics = pharmacodynamics, dose = recommended daily dosage range for geriatric patients, O = oral, P = parenteral, D = decreased, I = increased, NC = no change, * = conflicting data reported, ** = age-related alterations in sensitivity reported, and *** = dose to be individualized for particular patient.

References

1. Hazzard WR. Preventive gerontology. *Postgrad Med*. 1983; 74: 279–87.
2. Rowe JW, Kahn RL. Human aging: usual and successful. *Science*. 1987; 237:143–9.
3. Wynne HT, Cope LH, James OFW, et al. The effect of age and frailty upon acetanilide clearance in man. *Age and Ageing*. 1989; 18:415–6.
4. Williamson J, Chopin JM. Adverse reactions to prescribed drugs in the elderly: a multicenter investigation. *Age Ageing* 1980; 9:73–80.
5. Klein LE, German PS, Levine DM. Adverse drug reactions among the elderly: a reassessment. *J Am Geriatr Soc*. 1981; 29:525–30.
6. Nolan L, O'Malley K. Prescribing for the elderly Part I: sensitivity of the elderly to adverse drug reactions. *J Am Geriatr Soc*. 1988; 36:142–9.
7. Dawling S, Crome P. Clinical pharmacokinetic considerations in the elderly: an update. *Clin Pharmacokinet*. 1981; 17:236–63.
8. Evans MA, Triggs EJ, Broe GA, et al. Systemic availability of orally administered L-dopa in the elderly Parkinsonian patient. *Eur J Clin Pharmacol*. 1980; 17:215–21.
9. Bianchine JR, Calimlim LR, Morgan JP, et al. Metabolism and absorption of L-3,4 dihydroxyphenylalanine in patients with Parkinson's disease. *Ann NY Acad Sci*. 1971; 179:126–40.
10. Ochs HR, Greenblatt DJ, Allen MD, et al. Effect of age and Billroth gastrectomy on absorption of desmethyldiazepam from chlorazepate. *Clin Pharmacol Ther*. 1979; 26:449–56.
11. Lamy PP. Prescribing for the elderly. Littleton, MA: PSG Wright; 1980.
12. Kelly JG, McGarry K, O'Malley K, et al. Bioavailability of labetalol increases with age. *Br J Clin Pharmacol*. 1982; 14:304–5.
13. Storstein L, Larsen A, Saevareld L. Pharmacokinetics of calcium channel blockers in patients with renal insufficiency and in geriatric patients. *Acta Med Scand*. 1984; 681:25–30.
14. Greenblatt DJ. Reduced serum albumin concentration in the elderly: a report from the Boston Collaborative Drug Surveillance Program. *J Am Geriatr Soc*. 1979; 27:20–2.
15. Michalets EL. Update: Clinically significant cytochrome P-450 drug interactions. *Pharmacotherapy*. 1998; 18(1):84-112.
16. Wallace SM, Verbeek RO. Plasma protein binding of drugs in the elderly. *Clin Pharmacokinet*. 1987; 12:41–72.
17. Somerville K, Faulkner G, Langman M. Non-steroidal anti-inflammatory drugs and bleeding peptic ulcer. *Lancet*. 1986; 1:462–4.
18. Hayes MJ, Langman MJS, Short AH. Changes in drug metabolism with increasing age. *Br J Clin Pharmacol*. 1975; 2:73–9.
19. Mather LE, Tucker GT, Pflug AE, et al. Meperidine kinetics in man. *Clin Pharmacol Ther*. 1975; 17:21–30.
20. Dawling S, Lynn K, Rosser R, et al. Nortriptyline metabolism in chronic renal failure: metabolic elimination. *Clin Pharmacol Ther*. 1982; 32:322–9.

21. Abernathy DR, Greenblatt DJ, Shader RI. Imipramine and desipramine disposition in the elderly. *J Pharmacol Exp Ther*. 1985; 232:183–8.
22. Cohen BM, Sommer BR. Metabolism of thioridazine in the elderly. *J Clin Psychopharmacol*. 1988; 8:336–9.
23. Antal EJ, Kramer PA, Mercik SA, et al. Theophylline pharmacokinetics in advanced age. *Br J Clin Pharmacol*. 1981; 12:637–45.
24. Kinirons MT, Crome P. Clinical pharmacokinetic consideration in the elderly, an update. *Clin Pharmacokinet*. 1999; 33:302–12.
25. Smythe M, Hoffman J, Kizy K, et al. Estimating creatinine clearance in elderly patients with low serum creatinine concentrations. *AJHP*. 1994; 51:198–204.
26. Smith JM, Baldessarini RJ. Changes in prevalence, severity, and recovery in tardive dyskinesia with age. *Arch Gen Psychiatry*. 1980; 37:1368–73.
27. Feely J, Cloakley D. Altered pharmacodynamics in the elderly. *Clin Geriatr Med*. 1990; 6:269–83.
28. Stover KA. GAO reports elderly not taking drugs properly. *Pharmacy Today*. 1995; 1(14):8.
29. Beers MH, Ouslander JG, Fingold SF, et al. Inappropriate medication prescribing in skilled-nursing facilities. *Ann Intern Med*. 1992; 117:684–9.
30. Beers MH. Explicit criteria for determining potentially inappropriate medication use by the elderly, an update. *Arch Intern Med*. 1997; 157:1531-6.
31. Ritschel WA. Gerontokinetics—the pharmacokinetics of drugs in the elderly. Caldwell, NJ: Telford Press; 1988.
32. Tobias ED. Geriatric drug use. In: Knoben JE, Anderson PO, eds. Handbook of clinical drug data, 7th ed. Hamilton, IL: Drug Intelligence Publications; 1993:195–217.
33. Aronoff GR, Berns JS, Brier ME, et al. Drug prescribing in renal failure dosing guidelines for adults, 4th ed. Philadelphia, PA: ACP-ASIM; 1999.

Chapter 25
Sybelle Blakey

Dosing Concepts in Renal Dysfunction

Chapters 3 through 21 of this book describe drugs for which therapeutic drug monitoring (TDM) methods are directly used to guide dosage requirements. Pharmacokinetic principles can also be applied to the dosing of other (non-TDM) drugs, especially in patients with renal dysfunction. For drugs excreted renally, dosage modification may be necessary to prevent drug misadventures.

Patients with renal dysfunction may have alterations in drug bioavailability, distribution, protein binding, elimination, and excretion.[1] This chapter describes methods for modifying dosages of drugs that depend primarily on renal clearance for their elimination but for which TDM is not routinely used.

Renal Mechanisms of Drug Clearance

The kidneys clear parent drug compounds and metabolites (active and inactive) from the body via glomerular filtration, tubular secretion, and tubular reabsorption.[2] The net renal excretion (CL_r) of a drug can be

The contributions made by Victor Lampasona and William H. Asbury to this chapter are gratefully acknowledged.

summarized by the equation:

$$CL_r = (GFR \times f_u) + CL_{secretion} - CL_{reabsorption}$$

where GFR is the glomerular filtration rate and f_u is the fraction of drug unbound to plasma proteins.[3] Glomerular filtration is a passive process and accounts for the majority of a drug's renal clearance. The GFR can be approximated in most patients by evaluating their ability to clear the endogenous substance creatinine, a product of muscle metabolism (see chapter 1).

Tubular secretion is an active process that can be blocked by certain substances (e.g., probenecid, cimetidine, and trimethoprim). There is no endogenous substance that can be used in the clinical setting to assess tubular function in an individual patient. Therefore, creatinine clearance (CrCl) remains the most practical and commonly used measure of renal function in the clinical arena. The simple proportionality of renal clearance and CrCl is used as the basis for drug dosage regimen design for renally excreted drugs.[4]

A number of formulae can be used to calculate CrCl, each differing in accuracy and convenience (see chapter 1). Alternatively, CrCl may be directly measured by collecting a patient's urine over a specified period of time.

CrCl Limitations

Estimated CrCl values are heavily dependent on serum creatinine values, which reside in the denominator of most estimation equations. A number of factors may influence the CrCl determination (Table 1). Alterations in any of these factors may artificially overestimate or underestimate CrCl. Accurate estimation of CrCl from serum creatinine requires that creatinine production and excretion are at steady state. Rapid fluctuations in creatinine production or renal function may not be reflected by the serum creatinine concentration for several days. When serum creatinine fluctuates, quantitative estimations of

TABLE 1. Factors That May Alter Creatinine Clearance Determinations

Analytic (Falsely Increased Serum Creatinine)	Physiologic
Glucose	Age, weight, gender
Protein	Exercise
Pyruvate	Diurnal variation
Acetoacetate	Diet
Fructose	Drugs that inhibit tubular secretion of creatinine (cimetidine, trimethoprim, probenecid)
Uric acid	
Ascorbic acid	
Cephalosporins (cephalothin, cefazolin, cephalexin, cefoxitin, cefaclor, cephradine)	
Flucytosine	

Source: reproduced with permission from reference 2.

CrCl must be interpreted with caution. Elderly patients or patients with cachexia, malnutrition, low muscle mass, or amputation may have low serum creatinine concentrations relative to their actual GFR. Use of a low to normal serum creatinine value in the Cockcroft and Gault equation may result in overestimation of creatinine clearance. The ideal method for estimating creatinine clearance in these populations is uncertain.[5-7]

Direct measurement of CrCl may be more accurate than calculations using serum creatinine. Standard methods use a 24-hr collection period, although collection periods of 8 hours are as accurate and require less effort. Collection periods less than 8 hours are not accurate and should be discouraged.[8] Because of the time delay and problems with accurate and complete urine collection, the measured CrCl is not routinely used for initial drug dosage regimen design.

Although there is no universal agreement as to what CrCl value warrants dosage modification, clinicians and the medical literature often recommend dosage adjustments for parent drugs or active metabolites excreted primarily by the kidney according to the degree of renal impairment present. For most drugs, dose adjustment is not necessary when the CrCl is greater than 50 ml/min because mild reductions in renal function have little effect on the fate of a drug. Dose adjustment becomes necessary when the CrCl falls below 50 ml/min or when the patient is on dialysis.[9]

Relationship of CrCl to Drug Elimination

The overall elimination rate constant (K) of any drug is a sum of the renal (k_r) and nonrenal (k_{nr}) rate constants:

$$K = k_r + k_{nr}$$

The same can be said for overall drug clearance (CL_{total}) where $CL_{total} = CL_r + CL_{nr}$. For most drugs eliminated primarily by renal clearance processes, the renal rate constant and renal clearance can be represented as a function of CrCl:

$$k_r = \alpha(CrCl) \text{ or } CL_r = \alpha(CrCl)$$

where α defines the linear relationship between CrCl and k_r or CL_r. Therefore, the overall elimination rate constant or total clearance can be expressed as

$$K = \alpha(CrCl) + k_{nr} \text{ or } CL_{total} = \alpha(CrCl) + CL_{nr}$$

Once k_r and k_{nr} [or $\alpha(CrCl)$ and k_{nr}] are known, the Dettli[10] method can be used to calculate an individual's half-life ($t\frac{1}{2}$) for a drug with the following equation:

$$t\frac{1}{2} = 0.693/K$$

Modifying Drug Dosages

There are three basic methods for altering the dose of renally eliminated drugs:

1. Reduce the dose and use the dosage interval for normal renal function.
2. Use the dose for normal renal function and extend the dosage interval.
3. Adjust both dose and interval so that the overall dose per unit of time is decreased.

Depending on the drug in question, each method has advantages and disadvantages. A combination of changing the dose and the interval may be preferred for some drugs. The decision regarding which method to use depends on:

- Availability of specific drug pharmacokinetic data.
- Ability to increase the dosing interval to a logistically acceptable value for renal dysfunction.
- Availability of dosage forms for dosage reduction.
- Desire to maintain a steady concentration with little peak to trough fluctuation (Method 1 used) versus a high peak–low trough dosing format (Method 2 used).

Manufacturer package inserts often provide general recommendations for dosage adjustments in renal dysfunction. Since these guidelines are often produced from studies with small numbers of patients and a narrow range of renal dysfunction, the extrapolation of data to specific therapeutic situations should be evaluated on an individual drug basis. Many other guides for drug dosage adjustment in renal dysfunction are based on broad ranges of renal function (e.g., CrCl <10, = 10–50, or >50 ml/min) and may not be ideal for many patients whose renal function lies within the range.[11-13] Retrieving drug-specific data from the literature is a superior yet time-consuming method.

Individualizing a dosage regimen for a patient with renal dysfunction involves the calculation of a drug's half-life or clearance based on the patient's creatinine clearance (estimated or measured) relative to normal creatinine clearance.[3,14,15] The K and CL_{total} are calculated based on the relationship of the patient's CrCl and K or CL_{total} as previously described. The calculated drug half-life or clearance for a patient with renal dysfunction can be compared to the half-life or clearance for a patient with normal renal function, and the dose and/or dosing interval can then be adjusted empirically. Requirements for this method include

1. The desired dose and interval for a patient with normal renal function must be known.
2. The pharmacokinetic parameters of the drug have been determined in patients with normal renal function.
3. A reasonably accurate assessment of the patient's CrCl is available.

Using this method, the dosage regimen adjustment factor (DF) can be calculated as follows:

$$DF = 1 - [f_e(1 - KF)]$$

where f_e is the fraction of drug that is eliminated unchanged via the kidney in patients with normal renal function and KF is the ratio of the patient's CrCl ($CrCl_r$) to the presumed normal value of 120 ml/min/1.73 m² ($CrCl_n$).

$$KF = \frac{CrCl_r}{CrCl_n}$$

This procedure assumes that the decrease in total body clearance and elimination rate constant are proportional to CrCl, the drug's metabolism is not altered by renal disease, metabolites (if formed) are inactive and nontoxic, and the drug follows linear kinetic principles. After the DF is estimated, a maintenance dose (D_r) or adjusted dosage interval (τ_r) or both for the degree of reduced (r)

renal function can be calculated as follows:

Adjust Dose Only

$$D_r = D_n \times DF$$

Adjust Interval Only

$$\tau_r = \tau_n/DF$$

where D_n is the dose and τ_n is the dosage interval for patients with normal renal function, and D_r is the dose and τ_r is the dosage interval to be used in a patient with reduced renal function. The interval chosen must be reasonable (e.g., 4, 6, 8, 12, 24, or 48 hrs; 16, 18, and 36 hrs may be used, but the clinician should ensure that the schedule is carried out accurately) and the dose must be available.

In cases in which available dosage forms or logical interval adjustment prevents adjusting just the dose or interval, both the dose and interval can be altered. A feasible dosage interval may be first selected (τ_r) and a dose (D_r) then can be calculated based on that interval:

$$D_r = [D_n \times DF(\tau_r/\tau_n)]$$

Alternately, a different available dose may be chosen and a new interval calculated based on:

$$\tau_r = [(D_r/D_n) \times \tau_n]/DF$$

These methods are only valid when there are no significant changes in the volume of distribution, bioavailability, protein binding, or desired target concentrations in patients with either normal renal function or renal dysfunction.

Dialysis

For patients with chronic renal insufficiency, hemodialysis (HD) and continuous ambulatory peritoneal dialysis (CAPD) are the most commonly used dialysis modalities. Numerous factors affect the dialyz-

TABLE 2. Factors Affecting the Dialyzability of a Drug[16,17]

Physicochemical properties of the drug	Molecular weight Water solubility Lipid partition Ionization
Mechanical properties of the dialysis system	Surface area Porosity and thickness of dialysis membrane Dialysate type Dialysate flow rate Duration of dialysis procedure Type of membrane used (HD) Blood flow rate (HD) Presence/absence of peritonitis (CAPD) Peritoneal blood flow rate (CAPD) Dwell time (CAPD) Number of exchanges (CAPD)
Pharmacokinetic factors	Half-life Volume of distribution Protein binding Dialysis clearance Inherent metabolic clearance Red blood cell partition Drug recovery in the dialysate

ability of a drug (Table 2).[16,17] Removal of drugs during dialysis procedures is considered clinically significant only if the dialysis route increases body clearance by at least 30%.

Improved technology has resulted in a hemodialysis membrane called the high-flux membrane. While conventional membranes clear low molecular weight compounds (<500 D for low efficiency, <2000 D for high efficiency), high flux membranes clear larger molecules (<12000 D).[18,19] Many published guidelines for drug dosage regimen design are based on studies using conventional dialyzer membranes and are not applicable to the high-flux membranes.

For patients undergoing CAPD, a supplemental drug dose can be calculated by estimating the fraction of a dose that is removed by CAPD in a specified period. This calculated fraction can then be added to the usual dose for a patient with end-stage renal disease. The equation is

$$f_{pd} = (CL_{pd}/CL) \times f_u$$

where f_{pd} is the fraction of dose eliminated by CAPD in an unlimited period of time, CL_{pd} is the drug clearance by CAPD (dialysate outflow rate, approximately 10 L/day = 7 ml/min), CL is the body clearance of the drug (obtained from the literature), and f_u is the fraction of drug unbound to plasma proteins.[20] For most systemically or orally administered drugs, removal by CAPD is very low.

The total body clearance (CL_{total}) of a drug in a patient undergoing HD can be calculated as:

$$CL_{total} = CL + CL_{HD}$$

where CL is the total body clearance during the interdialytic period and CL_{HD} (obtained from the literature) is the dialyzer clearance. The half-life ($t\frac{1}{2}$) of the drug during the interdialytic period and during dialysis can be calculated from the following formulae by assuming a volume of distribution (V) (obtained from the literature):

$$t\frac{1}{2} \text{ off HD} = 0.693(V/CL)$$

$$t\frac{1}{2} \text{ on HD} = 0.693[V/(CL + CL_{HD})]$$

The CL, CL_{HD}, and V values obtained can then be used to determine the dose and interval of drug administration.[1]

While patients with chronic renal failure are treated mainly with HD and CAPD, patients with acute renal failure are frequently treated with a form of continuous renal replacement therapy (CRRT). These modalities include: continuous arteriovenous hemofiltration (CAVH), continuous venovenous hemofiltration (CVVH), continuous arteriovenous hemodialysis (CAVHD), and continuous venovenous hemodialysis (CVVHD). These modalities are slow but continuous and allow large volume and solute removal while maintaining hemodynamic stability. Drug disposition in patients receiving CRRT has not been thoroughly studied and dosage adjustments recommended for conventional HD and CAPD cannot be extrapolated to CRRT. In general, patients on CRRT receive the same loading dose of a drug as patients with normal renal function and receive an adjusted maintenance dose if removal of the drug via CRRT is significant. Dosing recommendations during CRRT should be based on actual CL data. If actual CL data is not available, estimation of drug CL can be made based on protein binding and V. The prototypic drug that will be removed by CRRT is one with low protein binding (<80%) and small V (<0.7 L/kg).[12,21]

Active or Toxic Metabolites

Active or toxic metabolites of drugs may accumulate in patients with renal dysfunction (Table 3).[22,23] Retention of these metabolites is particularly problematic when renal excretion contributes significantly to the overall elimination of the drug or active metabolite. In patients with significant renal dysfunction, clinicians should avoid drugs with active or toxic metabolites when possible.

Clinical Considerations

Some commonly used drugs that require dose adjustment in renal dysfunction are listed in Table 4. This

TABLE 3. Drugs with Active or Toxic Metabolites Excreted by the Kidneys[a,b]

Drug	Metabolite
Acebutolol	N-Acetyl analogue
Acetaminophen	p-Hydroxyacetanilid
Acetohexamide	Hydroxyhexamide
Allopurinol	Oxypurinol
Azathioprine	6-Mercaptopurine
Chlorpropamide	Hydroxy metabolites
Cyclophosphamide	4-Ketocyclophosphamide
Daunorubicin hydrochloride	Daunorubicinol
Doxorubicin hydrochloride	Adriamycinol
Meperidine hydrochloride	Normeperidine
Methyldopa	Methy-o-sulfate-α-methyldopamine
Morphine sulfate	6-Glucuronide morphine
Nitrofurantoin	Toxic metabolites
Phenylbutazone	Oxyphenbutazone
Propoxyphene	Norpropoxyphene
Propranolol	p-Hydroxypropranolol
Rifampin	Desacetylrifampin
Sodium nitroprusside	Thiocyanate
Sulfonamides	Acetylated metabolites

[a]Adapted, with permission, from Aweeka FT. Drug dosing in renal failure. In: Koda-Kimble MA, Young LY, eds. Applied therapeutics: the clinical use of drugs, 5th ed. Vancouver, WA: Applied Therapeutics; 1992:26–12 and references 20 and 21.
[b]TDM drugs are not included.

TABLE 4. Pharmacokinetic Parameters and Maintenance Dosages for Some Commonly Used Drugs in Patients with Renal Dysfunction [12,24,25]

Drug	V(L/kg)	PB(%)	fe(%)	Regimen for Normal Renal Function	Method	Dose and/or Interval Adjustment for Renal Dysfunction GFR (ml/min) >50	GFR 10-50	<10	Supplement for Dialysis HD	PD	CRRT
CARDIOVASCULAR											
Acebutolol	1.2	20	55	400–600mg q12–24h	D	100%	50%	30–50%	None	None	GFR 10-50
Atenolol	1.1	3	>90	50–100mg q24h	D,I	100% q24h	50% q48h	30–50% q96h	25–50mg	None	GFR 10-50
Benazepril	0.15	95	20	10mg q24h	D	100%	50–75%	25–50%	None	None	GFR 10-50
Bisoprolol	3	30–35	50	10mg q24h	D	100%	75%	50%	No data	No data	GFR 10-50
Enalapril	No data	50–60	43	5–10mg q12h	D	100%	75–100%	50%	20–25%	None	GFR 10-50
Hydralazine	0.5–0.9	87	25	2.5–50mg q8h	I	q8h	q8h	q8-16h	None	None	GFR 10-50
Lisinopril	0.13–0.15	0–10	80–90	5–10mg q24h	D	100%	50–75%	25–50%	20%	None	GFR 10-50

DOSING CONCEPTS IN RENAL DYSFUNCTION

Drug										
Methyldopa	0.5	<15	25-40	250-500mg q8h	I	q8h	q8-12h	q12-24h	250mg	None	GFR 10-50
Nadolol	1.9	28	90	80-120mg q24h	D	100%	50%	25%	40mg	None	GFR 10-50
Quinapril	1.5	97	30	10-20mg q24h	D	100%	75-100%	75%	25%	None	GFR 10-50
Ramipril	1.2	55-70	10-21	10-20mg q24h	D	100%	50-75%	25-50%	20%	None	GFR 10-50
Sotalol	1.3	<1	60	160mg q24h	D	100%	30%	15-30%	80mg	None	GFR 10-50
ANTIMICROBIAL AGENTS										
Acyclovir	0.7	15-30	40-70	5mg/kg q8h	D,I	5mg/kg q8h	5mg/kg q12-24h	2.5mg/kg q24h	Dose after HD	GFR <10	3.5mg/kg q24h
Amantadine	4-5	60	90	100mg q12h	I	q24-48h	q48-72h	q7d	None	None	GFR 10-50
Amoxicillin	0.26	15-25	50-70	250-500mg q8h	I	q8h	q8h-12h	q24h	Dose after HD	250mg q12h	NA
Amphotericin B	4	90	5-10	20-50mg q24h	I	q24h	q24h	q24-36h	None	GFR <10	GFR 10-50
Ampicillin	0.17-0.31	20	30-90	250mg-2g q6h	I	q6h	q6-12h	q12-24h	Dose after HD	250mg q12h	GFR 10-50

TABLE 4. (continued)

Drug	V(L/kg)	PB(%)	fe(%)	Regimen for Normal Renal Function	Method	GFR(ml/min) >50	GFR(ml/min) 10-50	GFR(ml/min) <10	Supplement for Dialysis HD	Supplement for Dialysis PD	Supplement for Dialysis CRRT
Aztreonam	0.5-1	45-60	75	2g q8h	D	100%	50-75%	25%	0.5g after HD	GFR <10	GFR 10-50
Cefazolin	0.13-0.22	80	75-95	1-2g q8h	I	q8h	q12h	q24-48h	0.5-1g after HD	0.5g q12h	GFR 10-50
Cefepime	0.3	16	85	2g q12h	I	q12h	q16-24h	q24-48h	1g after HD	GFR <10	Not-recommended
Cefotaxime	0.15-0.55	37	60	1g q6h	I	q6h	q8-12h	q24h	1g after HD	1g/day	1g q12h
Cefoxitin	0.2	41-75	80	1-2g q8h	I	q8h	q8-12h	q24-48h	1g after HD	1g/day	GFR 10-50
Ceftazidime	0.28-0.4	17	60-85	1-2g q8h	I	q8-12h	q24-48h	q48h	1g after HD	0.5g/d	GFR 10-50
Ceftizoxime	0.26-0.42	28-50	57-100	1-2g q8-12h	I	q8-12h	q12-24h	q24h	1g after HD	0.5-1g/d	GFR 10-50
Cefuroxime sodium	0.13-1.8	33	90	0.75-1.5g q8h	I	q8h	q8-12h	q12h	Dose after HD	GFR <10	1g q12h

DOSING CONCEPTS IN RENAL DYSFUNCTION 521

Drug											
Cephalexin	0.35	20	98	250–500mg q6h	I	q8h	q12h	q12h	Dose after HD	GFR <10	NA
Ciprofloxacin	2.5	20–40	50–70	400mg q12h	D	100%	50–75%	50%	200mg q12h	200mg q8h	200mg q12h
Clarithromycin	2–4	70	15–25	0.5–1g q12h	D	100%	75%	50–75%	Dose after HD	None	None
Didanosine	1	<5	40–69	200mg q12h (125mg if <60kg)	D,I	100%	200mg q24h	50% q24h	Dose after HD	GFR <10	GFR <10
Famciclovir	1.5	<25	50–65	500mg q8h	D,I	100%	250–500mg q24–48h	250mg q48h	Dose after HD	No data	GFR 10–50
Flucytosine	0.6	<10	90	37.5mg/kg q6h	I	q12h	q16h	q24h	Dose after HD	0.5–1g/day	GFR 10–50
Foscarnet	0.3–0.6	17	85	40mg/kg q8h–90mg/kg q12h	D	28mg/kg	15mg/kg	6mg/kg	Dose after HD	GFR <10	GFR 10–50
Ganciclovir	0.47	No data	90–100	5mg/kg q12h	I	q12h	q24–48h	q48–96h	Dose after HD	GFR <10	2.5mg/kg q24h
Imipenem†	0.17–0.3	13–21	20–70	0.5–1g q6h	D	100%	50%	25%	Dose after HD	GFR <10	GFR 10–50
Itraconazole	10	99	35	100–200mg q12h	D	100%	100%	50%	100mg q12–24h	100mg q12–24h	100mg q12–24h

TABLE 4. (continued)

Drug	V(L/kg)	PB(%)	fe(%)	Regimen for Normal Renal Function	Method	Dose and/or Interval Adjustment for Renal Dysfunction GFR(ml/min) >50	GFR(ml/min) 10-50	GFR(ml/min) <10	Supplement for Dialysis HD	PD	CRRT
Lamivudine	0.83	36	70–80	150mg q12h	D,I	100%	50–150mg q24h	25–50mg q24h	Dose after HD	GFR <10	GFR 10–50
Levofloxacin	1.1–1.5	24–38	67–87	500mg q24h	D,I	100%	250mg q24-48h	250mg q48h	GFR <10	GFR <10	GFR 10–50
Meropenem	0.35	2	65	0.5–1g q6h	D,I	500mg q6h	250–500mg q12h	250–500mg q24h	Dose after HD	GFR <10	GFR 10–50
Methicillin	0.31	35–60	2.5–80	1–2g q4h	I	q4–6h	q6–8h	q8–12h	None	None	GFR 10–50
Metronidazole	0.25–0.85	20	20	7.5mg/kg q6h	D	100%	100%	50%	Dose after HD	GFR <10	GFR 10–50
Ofloxacin	1.5–2.5	25	68–80	400mg q12h	D,I	100%	200–400mg q24h	200mg q24h	100–200mg after HD	GFR <10	300mg/d
Penicillin G	0.3–0.42	50	60–85	0.5–4 million units q6h	D	100%	75%	20–50%	Dose after HD	GFR <10	GFR 10–50
Pentamidine	3–4	69	<5	4mg/kg q24h	I	q24h	q24h	q24–36h	None	None	None

Drug						q4–6h	q6–8h	q8h	Dose after HD	GFR <10	GFR 10–50
Piperacillin	0.18–0.3	30	75–90	3–4g q4h	I	100%	50–75%	50% q48h	Dose after HD		
Sparfloxacin	4.5	35–55	10	400mg q24h	D,I	100%	50–75%	50% q48h	GFR <10	No data	GFR 10–50
Stavudine	0.5	<1	35–40	30–40mg q12h	D,I	100%	50% q12–24h	50% q24h	GFR <10 after HD	No data	GFR 10–50
Tetracycline	>0.7	55–90	48–60	250–500mg q6h	I	q8–12h	q12–24h	q24h	None	None	GFR 10–50
Trimethoprim	1–2.2	30–70	40–70	100–200mg q12h	I	q12h	q18h	q24h	Dose after HD	q24h	q18h
Zalcitabine	0.54	<4	75	0.75mg q8h	I	q8h	q12h	q24h	Dose after HD	No data	GFR 10–50
GASTROINTESTINAL											
Cimetidine	0.8–1.3	20	50–70	400mg q12h	D	100%	50%	25%	None	None	GFR 10–50
Cisapride	2.4	98	<5	5–10mg q8h	D	100%	100%	50%	None	No data	50–100%
Famotidine	0.8–1.4	15–22	65–80	20–40mg qhs	D	50%	25%	10%	None	None	GFR 10–50
Metoclopramide	2–3.4	40	10–22	10–15mg q6h	D	100%	75%	50%	None	No data	50–75%
Nizatidine	0.8–1.3	28–35	10–15	150–300mg qhs	D	75%	50%	25%	No data	No data	GFR 10–50

TABLE 4. (continued)

Drug	V(L/kg)	PB(%)	fe(%)	Regimen for Normal Renal Function	Method	Dose and/or Interval Adjustment for Renal Dysfunction GFR(ml/min) >50	GFR 10-50	<10	Supplement for Dialysis HD	PD	CRRT
Ranitidine	1.2–1.8	15	80	150–300mg qhs	D	75%	50%	25%	50%	None	GFR 10–50
ENDOCRINE											
Glyburide	0.16–0.3	99	50	1.25–20mg q24h	D	No data	Avoid	Avoid	None	None	Avoid
Glipizide	0.13–0.16	97	4.5–7	2.5–15mg q24h	D	100%	50%	50%	No data	No data	Avoid
Metformin‡	1–4	Negligible	90–100	500–850mg q12h	D	50%	25%	Avoid	No data	No data	Avoid
Insulin	0.15	5	None	Variable	D	100%	75%	50%	None	None	GFR 10–50
Lispro insulin	0.26–0.36	No data	No data	Variable	D	100%	75%	50%	None	None	None
CENTRAL NERVOUS SYSTEM											
Gapapentin	0.7	0	90	300–600mg q8h	D,I	400mg q8h	300mg q12–24h	300mg q48h	200–300mg after HD	300mg q48h	GFR 10–50

ANTIHISTAMINES

	V	PB	fe	Dose for normal renal function	D,I	100%	50%	25%			GFR 10–50
Cetirazine	0.4–0.6	93	60–70	5–20mg q24h	D	100%	50%	25%	None	No data	NA
Fexofenadine	5–6	70	10	60mg q12h	I	q12h	q12–24h	q24h	No data	No data	GFR 10–50

V = volume of distribution; PB = plasma protein binding; fe = percent excreted unchanged in the urine; D = dose reduction method; the percent of the dose for normal renal function to be given at the interval for normal renal function is listed; I = interval extension method; the interval to be used with the dose for normal renal function is listed; D,I = adjustment of both dose and interval; GFR = glomerular filtration rate (the range following GFR indicates the use of the dose that corresponds to that range of GFR in patients not on dialysis); HD = hemodialysis; PD = peritoneal dialysis; CRRT = continuous arteriovenous or venovenous hemofiltration;
† = seizures in end-stage renal disease;
‡ = contraindicated when serum creatinine is >1.5 mg/dl (males) or >1.4mg/dl (females).

is not a complete listing of all drugs requiring dose adjustment. This table includes selected pharmacokinetic parameters for drugs in patients with normal renal function or renal dysfunction, as well as recommendations for dosage adjustments in patients with renal dysfunction and those on dialysis. Data from these tables can also be used with the above equations to facilitate dosage adjustments in selec-ted patients. Prior to making dosage adjustments, however, the clinician should consider the reliability of renal function assessment (refer to Table 1). The clinician also should prioritize the need to adjust drug doses based on the agent's therapeutic index or cost, with drugs having narrower therapeutic indices or very high cost receiving the highest priority.

A drug's pharmacodynamic profile also should be considered. Patients with renal dysfunction may be more susceptible to the central nervous system (CNS) effects of some drugs.[26,27] Other drugs, such as loop diuretics, may have diminished effects.[28] With digoxin, the complex interaction between pharmacokinetic and pharmacodynamic parameters must be considered. Pharmacokinetic changes may lead to elevated digoxin concentrations and potential toxicity while elevated potassium concentrations seen in some patients with renal dysfunction can alter the pharmacodynamic profile by decreasing receptor occupancy.[29] Pharmacodynamic alterations may be difficult to quantify. When available, markers should be monitored before and after dose adjustments are made (e.g., pulse rate for beta-blockers). Some antibiotics have more efficacy with minimum fluctuations in serum concentrations, as long as concentrations exceed minimum inhibitory values (e.g., beta-lactams). Other antibiotics have better efficacy when high peak to trough ratios are maintained (e.g., quinolones). These considerations can help determine whether to adjust the dose, the interval, or both. Table 5 lists guiding princi-

TABLE 5. Guiding Principles to Enhance the Safe Use of Drugs in Patients with Renal Disease

---

Know the potential toxicity of any proposed diagnostic or therapeutic agent

Evaluate the potential drug interactions that alter the tolerability profile of the new therapy

Consider the potential risks and benefits of diagnostic and therapeutic alternatives

Adjust the drug therapy regimen on the basis of the patient's renal and hepatic function

Monitor for the development of adverse effects

Modify therapy if significant toxicity develops

Source: reproduced with permission from reference 3.

ples to enhance the safe use of drugs in patients with renal disease.

Conclusion

Dosage modifications in patients with renal dysfunction may be useful for agents primarily dependent on glomerular filtration or tubular secretion for clearance. Methods to accomplish this adjustment without TDM depend on the availability of pharmacokinetic data, such as the fraction of drug excreted unchanged in the urine. These methods are less precise and qualitative compared to TDM, but may be clinically useful.

Dosage regimen adjustments should be considered in patients on dialysis or when calculated CrCl values are less than or equal to 50 ml/min. Prior to adjusting drug therapy, clinicians must consider influences on renal function assessment, the drug's target range, pharmacodynamic profile, and significant drug interactions in patients with renal dysfunction.

References

1. Lam YWF, Banerji S, Hatfield C, et al. Principles of drug administration in renal insufficiency. *Clin Pharmacokinet.* 1997; 32(1):30–57.
2. Comstock TJ. Quantification of renal function. In: Pharmacotherapy: a pathophysiologic approach. 3rd ed. DiPiro JT, Talbert RL, Yee GC, et al., eds. Norwalk, CT: Appleton and Lange; 1997:867–85.
3. Matzke GR, Frye RF. Drug administration in patients with renal insufficiency: minimizing renal and extrarenal toxicity. *Drug Saf.* 1997; 16(3):205–31.
4. Aronoff GR. Drugs and the kidney. *Curr Opin Nephrol Hypertens.* 1993; 2(2):187–91.
5. Bertino JS. Measured versus estimated creatinine clearance in patients with low serum creatinine values. *Ann Pharmacother.* 1993; 27:1439–42.
6. O'Connell MB, Dwinell AM, Bannick-Mohrland SD. Predictive performance of equations to estimate creatinine clearance in hospitalized elderly patients. *Ann Pharmacother.* 1992; 26:627–35.
7. Robert S, Zarowitz BJ, Peterson EL, et al. Predictability of creatinine clearance estimates in critically ill patients. *Crit Care Med.* 1993; 21:1487–95.
8. O'Connell MB, Wong MO, et al. Accuracy of 2- and 8-hour urine collections for measuring CrCl in the hospitalized elderly. Pharmacotherapy. 1993; 13(2):135–42.
9. Fillastre J, Singlas E. Pharmacokinetics of newer drugs in patients with renal impairment (part I). *Clin Pharmacokinet.* 1991; 20(4):293–310.
10. Dettli L. Drug dosage in renal disease. *Clin Pharmacokinet.* 1976; 1:126–34.
11. McEvoy GK, ed. American hospital formulary service drug information 1999. Bethesda, MD: American Society of Health-System Pharmacists; 1999.
12. Aronoff GR, Bern JS, et al. Drug prescribing in renal failure: dosing guidelines for adults. 4th ed. Philadelphia, PA: American College of Physicians; 1999.
13. Arky R, ed. Physicians' Desk Reference 1999. Oradell, New Jersey: Medical Economics Co., Inc.; 1999.
14. Dettli L. Elimination kinetics and dosage adjustments of drugs in patients with kidney disease. *Prog Pharmacol.* 1977; 1:1–34.
15. Tozer TN. Nomogram for modification of dosage regimens in patients with chronic renal impairment. *J Pharmacokinet Biopharm.* 1974; 2:13–28.
16. Lee CC, Marbury TC. Drug therapy in patients undergoing hemodialysis: clinical pharmacokinetic considerations. *Clin Pharmacokinet.* 1984; 9:42–66.
17. Paton TW, Cornish WR, Manuel MA, et al. Drug therapy in patients undergoing peritoneal dialysis. *Clin Pharmacokinet.* 1985; 10:404–26.

18. Lanese DM, Alfrey PS, Molitoas BA. Markedly increased clearance of vancomycin during hemodialysis using polysulfone dialyzers. *Kidney Int.* 1989; 35:1409–12.
19. Matzke GR. Pharmacotherapeutic consequences of recent advances in hemodialysis therapy. *Ann Pharmacother.* 1994; 28:512–4.
20. Keller E, Reetze P, Schollmeyer P. Drug therapy in patients undergoing continuous ambulatory peritoneal dialysis: clinical pharmacokinetic considerations. *Clin Pharmacokinet.* 1990; 18(2):104–17.
21. Reetze-Bonorden, Böhler J, et al. Drug dosage in patients during continuous renal replacement therapy: pharmacokinetic and therapeutic considerations. *Clin Pharmacokinet.* 1993; 24(5):362–79.
22. Verbeeck RK, Branch RA, Wilkinson GR. Drug metabolites in renal failure: pharmacokinetic and clinical implications. *Clin Pharmacokinet.* 1981; 6:329–45.
23. Turnheim K. Pitfalls of pharmacokinetic dosage guidelines in renal insufficiency. *Eur J Clin Pharmacol.* 1991; 40:87–93.
24. Swan SK. Drug dosing guidelines in renal failure. *Curr Pract Med.* 1999; 2(8):1607–15.
25. St. Peter WL, Redic-Kill KA, et al. Clinical pharmacokinetics of antibiotics in patients with impaired renal function. *Clin Pharmacokinet.* 1992; 22:169–210.
26. Schmith VD, Piraino B, Smith RB, et al. Alprazolam in end stage renal disease. II. pharmacodynamics. *Clin Pharmacol Ther.* 1992; 51(5):533–40.
27. Bauer TM, Ritz R, Haberthur C, et al. Prolonged sedation due to accumulation of conjugated metabolite of midazolam. *Lancet.* 1995; 346:145–7.
28. Brater DC. Clinical pharmacology of loop diuretics. *Drugs.* 1991; 41:14–22.
29. Schwartz A, Lindenmayer GE, Allen JC. The sodium-potassium adenosine triphosphate: pharmacological, physiological, and biochemical aspects. *Pharmacol Res.* 1975; 27(1):3–134.

Appendix A
Nomogram for Determining Body Surface of Adults from Height and Mass

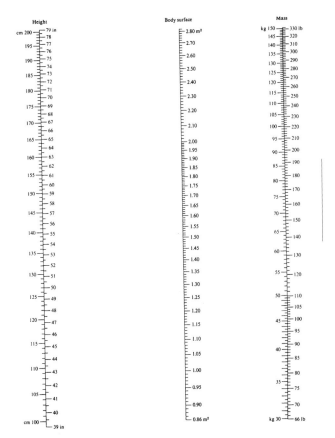

From the formula of DuBois and DuBois, *Arch Intern Med*, 17, 863 (1916): $S = M^{0.425} \times H^{0.725} \times 71.84$, or $\log S = \log M \times 0.425 + \log H \times 0.725 + 1.8564$ (S: body surface in cm^2, M: mass in kg, H: height in cm).

Reproduced, with permission, from Geigy scientific tables, vol 1, 8th ed. Lentner C, ed. Basle, Switzerland: CIBA-GEIGY Limited; 1993:227.

Appendix B
Nomogram for Determining Body Surface of Children from Height and Mass

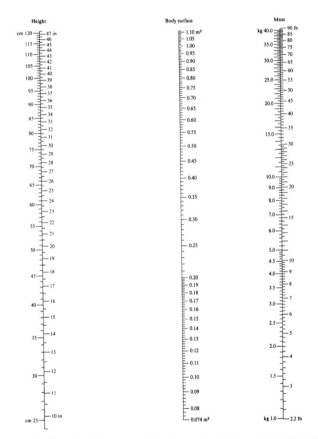

From the formula of DuBois and DuBois, *Arch Intern Med*, 17, 863 (1916): $S = M^{0.425} \times H^{0.725} \times 71.84$, or $\log S = \log M \times 0.425 + \log H \times 0.725 + 1.8564$ (S: body surface in cm^2, M: mass in kg, H: height in cm).

Reproduced, with permission, from Geigy scientific tables, vol 1, 8th ed. Lentner C, ed. Basle, Switzerland: CIBA-GEIGY Limited; 1993:226.

Appendix C
Therapeutic Ranges of Drugs in Traditional and SI Units[a]

Drug	Traditional Range	Conversion Factor[b]	SI Range
Acetaminophen	>5 mg/dL toxic	66.16	>330 µmol/L toxic
N-Acetylprocainamide	4–10 mg/L	3.606	14–36 µmol/L
Amitriptyline	75–175 ng/mL	3.605	180–720 nmol/L
Carbamazepine	4–12 mg/L	4.230	17–51 µmol/L
Chlordiazepoxide	0.5–5.0 mg/L	3.336	2–17 µmol/L
Chlorpromazine	50–300 ng/mL	3.136	150–950 nmol/L
Chlorpropamide	75–250 µg/mL	3.613	270–900 µmol/L
Clozapine	450–? ng/mL	0.003	1.38–? µmol/L
Cyclosporine	100–200 ng/mL[c]	0.832	80–160 nmol/L
Desipramine	100–160 ng/mL	3.754	170–700 nmol/L
Diazepam	100–250 ng/mL	3.512	350–900 nmol/L
Digoxin	0.9–2.2 ng/mL	1.281	1.2–2.8 nmol/L
Disopyramide	2–6 mg/L	2.946	6–18 µmol/L
Doxepin	50–200 ng/mL	3.579	180–720 nmol/L
Ethosuximide	40–100 mg/L	7.084	280–710 µmol/L
Fluphenazine	0.5–2.5 ng/mL	2.110	5.3–21 nmol/L
Glutethimide	>20 mg/L toxic	4.603	>92 µmol/L toxic
Gold	300–800 mg/L	0.051	15–40 µmol/L
Haloperidol	5–15 ng/mL	2.660	13–40 nmol/L
Imipramine	200–250 ng/mL	3.566	180–710 nmol/L
Isoniazid	>3 mg/L toxic	7.291	>22 µmol/L toxic
Lidocaine	1–5 mg/L	4.267	5–22 µmol/L
Lithium	0.5–1.5 mEq/L	1.000	0.5–1.5 µmol/L
Maprotiline	50–200 ng/mL	3.605	180–720 µmol/L
Meprobamate	>40 mg/L toxic	4.582	>180 µmol/L toxic
Methotrexate	>2.3 mg/L toxic	2.200	>5 µmol/L toxic
Nortriptyline	50–150 ng/mL	3.797	190–570 nmol/L
Pentobarbital	20–40 mg/L	4.419	90–170 µmol/L
Perphenazine	0.8–2.4 ng/mL	2.475	2–6 nmol/L
Phenobarbital	15–40 mg/L	4.306	65–172 µmol/L
Phenytoin	10–20 mg/L	3.964	40–80 µmol/L
Primidone	4–12 mg/L	4.582	18–55 µmol/L
Procainamide	4–8 mg/L	4.249	17–34 µmol/L
Propoxyphene	>2 mg/L toxic	2.946	>6 µmol/L toxic
Propranolol	50–200 ng/mL	3.856	190–770 nmol/L
Protriptyline	100–300 ng/mL	3.797	380–1140 nmol/L
Quinidine	2–6 mg/L	3.082	5–18 µmol/L
Salicylate (acid)	15–25 mg/dL	0.072	1.1–1.8 mmol/L
Theophylline	10–20 mg/L	5.550	55–110 µmol/L
Thiocyanate	>10 mg/dL toxic	0.172	>1.7 mmol/L toxic
Valproic acid	50–100 mg/L	6.934	350–700 µmol/L
Warfarin	1–3 mg/L	3.243	3.3–9.8 µmol/L

[a]*Source: Traub SL. Interpreting Laboratory Data. 2nd edition. Bethesda, MD: American Society of Health-System Pharmacists; 1996:p. 397.*
[b]*Traditional units are multiplied by conversion factor to get SI units.*
[c]*Whole blood assay.*

Appendix D
Nondrug Reference Ranges for Common Laboratory Tests in Traditional and SI Units[a]

Laboratory Test	Reference Range Traditional Units	Conversion Factor	Reference Range SI Units	Comment
Alanine aminotransferase (ALT)	0–30 IU/L	0.01667	0–0.50 μkat/L	SGPT
Albumin	3.5–5 g/dL	10.00	35–50 g/L	
Ammonia	30–70 μg/dL	0.587	17–41 μmol/L	
Aspartate aminotransferase (AST)	8–42 IU/L	0.01667	0.133–0.700 μkat/L	SGOT
Bilirubin (direct)	0.1–0.3 mg/dL	17.10	1.7–5 μmol/L	
Bilirubin (total)	0.3–1.0 mg/dL	17.10	5–17 μmol/L	
Calcium	8.5–10.8 mg/dL	0.25	2.1–2.7 mmol/L	
Carbon dioxide (CO_2)	24–30 mEq/L	1.000	24–30 mmol/L	Serum bicarbonate
Chloride	96–106 mEq/L	1.000	96–106 mmol/L	
Cholesterol (HDL)	>35 mg/dL	0.026	>0.91 mmol/L	desirable
Cholesterol (LDL)	<130 mg/dL	0.026	<3.36 mmol/L	desirable
Creatine kinase (CK)	40–200 IU/L 35–150 IU/L	0.01667	0.667–3.33 μkat/L 0.583–2.50 μkat/L	males females
Serum creatinine (SCr)	0.7–1.5 mg/dL	88.40	62–133 μmol/L	
Creatinine clearance (CrCl)	90–140 mL/min/1.73 m^2	0.017	1.53–2.38 mL/sec/1.73 m^2	
Folic acid	≥3.3 ng/dL	2.212	>7.3 nmol/L	
γ-glutamyl transpeptidase	0–30 U/L (but varies)	0.01667	0–0.50 μkat/L (but varies)	GGTP
Globulin	2–3 g/dL	10.00	20–30 g/L	
Glucose (fasting)	70–110 mg/dL	0.056	3.9–6.1 mmol/L	fasting
Hemoglobin (Hgb)	14–18 g/dL 12–16 g/dL	0.622	8.7–11.2 mmol/L 7.4–9.9 mmol/L	males females
Iron	50–150 μg/dL	0.179	9–26.9 μmol/L	
Iron-binding capacity	250–410 μg/dL	0.179	45–73 μmol/L	TIBC
Lactate dehydrogenase	100–210 IU/L	0.01667	1.67–3.50 μkat/L	LDH
Serum lactate (venous)	0.5–1.5 mEq/L	1.000	0.5–1.5 mmol/L	Lactic acid
Serum lactate (arterial)	0.5–2.0 mEq/L	1.000	0.5–2.0 mmol/L	
Magnesium	1.5–2.2 mEq/L	0.500	0.75–1.1 mmol/L	
5′ Nucleotidase	1–11 U/L (but varies)	0.01667	0.02–0.18 μkat/L (but varies)	
Phosphate	2.6–4.5 mg/dL	0.329	0.85–1.48 mmol/L	
Potassium	3.5–5.0 mEq/L	1.000	3.5–5.0 mmol/L	
Sodium	136–145 mEq/L	1.000	136–145 mmol/L	
Total serum thyroxine (T_4)	4–12 μg/dL	12.87	51–154 nmol/L	Total T_4
Triglycerides	<200 mg/dL	0.0113	<2.26 mmol/L	
Total serum triiodothyronine (T_3)	78–195 ng/dL	0.0154	1.2–3.0 nmol/L	Total T_3
Urea nitrogen, blood	8–20 mg/dL	0.357	2.9–7.1 mmol/L	BUN
Uric acid (serum)	3.4–7 mg/dL	59.48	202–416 μmol/L	

[a]*Source: Traub SL. Interpreting Laboratory Data. 2nd edition. Bethesda, MD: American Society of Health-System Pharmacists; 1996:p. 399. Note that some laboratories are maintaining traditional units for enzyme tests.*

Notes